Analysis and Evaluation of
Conceptual Models
of Nursing

Second Edition

Analysis and Evaluation of Conceptual Models of Nursing

Second Edition

Jacqueline Fawcett, Ph.D., F.A.A.N.

Associate Professor
University of Pennsylvania
School of Nursing
Philadelphia, Pennsylvania

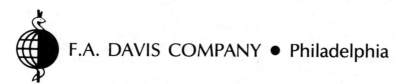

F.A. DAVIS COMPANY • Philadelphia

Printed in the United States of America

Last digit indicates print number: 10 9 8 7 6 5 4 3 2

LIBRARY OF CONGRESS
Library of Congress Cataloging-in-Publication Data

Fawcett, Jacqueline.
    Analysis and evaluation of conceptual models of nursing /
Jacqueline Fawcett.—2nd ed.
        p.   cm.
    Includes bibliographies and index.
    ISBN 0-8036-3410-2
    1. Nursing—Philosophy.   I. Title.
    [DNLM: 1. Models, Theoretical.   2. Nursing.   WY 100 F278a]
RT84.5.F38 1989
610.73′01—dc19
DNLM/DLC
for Library of Congress   86-16148
                                                                            CIP

Dedication

I dedicate this book to my husband, John S. Fawcett, who gave up so much during the 6 months it took to prepare this edition. My appreciation for his love, support, encouragement, and understanding is boundless.

Preface

    The second edition of this book was written for all nurses and nursing students who are interested in the development of nursing knowledge and the use of that knowledge to guide nursing practice, research, education, and administration. This edition represents a continuing attempt to clarify the confusion between conceptual models and theories still seen in the nursing literature. To that end, the second edition continues to focus on the global formulations of nursing knowledge that are called conceptual models of nursing, with added discussion of grand and middle range theories that have been derived from or linked with various conceptual models.

    The centrality of conceptual models of nursing to all nursing activities is attested to by the voluminous literature and anecdotal reports that have appeared since the first edition of this book went to press. Furthermore, many conferences on conceptual models of nursing, held in several of the United States and in Canada in recent years, have attracted thousands of nurses and nursing students. Indeed, conceptual models now are being used by nurses throughout the planet Earth, and consideration is being given to the use of conceptual models of nursing by future astronaut nurses.

    The continuing evolution of conceptual models of nursing is reflected in the revisions for the second edition of this book. Chapter 1 presents a detailed discussion of conceptual models and theories. This chapter has been revised to further clarify the distinctions between conceptual models and theories. The discussion of how conceptual models guide nursing research, nursing practice, nursing education, and nursing administration has been expanded to include lists of rules for research, practice, education, and administration that are inherent in the conceptual models.

    Chapter 2 presents a revised framework for analysis and evaluation of conceptual models of nursing. The discussion of appropriate comparisons of conceptual models has been revised to reflect current thinking, and the guidelines for selecting a conceptual model for use in clinical practice have been refined.

Chapters 3 through 9 present detailed and comprehensive analyses and evaluations of the most recent versions of works by Dorothy Johnson, Imogene King, Myra Levine, Betty Neuman, Dorothea Orem, Martha Rogers, and Callista Roy. Each of these chapters has been extensively revised to reflect the most recent refinements in each conceptual model and to present a comprehensive review of the most recent literature dealing with the use of each conceptual model in nursing research, nursing practice, nursing education, and nursing administration. The analysis and evaluation of each conceptual model were enhanced by materials not yet published by model authors that were made available to me for this edition of the book. These chapters clearly differentiate the work of each author that may be considered at the level of a conceptual model and that which is at the theory level.

Throughout these chapters, care was taken to present an accurate account of the conceptual model as it was developed by its author rather than to draw from secondary analyses and other interpretations of the author's work. Readers are, therefore, encouraged to use this book in combination with the original source material for each conceptual model.

Other works that fit the definition of conceptual model of nursing given in this book were not included in this edition. The works that are included continue, in my opinion, to be the major representatives of conceptual models of nursing in the contemporary nursing literature. Indeed, most of the other frequently cited works fit the definition of theory given in this book. Readers who are interested in understanding the content of other conceptual models are, however, encouraged to use the framework for analysis and evaluation of conceptual models, presented in Chapter 2 and used as a structure for the content of Chapters 3 through 9, to analyze and evaluate these other models. It is my sincere hope that this book will stimulate readers to continue their study of conceptual models of nursing and nursing theories and to adopt explicit conceptual-theoretical systems of knowledge for their nursing activities.

Chapter 10 is a new addition to the book, written in response to requests for a concluding chapter. This chapter expands the discussion of conceptual models and theories that began in Chapter 1. Emphasis is placed on implications of conceptual models for nursing practice. Issues related to numbers of conceptual models needed by the discipline of nursing and by individual schools of nursing and clinical agencies are explored, and consideration is given to matching conceptual models to clinical specialties, clinical agencies, and patients' views of health care. Methods to determine the credibility of conceptual models are explained, and the importance of credibility determination for the advancement of the discipline of nursing is underscored. This new chapter concludes with a discussion of directions for future work with conceptual models of nursing and nursing theories.

Each chapter of the book presents a list of key terms, which are defined and discussed in the chapter. Each chapter also includes an annotated bibliography of the literature related to the content of that chapter. The bibliographies for Chapters 1 through 9 are greatly expanded since the first edition owing to the substantial increase in the literature dealing with conceptual models of nursing. Given the marked increase in literature, the annotated bibliographies are limited to full journal articles and books. Abstracts, master's theses, doctoral dissertations, paper presentations, and audio and video productions are, however, cited in the narrative portions of the book. I am indebted to the model authors and to my students and colleagues for the many citations of relevant publications they shared with me. I also am indebted to the staffs of the University of Pennsylvania Biomedical Library and the University of Connecticut Wilbur Cross Library for all they did to make difficult to locate materials accessible to me.

An Appendix has been added to the second edition to enhance access to the audio and video productions related to conceptual models of nursing. Lists of audio and video tapes of conferences, interviews, and presentations about conceptual models are given with distribution sources.

J.F.

Acknowledgments_____

The writing of the second edition of this book was a consuming but stimulating experience. Its preparation is due to many people. First, I must continue to acknowledge Dorothy Johnson, Imogene King, Myra Levine, Betty Neuman, Dorothea Orem, Martha Rogers, and Callista Roy. Their continuing efforts to establish and refine the knowledge base for the discipline of nursing made this edition possible. I also acknowledge Bonnie Holladay, who provided additional information about the use of Johnson's conceptual model.

Next, I acknowledge the support, intellectual challenges, and constructive criticism offered by my colleagues, especially Carol P. Germain, with whom I teach a doctoral course on contemporary nursing knowledge at the University of Pennsylvania School of Nursing, and the members of the Nursing Theory Think Tank; my students; and participants at the many conferences and workshops at which I have had the honor to present my ideas. I also acknowledge Suzanne Bryer Levy, who assisted with the preparation of the annotated bibliographies for the first edition of the book, and Diane Fager Barger and Mary L. Botter, who prepared most of the annotations for the second edition. I also would like to acknowledge the encouragement given to me by Robert G. Martone, Senior Editor, and Ruth De George of F.A. Davis Company. Finally, I gratefully acknowledge all the people who contributed to the production of this edition of the book, especially Herbert J. Powell, Jr., who supervised the production; and John S. Fawcett, who provided consultation on all aspects of the book design.

The Author and Publisher would like to thank Appleton and Lange for allowing the use of extensive material from their nursing models books.

Contents

CHAPTER
1

Conceptual Models and Theories⎯⎯⎯⎯⎯⎯

This chapter lays the groundwork for the remainder of the book. Here, conceptual models and theories are defined, described, and placed in a structural hierarchy of knowledge. Then, the argument is advanced that conceptual models and theories are clearly distinguished by their levels of abstraction and thus must be used in different ways. The chapter concludes with a discussion of the conceptual-theoretical systems of nursing knowledge required for scientific and professional activities.

The key terms used in this chapter are listed below. Each term is defined and described in the chapter.

KEY TERMS⎯⎯⎯

Conceptual Model	World Views
Conceptual Framework	Mechanism and Organicism
Conceptual System	Change and Persistence
Paradigm	Categories of Conceptual
Disciplinary Matrix	Models of Nursing
Concept	Developmental
Proposition	Systems
Metaparadigm	Interaction
Nursing's Metaparadigm	Needs
Concepts	Outcomes
Person, Environment, Health,	Humanistic
Nursing	Energy Fields

1

Categories of Conceptual Models of Nursing—Cont.	Scope of Theories
Intervention	Grand Theory
Substitution	Middle Range Theory
Conservation	Partial Theory
Sustenance	Structural Hierarchy of Knowledge
Enhancement	Conceptual-Theoretical Systems of Nursing Knowledge for:
Theory	Research
Types of Theories	Clinical Practice
Descriptive Theory	Education
Explanatory Theory	Administration
Predictive Theory	

CONCEPTUAL MODELS

The term conceptual model, and synonymous terms such as conceptual framework, conceptual system, paradigm, and disciplinary matrix, refer to global ideas about the individuals, groups, situations, and events of interest to a discipline. Conceptual models are made up of concepts, which are words describing mental images of phenomena, and propositions, which are statements about the concepts. A conceptual model, therefore, is defined as a set of concepts and the propositions that integrate them into a meaningful configuration (Lippitt, 1973; Nye & Berardo, 1981).

The concepts of a conceptual model are highly abstract and general. Thus, they are not directly observed in the real world nor are they limited to any specific individual, group, situation, or event. Adaptation is an example of a conceptual model concept. It can refer to all types of individuals and groups, in a wide variety of situations.

The propositions of a conceptual model also are very abstract and general. Therefore, they are not amenable to direct empirical observation or test. Some propositions provide the foundation for further development of the model; these are the basic assumptions of the model. An example of this kind of proposition is: People are rational beings. Other propositions are broad definitions of the conceptual model concepts. Adaptation, for example, might be defined as the ability to adjust to changing situations. Because conceptual model concepts are so abstract, not all of them are defined, and those that are defined have rather loose definitions. Definitional propositions for conceptual model concepts, therefore, do not and cannot state how the concepts are observed or measured.

Still other propositions state the relationships between conceptual model concepts. This kind of proposition is exemplified by the following statement: Nursing intervention is directed toward management of environmental stressors.

The concepts and propositions of each conceptual model often are stated in a distinctive vocabulary. One model, for example, uses the terms adaptation and stress, and another uses the terms helicy and resonancy. Furthermore, the meaning of each term usually is connected to the particular focus of the model. Thus, the same or similar terms may have different meanings in different conceptual models. For example, stressor may be defined as a negative stimulus in one model and as a positive, growth-promoting force in another.

In summary, a conceptual model is composed of abstract and general concepts and propositions. These global ideas and statements are expressed in a distinctive manner in each model.

Uses of Conceptual Models

A conceptual model provides a distinctive frame of reference for its adherents, telling them what to look at and speculate about. Most importantly, a conceptual model determines how the world is viewed and what aspects of that world are to be taken into account (Redman, 1974; Rogers, 1973). Conceptual models thus have the "basic purpose of focusing, ruling some things in as relevant, and ruling others out due to their lesser importance" (Williams, 1979, p. 96). For example, one conceptual model may focus on interventions designed to help the person adapt to stressors, and another may emphasize the person's capacity for self-care.

The utility of conceptual models comes from the organization they provide for thinking, for observations, and for interpreting what is seen. Conceptual models also provide a systematic structure and a rationale for activities. Furthermore, they give direction to the search for relevant questions about phenomena and they point out solutions to practical problems. Conceptual models also provide general criteria for knowing when a problem has been solved. These features of conceptual models are illustrated in the following example: Suppose that a conceptual model focuses on adaptation of the person to external stressors, and proposes that management of the stressor most obvious to the person leads to adaptation. Here, a relevant question might be: What is the most obvious stressor in a given situation? Anyone interested in solutions to problems in adaptation would focus on the various ways of managing stressors. And, one would be led to look for manifestations of adaptation when seeking to determine if the problem has been solved.

Development of Conceptual Models

Conceptual models have existed since people began to think about themselves and their surroundings. Lippitt (1973) identified examples of conceptual models in the early Egyptian and Chinese civilizations; in early sciences such as physics and medicine; in later sciences such as mathematics, chemistry, and biology; and in all modern sciences. He noted that many of the models were influential in shaping the world. For example,

> The thinking of Karl Marx, Albert Einstein and Sigmund Freud is paramount in the shaping of the 20th-century world. Each had a conceptual model. Marx's was a political, philosophic, social, and economic model forming the framework of communist ideology. Einstein's model of relativity paved the way to the atomic era. His model helped break an adherence to inflexible laws of physics and mathematics which hindered the development of science and technology. Freud's model was a tri-dimensional structure for the understanding of man which he called psychoanalysis. (Lippitt, 1973, p. 14)

In each instance, the conceptual model evolved from empirical observations and intuitive insights of scholars and/or from deductions that creatively combined ideas from several fields of inquiry. A conceptual model is inductively developed when generalizations about various observed events are formulated and is deductively developed when specific situations are seen as examples of other more general events. For example, Freud induced his concepts of the ego, id, and superego from observations of his patients' behavior. In contrast, much of Einstein's model of relativity was deduced from previous work dealing with the physical world.

Conceptual models present diverse views of certain phenomena in the world that have profound influences on our perceptions of that world. A model is, however, only an approximation or simplification of reality, a representation of the world that includes only those concepts that the model builder considers relevant and as aids to understanding (Lippitt, 1973; Reilly, 1975). Each conceptual model is a unique combination or a synthesis of many concepts, and, therefore, presents a distinctive perspective for the phenomena of interest to a discipline (Phillips, 1977; Reilly, 1975). Such a combination or synthesis, however, must adhere to the criterion of logical congruence of ideas. A detailed discussion of logically incompatible world views is presented later in this chapter. Suffice it to say now that a model would not be logically congruent if it combined an emphasis on the person as passively reacting to the environment with a focus on the person as actively interacting with the environment.

Metaparadigms and Conceptual Models

Now that conceptual models have been defined and their use and development have been described, they may be placed within the structural hierarchy of knowledge within disciplines. This will be done by introducing the idea of the metaparadigm. Later in the chapter, the relation of metaparadigms and conceptual models to theories will be explained.

Each discipline singles out certain phenomena with which it will deal in a unique manner. The concepts and propositions that identify and interrelate these phenomena are even more abstract and general than those of conceptual models, and comprise the metaparadigm of the discipline (Kuhn, 1977). The metaparadigm, therefore, is the most global perspective of a discipline and "acts as an encapsulating unit, or framework, within which the more restricted . . . structures develop" (Eckberg & Hill, 1979, p. 927). The metaparadigm of sociology, for example, tells the sociologist to look at the social behavior of human beings.

Disciplines are differentiated from each other by virtue of the phenomena of concern to each. The metaparadigm of each discipline, therefore, is the first level of distinction between disciplines. It is not unusual, however, to find that more than one discipline is interested in the same or similar concepts. The unique perspective of each discipline with regard to the concepts is specified by its metaparadigm. For example, both sociology and psychology are concerned with behavior, but sociology focuses on social behavior and psychology focuses on psychological behavior.

Most disciplines have a single metaparadigm, but multiple conceptual models. These are derived from the metaparadigm and, therefore, incorporate the most global concepts and propositions in a more restrictive, yet still abstract manner. Each conceptual model, then, provides a different view of the metaparadigm concepts. As Kuhn (1970) explained, although adherents of different models are looking at the same phenomena, "in some areas they see different things, and they see them in different relations to one another" (p. 150). Nye and Berardo (1981), for example, identified 16 different conceptual models of the family derived from the metaparadigm of sociology.

The content of each conceptual model reflects the philosophical stance, cognitive orientation, research tradition, and practice modalities of a particular group of scholars within a discipline, rather than the beliefs, values, thoughts, research methods, and approaches to practice of all members of the discipline. The adherents of each conceptual model, then, comprise a subculture or community of scholars within a discipline (Eckberg & Hill, 1979). The conceptual model maps and categorizes the activities of its adherents and, therefore, distinguishes one group of researchers, clinicians, educators, and administrators from another group (Nye & Berardo, 1981). One conceptual model, for example, may lead its adherents to study stress and adaptation, and another conceptual model will lead its adherents to look at structure and function.

Furthermore, conceptual models move beyond metaparadigms to provide a second level of distinction between disciplines (Aggleton & Chalmers, 1986; Nye & Berardo, 1981). This is especially so when more than one discipline is interested in a particular concept. Stress is a prominent example of a concept that is of interest to many disciplines. Close examination of the focus of each discipline, however, reveals that ideas and statements about stress are quite different. Consider, for example, the meaning of stress to the engineers who build bridges versus its meaning to psychologists who study intrapsychic reactions to noxious stimuli.

Metaparadigm of Nursing

Considerable agreement now exists that the central concepts of the discipline of nursing are: person, environment, health, and nursing. Person refers to the recipient of nursing actions, who may be an individual, a family, a community, or a particular group. Environment refers to the recipient's significant others and surroundings, as well as to the setting in which nursing actions occur. Health refers to the wellness and/or illness state of the recipient. And, nursing refers to the actions taken by nurses on behalf of or in conjunction with the recipient.

The connections among the four metaparadigm concepts are clearly made in the following statement: "Nursing studies the wholeness or health of humans, recognizing that humans are in continuous interaction with their environments" (Donaldson & Crowley, 1978, p. 119). This statement may be considered the major proposition of nursing's metaparadigm, reflecting as it does the overall focus of the discipline of nursing.

Three other propositions state relationships between and among the metaparadigm concepts. These statements, which reflect the major areas of interest to the discipline of nursing, are:

- The principles and laws that govern the life-process, well-being, and optimum function of human beings, sick or well
- The patterning of human behavior in interaction with the environment in normal life events and critical life situations
- The processes by which positive changes in health status are effected (Donaldson & Crowley, 1978; Gortner, 1980)

Nursing's metaparadigm has been evolving since Nightingale

(1859) first wrote of nurses' actions in relation to environmental influences on the person's health. Explicit formalization of the metaparadigm, however, has occurred only recently (Fawcett, 1983, 1984).

Conway (1985) raised the question of whether nursing should be considered a concept within the metaparadigm of nursing. She regarded nursing as the discipline and did not accept the view of nursing as action or activity of discipline members as an appropriate metaparadigm concept. Contemporary works by Meleis (1985) and Kim (1987), however, do underscore the centrality of person, environment, health, and nursing (as activity or action), but present slight variations of the metaparadigm. Meleis's list includes nursing client, transitions, interaction, nursing process, environment, nursing therapeutics, and health. She proposed that

> The nurse interacts (interaction) with a human being in a health/illness situation (nursing client) who is in an integral part of his sociocultural context (environment) and who is in some sort of transition or is anticipating a transition (transition); the nurse/patient interactions are organized around some purpose (nursing process) and the nurse uses some actions (nursing therapeutics) to enhance, bring about, or facilitate health (health). (Meleis, 1985, p. 184)

Kim (1987) identified four domains of nursing knowledge. The client domain is concerned with the client's development, problems, and health care experiences. The client-nurse domain focuses on encounters between client and nurse and the interactions between the two in the process of providing nursing care. The practice domain emphasizes the cognitive, behavioral, and social aspects of nurses' professional actions. The domain of environment is concerned with time, space, and quality variations of the client's environment.

Hinshaw (1987) pointed out that Kim's work does not include the concept of health, and asked: "Is health a strand that permeates each of the . . . domains . . . rather than a major separate domain?" (p. 112). Kim (personal communication, October 31, 1986) has indicated that the client domain could encompass health.

Conceptual Models of Nursing

Peterson (1977) and Hall (1979) linked the proliferation of conceptual models of nursing with interest in conceptualizing nursing as a distinct discipline and to the concomitant introduction of ideas about nursing theory. Meleis (1985) reached the same conclusion in her historiography of nursing knowledge development. Readers who are especially interested in the progression of nursing knowledge are referred to her excellent work, for a comprehensive historic review is beyond the scope of this book.

The works of several nurse scholars currently are recognized as conceptual models. Among the best known are Johnson's (1980) Behavioral System Model, King's (1981) Interacting Systems Framework, Levine's (1973, in press) Conservation Model, Neuman's (in press) Systems Model, Orem's (1985) Self-Care Framework, Rogers's (1986) Science of Unitary Human Beings, and Roy's (1984) Adaptation Model.

As with conceptual models and metaparadigms of other disciplines, the conceptual models of nursing represent various paradigms derived from the metaparadigm of the discipline of nursing. Thus, it is not surprising that each defines the four metaparadigm concepts differently and links these concepts in diverse ways.

Examination of conceptual models of nursing reveals that person usually is identified as an integrated bio-psycho-social being, but is defined in diverse ways, such as an adaptive system, a behavioral system, a self-care agent, or an energy field. Environment frequently is identified as internal structures and external influences, including family members, the community, and society, as well as the person's physical surroundings. The environment is seen as a source of stressors in some models, but a source of resources in others. Health is presented in various ways, such as a continuum from adaptation to maladaptation, a dichotomy of behavioral stability or instability, or a value identified by each cultural group. The conceptual models also present descriptions of the concept of nursing, usually by defining nursing and then specifying goals of nursing actions and a nursing process. The goals of nursing action frequently are derived directly from the definition of health given by the model. For example, a nursing goal might be to assist people to attain, maintain, or regain the ability to care for themselves, with health equated with self-care ability. The nursing process described in each model emphasizes assessing the person's health status, setting goals for nursing action, implementing nursing actions, and evaluating the person's health status after nursing intervention. The steps of the process, however, frequently differ from model to model. Later chapters in this book present detailed descriptions of several conceptual models of nursing and discuss the connections among the concepts of each model.

Conceptual models are not really new to nursing, as they have existed since Nightingale (1859) first advanced her ideas about nursing. Most early conceptualizations of nursing, however, were not presented in the formal manner of models. It remained for the Nursing Development Conference Group (1973, 1979), Johnson (1974), Riehl and Roy (1974, 1980), and Reilly (1975) to explicitly label various perspectives of nursing as conceptual models.

The development of conceptual models and labeling them as such is an important advance for the discipline of nursing. Reilly's (1975) comments help to underscore this point.

We all have a private image (concept) of nursing practice. In turn, this private image influences our interpretation of data, our decisions, and our actions. But can a discipline continue to develop when its members hold so many differing private images? The proponents of conceptual models of practice are seeking to make us aware of these private images, so that we can begin to identify commonalities in our perceptions of the nature of practice and move toward the evolution of a well-ordered concept. (p. 567)

Johnson (1987) also pointed out that nurses always use some frame of reference for their activities and explained the drawbacks of implicit frameworks. She stated,

It is important to note that some kind of implicit framework is used by every practicing nurse, for we cannot observe, see, or describe, nor can we prescribe anything for which we do not already have some kind of mental image or concept. Unfortunately, the mental images used by nurses in their practice, images developed through education and experience and continuously governed by the multitude of factors in the practice setting, have tended to be disconnected, diffused, incomplete and frequently heavily weighted by concepts drawn from the conceptual schema used by medicine to achieve its own social mission. (p. 195)

Conceptual models of nursing, then, are the formal presentations of some nurses' private images of nursing. The proponents of nursing models maintain that use of a conceptual model facilitates communication among nurses and provides a systematic approach to nursing practice, education, administration, and research.

The importance of conceptual models of nursing was highlighted by Johnson (1987), who commented,

Conceptual models are important for the . . . nurse as they provide philosophical and pragmatic orientations to the service nurses provide patients—a service which only nurses can provide—a service which provides a dimension to total care different from that provided by any other health professional. (p. 195)

Conceptual models of nursing provide explicit orientations not only for nurses but also for the general public. They identify the purpose and scope of nursing and provide frameworks for objective records of the effects of nursing. Johnson (1987) explained, "Conceptual models specify for nurses and society the mission and boundaries of the profession. They clarify the realm of nursing responsibility and accountability, and they allow the practitioner and/or the profession to document services and outcomes" (pp. 196–197).

World Views of Conceptual Models of Nursing

Conceptual models of nursing, like the conceptual models of other disciplines, reflect different and logically incompatible views of the world. As used here, world view refers to philosophical beliefs about the nature of person-environment relationships underlying each conceptual model. Watson (1981) pointed out that such beliefs clearly influence the focus of inquiry and the approach to development of nursing knowledge. The contrasting world views of mechanism and organicism and of change and persistence are appropriate when considering conceptual models of nursing.

Mechanism and Organicism

The metaphor for the mechanistic world view is the machine, and that for the organismic world view is the living organism. The elements of each of these contrasting world views are listed in Table 1–1.

The mechanistic world view proposes that the person, much like a machine, is inherently at rest, responding in a reactive manner to external forces. Behavior is then considered a linear chain of causes and effects, or stimuli and responses.

Mechanism assumes elementarism, such that the whole of any phenomenon, living or nonliving, is the sum of its discrete parts. This world view also assumes reductionism, "a doctrine that maintains that all objects and events, their properties, and our experience and knowledge of them are made up of ultimate elements, indivisible parts" (Ackoff, 1974, p. 8). Reductionism is associated with the notion that behavior is objective and predictable by reducing it to its component parts. This is a deterministic view, such that if enough is known about the parts, then behavior is completely predictable. Furthermore, changes in the person are described as quantitative, an adding or subtracting of a certain number of parts (Battista, 1977; Looft, 1973; Reese & Overton, 1970).

The organismic world view contrasts sharply with mechanism. This world view proposes that the person is inherently and spontaneously active, the source of acts. The person engages in interactions with the environment, rather than reacting to it. Here, cause and effect are denied and complete prediction is rejected. Rather, behavior is understood only in a probabilistic sense.

TABLE 1–1. Elements of Organicism and Mechanism

Organicism	Mechanism
Metaphor is the living organism	Metaphor is the machine
Human being is active	Human being is reactive
Behavior is probabilistic	Behavior is a predictable linear chain
Holism and expansionism assumed—focus on wholes	Elementarism and reductionism assumed—focus on parts
Change is qualitative and quantitative	Change is quantitative

Organicism assumes holism, such that the living organism is postulated to be an integrated, organized entity who is not reducible to discrete parts. Although parts of the organism are acknowledged, they have meaning only within the context of the whole. Ackoff (1974) explained that this doctrine, which is called expansionism, "maintains that all objects, events, and experiences of them are parts of larger wholes. It does not deny that they have parts but focuses on the wholes of which they are part" (p. 12). Kahn (1988) has identified two interpretations of the phrase associated with holism, "the whole is more than the sum of its parts." One interpretation, which Kahn called emergent holism, maintains that the whole has a property not found in any of its parts; the new property emerged from the part. The other interpretation, called connected holism, maintains that the whole forms different relationships with other objects than do the separate parts. Thus, a simple sum of the relationships of each part with another object, such as the environment, does not yield an accurate understanding of the relationship of the whole with the other object.

Organicism also proposes that behavior is associated with structural changes in the organism. These changes are qualitative as well as quantitative, such that one stage of life is completely distinct from another (Battista, 1977; Looft, 1973; Reese & Overton, 1970).

Parse (1987) proposed two world views that are related to mechanism and organicism. The description of what she calls the simultaneity paradigm reflects the organismic world view. Simultaneity regards the person as "more than and different from the sum of the parts . . . an open being free to choose in mutual rhythmical interchange with the environment" (p. 136). Parse's totality paradigm, however, does not seem to reflect the mechanistic world view, as she claims, but rather has elements of both mechanism and organicism. Totality regards the person as the sum of bio-psycho-socio-spiritual parts. The person adapts to the environment, which in turn can be manipulated to maintain or promote balance. Furthermore, the person "interacts with the environment, establishes transactions, and plans toward goal attainment" (p. 32). Although the sum of parts and adaptation to environment notions reflect a mechanistic view, interaction, transaction, and planning to attain goals imply a much more active organism than the passively reacting person of mechanism. The totality world view, then, may be regarded as a bridge between the mechanistic and organismic views of the world.

In summary, from a mechanistic view of the world, the person, who is composed of discrete parts, is passive and reacts when external environmental forces provide the necessary stimulation. In contrast, from an organismic world view, the person, who is seen as an integrated whole, is active and interacts with the environment. These two world views, then, are not logically compatible.

Change and Persistence

The world view of change uses the growth metaphor, and the persistence world view focuses on stability. The elements of these contrasting world views are presented in Table 1–2.

Hall (1981) explained that the change world view holds that "change processes are an inherent and natural part of life" (p. 2). This view also maintains that change is continuous, such that the person always is in a state of transition. Change may be thought of as continual intraindividual variance (Thomae, 1979). Here, progress is valued, and realization of one's potential is emphasized.

In contrast, the persistence world view maintains that stability is natural and normal, "the certain, secure, and healthy condition" (Hall, 1983, p. 19). Persistence is endurance in time and is produced by a synthesis of growth and stability. The focus is on continuation and maintenance of patterns and routines in human behavior through socialization and the commitment of support systems. People are viewed as becoming more like themselves throughout their lifetimes. Furthermore, persistence assumes that people have the power to shape their own lives. Change occurs only when necessary for survival, and is regarded as creative invention of new routines to avoid the disaster of extinction.

Persistence may be thought of as intraindividual invariance (Thomae, 1979). Here, solidarity and stability are valued, and conservation and retrenchment are emphasized.

Thomae (1979) presented evidence for both change and persistence throughout the life cycle. He stated that research supports the proposition that behavior during all periods of life "can be ordered along a dimension running from low to high change or from high to low stability. It is a matter of convenience whether we prefer 'change' or 'stability' as the label" (p. 288).

In summary, from the change view of the world, change and growth are desirable and continual throughout the person's life. From the persistence world view, to the contrary, stability is the natural state. These two world views, then, also are not logically compatible.

TABLE 1–2.   Elements of Change and Persistence

Change	Persistence
Metaphor is growth	Metaphor is stability
Change is inherent and natural	Stability is natural and normal
Change is continuous	Change occurs only for survival
Intraindividual variance	Intraindividual invariance
Progress valued	Conservation and retrenchment emphasized
Realization of potential emphasized	Solidarity valued

Categories of Conceptual Models of Nursing

Conceptual models of nursing reflect not only different world views, but also different broad classifications. Nursing models have been categorized according to the discipline or anthropology from which they were derived and most often are labeled developmental, systems, or interaction models (Johnson, 1974; Reilly, 1975; Riehl & Roy, 1980). Additional categories mentioned in the nursing literature are needs and outcomes (Meleis, 1985); humanistic and energy fields (Marriner, 1986); and intervention, substitution, conservation, sustenance, and enhancement (Stevens, 1984).

The various categories of nursing models are "different classes of approaches to understanding the person who is a patient, [so that they] not only call for differing forms of practice toward different objectives, but also point to different kinds of phenomena, suggest different kinds of questions, and lead eventually to dissimilar bodies of knowledge" (Johnson, 1974, p. 376).

Developmental Models

Developmental models emphasize processes of growth, development, and maturation. Emphasis also is placed on identification of actual and potential developmental problems and delineation of intervention strategies that foster maximum growth and development of people and their environments.

The major thrust of this type of model is change, with the assumption made "that there are noticeable differences between the states of a system at different times, that the succession of these states implies the system is heading somewhere, and that there are orderly processes that explain how the system gets from its present state to wherever it is going" (Chin, 1980, p. 30). Following from the assumption of change are the characteristics of direction, identifiable state, form of progression, forces, and potentiality.

Developmental models postulate that changes are directional, that the individuals, groups, situations, and events of interest are headed in some direction. Chin (1980) outlined the direction of change as: "(a) some goal or end state (developed, mature), (b) the process of becoming (developing, maturing), or (c) the degree of achievement toward some goal or end state (increased development, increase in maturity)" (p. 31).

The characteristic of identifiable state refers to the different states of the person seen over time. These states frequently are termed stages, levels, phases, or periods of development. Such states may be quantitatively or qualitatively differentiated from one another. And, as Chin (1980) pointed out, shifts in state may be either small, nondiscernible steps that eventually are recognized as change, or sudden, cataclysmic changes.

Developmental change, according to Chin (1980), is possible through four different forms of progression. First, unidirectional development may be postulated, such that "once a stage is worked through, the client system shows continued progression and normally never turns back" (p. 31). Second, developmental change may take the form of a spiral, so that while return to a previous problem may occur, the problem is dealt with at a higher level. Third, development may be seen as "phases which occur and recur . . . where no chronological priority is assigned to each state; there are cycles" (p. 32). And fourth, development may take the form of "a branching out into differentiated forms and processes, each part increasing in its specialization and at the same time acquiring its own autonomy and significance" (p. 32).

The developmental models postulate the existence of forces, defined by Chin (1980) as "causal factors producing development and growth" (p. 32). These forces may be viewed as a natural component of the person undergoing change, a coping response to new situations and environmental factors that leads to growth and development; or internal tensions within the person that at some time reach a peak and cause a disruption that leads to further growth and development.

Developmental models also postulate that people have the inherent potential for change. Potentiality may be overt or latent, triggered by internal states or by certain environmental conditions.

The characteristics of developmental models are listed in Table 1–3.

Systems Models

Systems models treat phenomena "as if there existed organization, interaction, interdependency, and integration of parts and elements" (Chin, 1980, p. 24). This type of model emphasizes identification of actual and potential problems in the function of systems and delineation of intervention strategies that maximize efficient and effective system operation. The focus of this category of models, then, is the examination of the system, its parts, and their relation-

TABLE 1–3.   Characteristics of Developmental Models

Growth, Development, and Maturation
Change
Direction of Change
Identifiable State
Form of Progression
Forces
Potentiality

ships at a given time. In contrast to developmental models, change is of secondary importance in systems models.

The major features of systems models are the system and its environment. Hall and Fagen (1968) defined system as "a set of objects together with relationships between the objects and between their attributes" (p. 83). They defined environment as "the set of all objects a change in whose attributes affect the system and also those objects whose attributes are changed by the behavior of the system" (p. 83). When viewing any particular phenomenon, the designation of what is system and what is environment depends on the situation. Thus, a system could be the person whose parts are body organs, and whose environment is the family. Or the system might be the community, whose parts are families and whose environment is the state in which the community is located.

Systems are open or closed. An open system "maintains itself in a continuous inflow and outflow, a building up and breaking down of components," but a closed system is "considered to be isolated from [its] environment" (Bertalanffy, 1968, p. 39). Moreover, open systems continuously import energy in a process called negative entropy or negentropy, so that the system may become more differentiated, more complex, and more ordered. Conversely, closed systems exhibit entropy, such that they move toward increasing disorder.

According to Bertalanffy (1968), all living organisms are open systems. Although closed systems therefore do not exist in nature, it sometimes is convenient to view a system as if it had no interaction with its environment (Chin, 1980). The artificiality of such a view, however, must be taken into account.

Important characteristics of the systems models are boundary; tension, stress, strain, and conflict; equilibrium and steady state; and feedback. Boundary refers to the line of demarcation between a system and its environment. The placement of the boundary must take all relevant system parts into account. Thus, boundary is "the line forming a closed circle around selected variables, where there is less interchange of energy . . . across the line of the circle than within the delimiting circle" (Chin, 1980, p. 24). Boundaries may be thought of as more or less permeable. The greater the boundary permeability, the greater the interchange of energy between the system and its environment.

Tension, stress, strain, and conflict are terms that refer to the forces that alter system structure. Chin (1980) explained that the differences in system parts, as well as the need to adjust to outside disturbances, lead to different amounts of tension within the system. He further noted that internal tensions arising from the system's structural arrangements are called the stresses and strains of the system. Conflict occurs when tensions accumulate and become opposed along the lines of two or more components of the system. Change then occurs to resolve the conflict.

Systems are assumed to tend to move toward a balance between internal and external forces. Chin (1980) explained that "when the balance is thought of as a fixed point or level, it is called 'equilibrium.' 'Steady state,' on the other hand, is the term . . . used to describe the balanced relationship of parts that is not dependent upon any fixed equilibrium point or level" (p. 25). Bertalanffy (1968) maintained that steady state, which also is referred to as a dynamic equilibrium, is characteristic of living open systems. He further commented that the steady state is maintained by a continuous flow of energy within the system and between the system and its environment.

The flow of energy between a system and its environment is called feedback. Chin (1980) described feedback as a series of outputs and inputs across the system-environment boundary. He claimed that systems

> are affected by and in turn affect the environment. While affecting the environment, a process we call output, systems gather information about how they are doing. Such information is then fed back into the system as input to guide and steer its operations. (p. 27)

The feedback process works so that as open systems interact with their environments, any change in the system is associated with a change in the environment, and vice versa.

The characteristics of systems models are listed in Table 1–4.

Interaction Models

Interaction models emphasize social acts and relationships between people. The focus, therefore, is on identification of actual and potential problems in interpersonal relationships and delineation of intervention strategies that promote optimal socialization.

This type of model is derived from symbolic interactionism, which "sees human beings as creatures who define and classify situations, including themselves, and who choose ways of acting toward

---

TABLE 1–4. Characteristics of Systems Models

Integration of Parts
System
Environment
Open and Closed Systems
Boundary
Tension, Stress, Strain, Conflict
Equilibrium and Steady State
Feedback

and within them" (Benoliel, 1977, p. 110). Symbolic interactionism "postulates that the importance of social life lies in providing the [person] with language, self-concept, role-taking ability, and other skills" (Heiss, 1976, p. 467). The major characteristics of this category of models are perception, communication, role, and self-concept.

The person's perceptions of other people, the environment, situations, and events—that is, the awareness and experience of phenomena—depend on meanings attached to these phenomena. These meanings, or definitions as they sometimes are called, determine how the person behaves in a given situation. Thus, the key data to be gathered when working in the context of interaction models are the person's perceptions, that is, his or her definition of the situation. Heiss (1981) explained,

> The fact that an other is, in fact, kindly or cruel may not be very significant. The fact that we define him or her as one or the other is important, because—regardless of the facts—we will act on that belief. (p. 3)

The person's perceptions are derived from social interactions with others. People may adopt fully, modify, or reject others' definitions of phenomena, but they always are influenced in some way by others. This is especially so when the other is significant to the person.

During social interactions, people communicate with one another. Communication is through language, "a system of significant symbols" (Heiss, 1981, p. 5). Communication, therefore, involves the transfer of arbitrary meanings of things from one person to another. Thus, people must communicate with one another to find out each other's perceptions of the particular situation.

Communication is important in learning roles, which are "prescriptions for behavior which are associated with particular actor-other combinations. They are the ways we think people of a particular kind ought to act toward various categories of others" (Heiss, 1981, p. 65). Each person has many different roles, each one providing a behavioral repertoire. We adopt the behaviors associated with a given role, when, through communication, we determine that a given role is called for in a particular situation.

The person's ability to perform roles, and to perform them according to self-imposed and societal standards, influences self-concept. "The self-concept is the individual's thoughts and feelings about himself" (Heiss, 1981, p. 83). An important aspect of self-concept is self-evaluation, which refers to "our view of how good we are at what we think we are" (Heiss, 1981, p. 83).

An especially important feature of interaction models is their emphasis on the person as an active participant in interactions. People are thought to actively evaluate communication from others, rather than passively accept their ideas. Moreover, they actively set goals on the basis of their perceptions of the relevant factors in a given situation.

The characteristics of interaction models are listed in Table 1–5.

Other Categories of Conceptual Models

Other categories of conceptual models of nursing have been identified in recent years. The little that has been written about these categories is summarized below. The characteristics of these categories are listed in Table 1–6.

Needs and Outcomes Models

The needs and outcomes categories of conceptual models were developed by Meleis (1985), who also included an interaction category in her classification scheme. The needs category of conceptual models focuses on nurses' functions and consideration of the patient in terms of a hierarchy of needs. When patients cannot fulfill their own needs, nursing care is required. The function of the nurse is to provide the necessary action to help patients meet their needs. This category reduces the human being to a set of needs, and nursing, to a set of functions. Nurses are portrayed as the final decision makers for nursing care.

The outcomes category of conceptual models is not well described by Meleis (1985), who commented only that emphasis is placed on the outcomes of nursing care and comprehensive descriptions of the recipient of care. No one perspective of the care recipient was noted.

Humanistic and Energy Fields Models

Marriner (1986) identified two other categories of nursing models, the humanistic and energy fields. Her classification scheme also included an interpersonal relationships category, which is similar to the interaction category already discussed in this chapter. Marriner mentioned that humanistic models view nursing as an art and science, and

TABLE 1–5. Characteristics of Interaction Models

Social Acts and Relationships
Perception
Communication
Role
Self-Concept

TABLE 1–6.   Characteristics of Other Categories of Models

Category	Characteristics
Needs	Nursing as set of functions to help patients meet their needs
Outcomes	Outcomes of nursing care
Humanistic	Nursing as art and science
Energy fields	Energy
Intervention	Manipulation of patient or environmental variables to effect change
Substitution	Provision of substitutes for lost or impaired patient capabilities
Conservation	Preservation of beneficial aspects of patient's situation
Sustenance	Helping patient endure insults to health
Enhancement	Improvement of quality of patient's existence

she implied that energy field models incorporate the concept of energy. The bulk of her discussion, however, focused on an overview of various models within the categories, rather than on identification of specific characteristics of each category.

Intervention, Substitution, Conservation, Sustenance, and Enhancement Models

Stevens (1984) developed a substantially different classification scheme for conceptual models of nursing. This scheme is based on "the character of the nursing act in relation to the patient" (p. 257). The intervention category emphasizes the nurse's professional actions and decisions and regards the patient as an object of nursing rather than a participant in nursing care. Agency rests with the nurse, who makes the care decision and manipulates selected patient or environmental variables to bring about change.

Substitution models focus on provision of substitutes for patient capabilities that cannot be enacted or have been lost. Agency rests with the patient, in that the patient exercises his or her will and physical control to the greatest possible extent. In contrast, conservation models emphasize preservation of beneficial aspects of the patient's situation that are threatened by illness or actual or potential problems. This category bridges the polarity of agency seen in the intervention and substitution categories in that agency rests with nurses, but they conserve the existing capabilities of the patient.

The sustenance category of models emphasizes helping the patient endure insults to health. The focus is on supporting the patient and building psychological and physiological coping mechanisms. The enhancement category regards nursing as a way to improve the quality of the patient's existence following a health insult.

In summary, each category of model emphasizes different phenomena and leads to different questions about the nurse–patient situation. It is anticipated that each category of nursing models will foster development of a different body of knowledge about the person, the environment, health, and nursing.

THEORIES

A theory may be defined as "a statement that purports to account for or characterize some phenomenon" (Stevens, 1984, p. 1). Theories, like conceptual models, are made up of concepts and propositions. Theories, however, address phenomena with much greater specificity than do conceptual models (Reese & Overton, 1970; Reilly, 1975).

The specificity of a theory requires that its concepts be more specific and concrete than those of a conceptual model. Therefore, they are tied more closely to particular individuals, groups, situations, or events. Examples of such concepts are temperature, pulse, blood pressure, distress, social support.

The propositions of a theory also are more specific than those of a conceptual model. Some statements, called nonrelational propositions, define or describe the concepts of a theory. One type of nonrelational proposition states the existence of a concept. An example is: There is a phenomenon known as social support. Another type of nonrelational proposition is the definition. Definitional propositions are required for all theory concepts. Indeed, though the concepts of a conceptual model may not be defined at all, or may be only loosely defined, the concepts of a theory must be constitutively defined. Such definitions, which also are called theoretical definitions, provide meaning for concepts by defining them in terms of other concepts; they are circular in nature. An example of a constitutive definition is: Social support is defined as supportive transactions that include expression of positive affect of one person toward another; affirmation of another's behavior, perceptions, or views; and provision of symbolic or material aid to another (Norbeck, Lindsey, & Carrieri, 1981). The concepts of a theory also must be operationally defined, so that the theory may be empirically tested. These definitions specify the way in which the concept is to be measured. An example of an operational definition is: In this study, social support was measured by the Norbeck Social Support Questionnaire. Operational definitions, then, connect constitutively defined concepts to the real world.

Other statements that may be part of a theory are called relational propositions. These propositions link two or more concepts; they express an association between concepts or identify the effect of one concept on another. An example of a relational proposition is: Social support is positively related to well-being. Another example is: Psychoeducational information given prior to surgery has a positive effect on postoperative recovery.

The hypothesis is a special type of proposition that states a conjecture about one or more concepts in empirically testable form. More specifically, a hypothesis is a prediction about the scores obtained from the measures of concepts. Suppose, for example, that social support was measured by the Norbeck Social Support Questionnaire (NSSQ) and well-being was measured by a Well-Being Inventory (WBI). Given the relational proposition about social support and well-being presented above, the hypothesis would state: As scores on the NSSQ increase, scores on the WBI will increase.

Types of Theories

A theory may be a description of a particular phenomenon, an explanation of the relations between phenomena, or a prediction of the effects of one phenomenon on another. Theories are developed by means of research, which may be defined as "a systematic, formal, rigorous, and precise process employed to gain solutions to problems and/or to discover and interpret new facts and relationships" (Waltz & Bausell, 1981, p. 1).

Descriptive theories describe or classify specific dimensions or characteristics of individuals, groups, situations, or events by summarizing the commonalities found in discrete observations. They are generated and tested by descriptive research. For example, Patterson, Freese, and Goldenberg (1986) conducted a descriptive study to generate a theory of self-diagnosis of pregnancy.

Explanatory theories specify relations among the dimensions or characteristics of individuals, groups, situations, or events. They are developed by correlational research. Rutledge (1987), for example, used correlational procedures to test a theory of the relationship of perceived susceptibility, perceived benefits, perceived barriers, self-concept, and age to frequency of breast self-examination.

Predictive theories move beyond explanation to the prediction of precise relationships between the dimensions or characteristics of a phenomenon or differences between groups. Experimental research is used to generate and test predictive theories. For example, an experimental study was designed by King and her associates (1987) to test a theory of the effects of a personal control intervention—self-administered versus nurse-administered medication—on patients' desire for control, pain intensity, disruption in daily activities, emotional responses, and use of pain medication over time.

Regardless of whether a theory is a description, an explanation, or a prediction, its strength "is its ability to bring a great deal of thought and information to bear on a specific problem or set of problems, and thereby go far beyond unsystematic thought" (Skidmore, 1975, p. 2). Inasmuch as each theory deals only with very specific problems, many theories are needed to deal with all phenomena of interest to a discipline. Mennell's (1974) comment helps to underscore this point: "Reality is so immense and complex that no theory, however well authenticated, ever represents more than a drop in the ocean. Some theories are broader in scope than others, but no theory can ever explain everything" (p. 1).

Scope of Theories

Theories that are broadest in scope are called grand theories. These theories frequently lack operationally defined concepts, because the concepts are quite abstract. Thus, they are not amenable to direct empirical testing. Indeed, grand theories rarely are developed by means of empirical research, but rather through thoughtful and insightful appraisal of existing ideas or creative leaps beyond existing knowledge. Some nurse scholars consider conceptual models and grand theories to be synonymous (e.g., Kim, 1983; Stevens, 1984). Although it is recognized that the line between a conceptual model and a grand theory is sometimes difficult to discern, it seems more accurate to separate the two. Furthermore, grand theories are beginning to appear in the nursing literature, and clearly demonstrate the differences between conceptual models and theories. For example, Newman's (1979, 1986) theory of health as expanding consciousness was derived from Rogers's (1970) conceptual model of nursing. Rogers's conceptual model was developed to deal with all that is of interest to nursing, whereas Newman's grand theory focuses primarily on health, albeit in an abstract manner. This example illustrates the fact that although a grand theory is quite abstract, it still is more circumscribed than a conceptual model.

Theories of the middle range are narrower in scope than grand theories, encompassing a limited number of concepts and a limited aspect of the real world. Merton (1957) contended that middle range theories are the most useful, because they can be empirically tested in a direct manner. The examples of descriptive, explanatory, and predictive theories cited earlier in this chapter are middle range theories. In fact, most research reported in the contemporary nursing literature is directed toward the generation and testing of middle range theories.

Partial theories, which also are called micro theories or empirical generalizations, are the most limited in scope and utility. They are summary statements of isolated observations dealing with an extremely narrow range of phenomena. Though partial theories frequently are regarded as trivial due to their limited scope, they do have heuristic value, and some may be developed into middle range theories through further research. For example, case studies, such as Durand's (1975) description of the impact of nursing care on a child with Down's syndrome, may yield partial theories that can be developed into middle range theories with additional study.

These examples illustrate the fact that theories deal with a limited number of concepts and propositions, and that these components of theories are quite specific and concrete. The examples also show the relation of theory to research. Inasmuch as the purpose of this book is to examine conceptual models, the discussion of theory development is necessarily limited. Readers who are interested in a detailed discussion of theory construction strategies are referred to the seminal work by Walker and Avant (in press).

Nursing Theories

A nursing theory may be defined as a relatively specific and concrete set of concepts and propositions that purports to account for or characterize phenomena of interest to the discipline of nursing. Theories that may be considered unique to nursing are being developed at the present time. Many unique nursing theories have been derived from the conceptual models that are discussed in this book. These theories are presented in later chapters.

Many other theories used by nurses have been borrowed from other disciplines. Theories of role, change, development, stress, and coping are just a few examples. Unfortunately, these theories sometimes are used with no consideration given to their credibility for the nursing situation. There is, however, increasing awareness of the need to test borrowed theories to determine if they are credible in nursing situations. The theory testing work by Lowery and her associates (1987) is an outstanding example of what can happen when a theory, borrowed in this case from psychology, is tested in the real world of acute and chronic illness. These investigators have determined that a basic proposition of attribution theory, stating that people search for causes to make sense of their lives, has not been fully supported in their research with patients with arthritis, diabetes, hypertension, or myocardial infarction. This result means that attribution theory cannot be considered a shared theory, that is, a theory that is borrowed from another discipline but found to be credible in the nursing milieu (Stevens, 1984). Further research should determine whether a modification of attribution theory is credible in nursing situations or if an entirely new theory is required.

An example of a borrowed theory that has become a shared theory is that of social support. This theory was developed initially in other disciplines, and many of its propositions have been supported in several nursing situations (Barnard, Brandt, Raff, & Carroll, 1984).

Many nurses continue to claim that there are few, if any, nursing theories. It is likely, however, that the apparent paucity of recognizable nursing theories is due to investigators' failure to be explicit about the theoretical components of their studies. Thus, the ideas presented by nurses in books and articles should be closely examined for evidence of the specific concepts and propositions that comprise theories. Identification of the components of a theory is accomplished by the technique of theory formalization, also called theoretical substruction. Discussion of this technique is beyond the scope of this book. Readers who are interested in theory formalization are, therefore, referred to Hinshaw's (1979) pioneering work and Fawcett and Downs's (1986) more recent work.

Metaparadigms, Conceptual Models, and Theories

Earlier in this chapter, the discussion of the structural hierarchy of knowledge within disciplines was begun. It was explained that most disciplines have a single metaparadigm and multiple conceptual models. Theories will now be placed within the structural hierarchy.

It already has been noted that the multiple conceptual models of each discipline specify the metaparadigm phenomena in diverse ways. Theories provide still greater specification of these phenomena. Theories are derived from or linked with conceptual models, as Reese and Overton (1970) explained:

> Any theory presupposes a more general model according to which the theoretical concepts are formulated. At the more general levels, the concepts are generally less explicitly formulated, but they nonetheless necessarily determine the concepts at the lower levels. (p. 117)

The abstract nature of conceptual models requires many theories to fully describe, explain, and predict phenomena within the domain of the model. Thus, the structural hierarchy of knowledge progresses from a single metaparadigm to multiple conceptual models and multiple theories derived from each model. This progression is depicted in Figure 1–1.

Although all theories are derived from conceptual models, the parent model is not always identified in reports of the theory development work. This omission has created difficulties in classifying theory development efforts and evaluating the state of knowledge development in a discipline. Nurse authors, however, are beginning to be more explicit about the conceptual models upon which their works are based. Silva (1986, 1987), for example, was able to identify many published research reports and doctoral dissertations associated with Johnson's, Orem's, Rogers's and Roy's conceptual models, and Newman's grand theory. Many of these studies, as well as other work

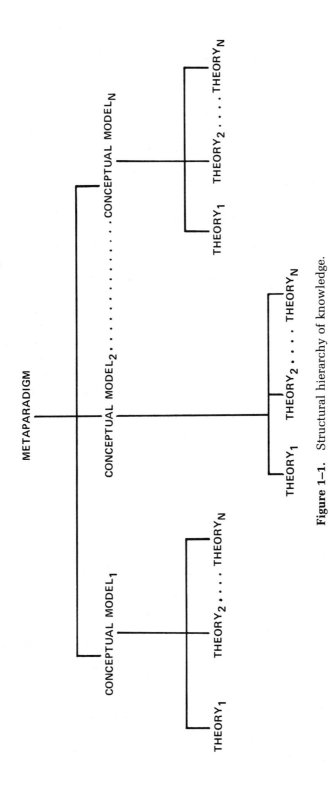

Figure 1–1. Structural hierarchy of knowledge.

based on the conceptual models presented in this book, are discussed in later chapters.

Distinctions Between Conceptual Models and Theories

Throughout this chapter, emphasis has been placed on the point that a conceptual model is not a theory, nor is a theory a conceptual model. This point requires further discussion because there still is considerable confusion about these two levels of knowledge in the nursing literature. Although some writers consider distinctions between conceptual models and theories a semantic point (e.g., Flaskerud & Halloran, 1980; Meleis, 1985), this issue should not be dismissed so easily. The distinction should be made because of the differences in the way that conceptual models and theories are used. Indeed, if one is to know what to do next, then one must know whether the starting point is a conceptual model or a theory.

The primary distinction between a conceptual model and a theory is the level of abstraction. A conceptual model is an abstract and general system of concepts and propositions. A theory, in contrast, deals with one or more relatively specific and concrete concepts and propositions. Conceptual models are only general guides that must be specified further by relevant and logically congruent theories before action can occur. Thus, all pragmatic activities of members of a discipline are finally directed by conceptual-theoretical systems of knowledge.

Distinguishing between conceptual models and theories on the basis of level of abstraction raises the question of how abstract is abstract enough for a work to be considered a conceptual model. Although the decision in a few cases may be somewhat arbitrary, the following rule serves as one guideline for classification of conceptual models and theories. This rule requires determination of the purpose of the work. If the purpose was to describe, explain, or predict specific phenomena, the work most likely is a theory. For example, works by Peplau (1952), Orlando (1961), and Travelbee (1966) focused on the interpersonal relationship between nurse and patient. There was no obvious intent on the part of these authors to address the entire domain of nursing. The specificity of these works, therefore, leads to their classification as theories. Conversely, if the purpose of the work was to articulate a body of distinctive knowledge for the discipline of nursing, the work most likely is a conceptual model. Given that this was the explicitly stated purpose of authors such as Johnson (1980), King (1981), Levine (1973, in press), Neuman (in press), Orem (1985), Rogers (1986), and Roy (1984), their works are classified as conceptual models. In summary, if a given work is an abstract, general, and comprehensive perspective of the metaparadigm of nursing, it is a conceptual model. If the work is more specific, concrete, and restricted to a more limited range of phenomena than that identified by the metaparadigm, it is a theory.

Another important distinction between conceptual models and theories is the number of steps required before the work can be used for pragmatic activities such as clinical practice or research. This distinction leads to another rule for classification of conceptual models and theories. This rule requires determination of how many levels of knowledge are needed before the work may be applied in particular nursing situations. If, for example, the work identifies physiologic needs as an assessment parameter, but does not explain the differences between normal and pathological functions of body systems, it most likely is a conceptual model. As such, the work is not directly applicable in clinical practice. A theory of normal and pathological functions must be linked with the conceptual model so that judgments about the functions of body systems may be made. Conversely, if the work includes a detailed description of behavior, or an explanation of how particular factors influence particular behaviors, it most likely is a theory. In this case, the work may be directly applied in clinical practice.

This rule also is exemplified by the number of steps required before empirical testing can occur (Reilly, 1975). A conceptual model cannot be tested directly, because its concepts are not operationally defined nor are the relationships between concepts observable. More specific concepts and propositions have to be derived from the conceptual model; that is, a theory must be formulated. These more specific concepts then must be defined in measurable ways, and hypotheses stating observable relationships must be derived from the propositions of the theory. Three steps, therefore, are required before a conceptual model can be tested, albeit indirectly. First, the conceptual model must be formulated; second, a theory must be derived from the conceptual model; and third, operational definitions must be given to the theory concepts, and hypotheses must be derived. In contrast, only two steps are required for empirical testing of a theory. First, the theory must be stated. Second, as above, the theory concepts must be operationally defined, and hypotheses must be formulated from the propositions.

 Failure to distinguish between a conceptual model and a theory leads to considerable misunderstanding and inappropriate expectations about the work. When a conceptual model is labeled a theory, expectations regarding empirical testing immediately arise. When such expectations cannot be met, the work frequently is regarded as inadequate. Similarly, when a theory is labeled a conceptual model, expectations regarding comprehensiveness arise. When those expectations cannot be met, that work also may be regarded as inadequate.

The distinctions between conceptual models and theories described here are in keeping with Johnson's (1974) and Reilly's (1975) statements about these two levels of knowledge. The meaning given to conceptual models in this book should not be confused with the meaning of model found in the philosophy of science literature and some nursing literature. The latter refers to representations of testable theories. Rudner (1966), for example, defined a model for a theory as "an alternative interpretation of the same calculus of which the theory itself is an interpretation" (p. 24). This kind of a model is made up of ideas or diagrams that are more familiar to the novice than are the concepts and propositions of the theory. Thus, the model is a heuristic device that facilitates understanding of the theory. Rudner illustrated this by the analogy of the flow of water through pipes as a model for a theory of electric current wires.

In summary, a conceptual model cannot be used directly, whether in research, clinical practice, education, or administration. Rather, a conceptual model must be linked with one or more theories to form the conceptual-theoretical systems of knowledge needed for action.

CONCEPTUAL-THEORETICAL SYSTEMS OF NURSING KNOWLEDGE

In nursing, conceptual models now are used as general guides for the organization of nursing knowledge and the design and implementation of research projects, clinical nursing practice, educational programs, and administrative systems. Currently, many theories used to amplify the concepts and propositions of any nursing model are borrowed from other disciplines, including psychology, sociology, biology, physics, and chemistry. When borrowed theories are linked with conceptual models, care must be taken to ensure logical congruence. Whall (1980) presented the first substantial discussion in the nursing literature of elements to consider when assessing congruence between conceptual models of nursing and borrowed theories. She proposed that conceptual models and theories must be examined for their stands on holism and linearity. Holism is the major focus of the organismic world view, and linearity is encompassed by the mechanistic world view. Both world views were discussed earlier in this chapter. Whall's discussion suggested that if the conceptual model and theory are not congruent with regard to mechanism or organicism, the theory should be discarded and another more congruent one chosen, or the theory should be reformulated so that it is congruent with the model. Inasmuch as the conceptual model is the more abstract starting point, the theory—not the model—is reformulated to ensure congruence. Examples of construction of logically congruent conceptual-theoretical systems of nursing knowledge using borrowed theories are given in Fitzpatrick, Whall, Johnston, and Floyd (1982), and in Whall (1986). The same care to ensure logical congruence must be taken if a shared nursing theory is to be linked with a conceptual model of nursing, or if a unique nursing theory not derived from an explicit conceptual model is to be linked with a model.

The following discussion focuses on general considerations in constructing conceptual-theoretical systems of nursing knowledge in the areas of research, clinical practice, education, and administration. Later chapters will document the use of conceptual models of nursing and related theories in various situations.

Nursing Research

The function of nursing research is to generate or test nursing theories. A fully developed conceptual model reflects a particular research tradition that includes the following six rules that guide theory generation and testing through all phases of a study:

- The first rule identifies the distinctive nature of the problems to be studied and the purposes to be fulfilled by the research.
- The second rule identifies the phenomena that are to be studied.
- The third rule identifies the research techniques that are to be employed and the research tools that are to be used.
- The fourth rule identifies the settings in which data are to be gathered and the subjects who are to provide the data.
- The fifth rule identifies the methods to be employed in reducing and analyzing the data.
- The sixth rule identifies the nature of contributions that the research will make to the advancement of knowledge. (Laudan, 1981; Schlotfeldt, 1975)

Thus, a conceptual model identifies the concepts from which specific variables are derived for the research. The model also presents the general propositions from which testable hypotheses eventually are derived. The subject matter of the study might be one concept or the relations between two or more concepts. Theories borrowed from other disciplines may be linked with the conceptual model in order to test the credibility of such knowledge in nursing situations. Or a study may involve generation or testing of a unique nursing theory.

The findings of research based on explicit conceptual-theoretical systems of nursing knowledge are, of course, used to evaluate the credibility of the theory. These findings, which constitute indirect evidence regarding the conceptual model, also should be used to evaluate its credibility (Fawcett & Downs, 1986; Silva, 1986). Thus, the credibility of the conceptual model should be considered as well as that of the theory whenever research is conducted. The empirical data, therefore, serve as a direct test of the theory and an indirect test of the conceptual model.

Clinical Nursing Practice

Conceptual models of nursing provide general guidelines for nursing practice. More specifically, a fully developed conceptual model represents a particular view of and approach to nursing practice. The domain of nursing practice and nursing processes are specified in the following four rules that are inherent in the conceptual model:

- The first rule identifies the general nature of the clinical problems to be considered and the purposes to be fulfilled by nursing practice.
- The second rule identifies the settings in which nursing practice occurs and the characteristics of legitimate recipients of nursing care.
- The third rule identifies the nursing process to be employed and the technologies to be used, including assessment format, diagnostic taxonomy, intervention typology, and evaluation methods.
- The fourth rule identifies the nature of contributions that nursing practice makes to the well-being of recipients of nursing care.

Thus, a conceptual model guides all aspects of clinical practice. The model tells the clinician what to look at when interacting with clients and how to interpret observations. It also tells the clinician how to plan interventions in a general manner, and provides beginning criteria for evaluation of intervention outcomes.

The specifics of nursing assessment, diagnosis, intervention, and evaluation, however, must come from theories. Although the conceptual model may, for example, direct the clinician to look for certain categories of problems in adaptation, theories of adaptation are needed to describe, to explain, and to predict manifestations of actual or potential patient problems in particular situations. Similarly, theories are needed to direct the particular nursing interventions required in such situations.

Nursing Education

In nursing education, the conceptual model, or conceptual framework as it usually is called, provides the general outline for curriculum content and teaching-learning activities. More specifically, a fully developed conceptual model represents a particular view of and approach to nursing education. The curricular structure and educational processes are specified in the following four rules inherent in each conceptual model:

- The first rule identifies the distinctive focus of the curriculum and the purposes to be fulfilled by nursing education.
- The second rule identifies the general nature and sequence of the content to be presented.
- The third rule identifies the settings in which nursing education occurs and the characteristics of the students.
- The fourth rule identifies the teaching-learning strategies to be employed.

When a conceptual model is used for curriculum construction, it must be linked with theories about education and the teaching-learning process, as well as with substantive theoretical content from nursing and other disciplines (Fawcett, 1985). The resulting conceptual-theoretical system then applies to the patient, the student, and the educator.

Nursing Administration

When a conceptual model is used in nursing administration, it provides a systematic structure for thinking about administrative matters, for observations of the administrative situation, and for interpreting what is seen in administrative settings. Each fully developed conceptual model, then, represents a particular view of and approach to administration of nursing services. The administrative structure and management practices are specified in the following three rules that are inherent in each conceptual model:

- The first rule identifies the distinctive focus of nursing in the clinical agency and the purpose to be fulfilled by nursing services.
- The second rule identifies the characteristics of nursing personnel and the settings in which nursing services are delivered.
- The third rule identifies the management strategies to be employed.

When a conceptual model is used to guide administrative practices, it must be linked with theories of organization and management developed in nursing and other disciplines. The resulting conceptual theoretical structure then is applicable to the patient, the nursing staff, and the nurse administrator.

CONCLUSION

This chapter discussed the definitions and distinctions between conceptual models and theories, as well as the formation of conceptual-theoretical systems of nursing knowledge. The distinctions between conceptual models and theories mandate separate criteria for analysis and evaluation of each of these levels of knowledge. Analysis and evaluation of theories have been discussed by many authors, including Chinn and Jacobs (1987), Fawcett and Downs (1986), and Walker and Avant (in press). Chapter 2 will present a framework expressly designed for the analysis and evaluation of conceptual models of nursing.

REFERENCES

Ackoff, R.L. (1974). Redesigning the future. A systems approach to societal problems. New York: John Wiley & Sons.

Aggleton, P., & Chalmers, H. (1986). Nursing research, nursing theory and the nursing process. Journal of Advanced Nursing, 11, 197–202.

Barnard, K.E., Brandt, P.A., Raff, B.S., & Carroll, P. (Eds.) (1984). Social support and families of vulnerable infants (Birth Defects: Original Article Series, Vol. 20, No. 5). White Plains, NY: March of Dimes Birth Defects Foundation.

Battista, J.R. (1977). The holistic paradigm and general system theory. General Systems, 22, 65–71.

Benoliel, J.Q. (1977). The interaction between theory and research. Nursing Outlook, 25, 108–113.

Bertalanffy, L. von (1968). General system theory. New York: George Braziller.

Chin, R. (1980). The utility of systems models and developmental models for practitioners. In J.P. Riehl and C. Roy, Conceptual models for nursing practice (2nd ed., pp. 21–37). New York: Appleton-Century-Crofts.

Chinn, P.L., & Jacobs, M.K. (1987). Theory and nursing. A systematic approach (2nd ed.). St. Louis: CV Mosby.

Conway, M.E. (1985). Toward greater specificity in defining nursing's metaparadigm. Advances in Nursing Science, 7(4), 73–81.

Donaldson, S.K., & Crowley, D.M. (1978). The discipline of nursing. Nursing Outlook, 26, 113–120.

Durand, B. (1975). Failure to thrive in a child with Down's syndrome. Nursing Research, 24, 272–286.

Eckberg, D.L., & Hill, L., Jr. (1979). The paradigm concept and sociology: A critical review. American Sociology Review, 44, 925–937.

Fawcett, J. (1983). Hallmarks of success in nursing theory development. In P.L. Chinn (Ed.), Advances in nursing theory development (pp. 3–17). Rockville, MD: Aspen.

Fawcett, J. (1984). The metaparadigm of nursing. Current status and future refinements. Image. The Journal of Nursing Scholarship, 16, 84–87.

Fawcett, J. (1985). Theory: Basis for the study and practice of nursing education. Journal of Nursing Education, 24, 226–229.

Fawcett, J., & Downs, F.S. (1986). The relationship of theory and research. Norwalk, CT: Appleton-Century-Crofts.

Feldman, H.R. (1980). Nursing research in the 1980s: Issues and implications. Advances in Nursing Science, 3(1), 85–92.

Fitzpatrick, J.J., Whall, A.L., Johnston, R.L., & Floyd, J.A. (1982). Nursing models and their psychiatric mental health applications. Bowie, MD: Brady.

Flaskerud, J.H., & Halloran, E.J. (1980). Areas of agreement in nursing theory development. Advances in Nursing Science, 3(1), 1–7.

Gortner, S.R. (1980). Nursing science in transition. Nursing Research, 29, 180–183.

Hall, B.A. (1981). The change paradigm in nursing: Growth versus persistence. Advances in Nursing Science, 3(4), 1–6.

Hall, B.A. (1983). Toward an understanding of stability in nursing phenomena. Advances in Nursing Science, 5(3), 15–20.

Hall, K.V. (1979). Current trends in the use of conceptual frameworks in nursing education. Journal of Nursing Education, 18(4), 26–29.

Hall, A.D., & Fagen, R.E. (1968). Definition of system. In W. Buckley (Ed.), Modern systems research for the behavioral scientist (pp. 81–92). Chicago: Aldine.

Heiss, J. (1976). Family roles and interaction (2nd ed.). Chicago: Rand McNally.

Heiss, J. (1981). The social psychology of interaction. Englewood Cliffs, NJ: Prentice-Hall.

Hinshaw, A.S. (1979). Theoretical substruction: An assessment process. Western Journal of Nursing Research, 1, 319–324.

Hinshaw, A.S. (1987). Response to "Structuring the nursing knowledge system: A typology of four domains." Scholarly Inquiry for Nursing Practice, 1, 111–114.

Johnson, D.E. (1974). Development of theory: A requisite for nursing as a primary health profession. Nursing Research, 23, 372–377.

Johnson, D.E. (1980). The behavioral system model for nursing. In J.P. Riehl and C. Roy, Conceptual models for nursing practice (2nd ed., pp. 207–216). New York: Appleton-Century-Crofts.

Johnson, D.E. (1987). Guest Editorial: Evaluating conceptual models for use in critical care nursing practice. Dimensions of Critical Care Nursing, 6, 195–197.

Kahn, S.M. (1988). Holism in nursing. Manuscript submitted for publication.

Kim, H.S. (1983). The nature of theoretical thinking in nursing. Norwalk, CT: Appleton-Century-Crofts.

Kim, H.S. (1987). Structuring the nursing knowledge system: A typology of four domains. Scholarly Inquiry for Nursing Practice, 1, 99–110.

King, I.M. (1981). A theory for nursing. Systems, concepts, process. New York: John Wiley & Sons.

King, K.B., Norsen, L.H., Robertson, R.K., & Hicks, G.L. (1987). Patient management of pain medication after cardiac surgery. Nursing Research, 36, 145–150.

Kuhn, T.S. (1970). The structure of scientific revolutions (2nd ed.). Chicago: University of Chicago Press.

Kuhn, T.S. (1977). Second thoughts on paradigms. In F. Suppe (Ed.), The structure of scientific theories (2nd ed., pp. 459–517). Chicago: University of Illinois Press.

Laudan, L. (1981). A problem-solving approach to scientific progress. In I. Hacking (Ed.), Scientific revolutions (pp. 144–155). Fair Lawn, NJ: Oxford University Press.

Levine, M.E. (1973). Introduction to clinical nursing (2nd ed.). Philadelphia: FA Davis.

Levine, M.E. (in press). The four conservation principles: Twenty years later. In J.P. Riehl-Sisca (Ed.), Conceptual models for nursing practice (3rd ed.). Norwalk, CT: Appleton and Lange.

Lippitt, G.L. (1973). Visualizing change. Model building and the change process. Fairfax, VA: NTL Learning Resources.

Looft, W.R. (1973). Socialization and personality throughout the life span: An examination of contemporary psychological approaches. In P.B. Baltes & K.W. Schaie (Eds.), Life span developmental psychology. Personality and socialization (pp. 25–52). New York: Academic Press.

Lowery, B.J., Jacobsen, B.S., & McCauley, K. (1987). On the prevalence of causal search in illness situations. Nursing Research, 36, 88–93.

Marriner, A. (1986). Nursing theorists and their work. St. Louis: CV Mosby.

Meleis, A.I. (1985). Theoretical nursing: Development and progress. Philadelphia: JB Lippincott.

Mennell, S. (1974). Sociological theory. Uses and unities. New York: Praeger.

Merton, R.K. (1957). Social theory and social structure (rev. ed.). New York: Free Press.

Neuman, B. (in press). The Neuman systems model: A holistic approach to client care. In B. Neuman, The Neuman systems model. Application to nursing education and practice (2nd ed.). Norwalk, CT: Appleton and Lange.

Newman, M.A. (1979). Theory development in nursing. Philadelphia: FA Davis.

Newman, M.A. (1986). Health as expanding consciousness. St. Louis: CV Mosby.

Nightingale, F. (1859). Notes on nursing: What it is, and what it is not. London: Harrison. (Reprinted by Lippincott, 1946.)

Norbeck, J.S., Lindsey, A.M., & Carrieri, V.L. (1981). The development of an instrument to measure social support. Nursing Research, 30, 264–269.

Nursing Development Conference Group. (1973). Concept formalization in nursing. Process and product. Boston: Little, Brown & Co.

Nursing Development Conference Group. (1979). Concept formalization in nursing. Process and product (2nd ed.). Boston: Little, Brown & Co.

Nye, F.I., & Berardo, F.N. (Eds.). (1981). Emerging conceptual frameworks in family analysis. New York: Macmillan.

Orem, D.E. (1985). Nursing: Concepts of practice (3rd ed.). New York: McGraw-Hill.

Orlando, I.J. (1961). The dynamic nurse-patient relationship. New York: GP Putnam's Sons.

Parse, R.R. (1987). Nursing science. Major paradigms, theories, and critiques. Philadelphia: WB Saunders.

Patterson, E.T., Freese, M.P. & Goldenberg, R.L. (1986). Reducing uncertainty: Self-diagnosis of pregnancy. Image. The Journal of Nursing Scholarship, 18, 105–109.

Peplau, H.E. (1952). Interpersonal relations in nursing. New York: GP Putnam's Sons.

Peterson, C.J. (1977). Questions frequently asked about the development of a conceptual framework. Journal of Nursing Education, 16(4), 22–32.

Phillips, J.R. (1977). Nursing systems and nursing models. Image, 9, 4–7.

Redman, B.K. (1974). Why develop a conceptual framework? Journal of Nursing Education, 13(3), 2–10.

Reese, H.W., & Overton, W.F. (1970). Models of development and theories of development. In L.R. Goulet & P.B. Baltes (Eds.), Life span developmental psychology. Research and theory (pp. 115–145). New York: Academic Press.

Reilly, D.E. (1975). Why a conceptual framework? Nursing Outlook, 23, 566–569.

Riehl, J.P., & Roy, C. (1974). Conceptual models for nursing practice. New York: Appleton-Century-Crofts.

Riehl, J.P., & Roy, C. (1980). Conceptual models for nursing practice (2nd ed.). New York: Appleton-Century-Crofts.

Rogers, C.G. (1973). Conceptual models as guides to clinical nursing specialization. Journal of Nursing Education, 12(4), 2–6.

Rogers, M.E. (1970). An introduction to the theoretical basis of nursing. Philadelphia: FA Davis.

Rogers, M.E. (1986). Science of unitary human beings. In V.M. Malinski (Ed.), Explorations on Martha Rogers' science of unitary human beings. Norwalk, CT: Appleton-Century-Crofts.

Roy, C. (1984). Introduction to nursing: An adaptation model (2nd ed.). Englewood Cliffs, NJ: Prentice-Hall.

Rudner, R.S. (1966). Philosophy of social science. Englewood Cliffs, NJ: Prentice-Hall.

Rutledge, D.N. (1987). Factors related to women's practice of breast self-examination. Nursing Research, 36, 117–121.

Schlotfeldt, R.M. (1975). The need for a conceptual framework. In P.J. Verhonick (Ed.), Nursing Research I (pp. 3–24). Boston: Little, Brown & Co.

Silva, M.C. (1986). Research testing nursing theory: State of the art. Advances in Nursing Science, 9(1), 1–11.

Silva, M.C. (1987). Conceptual models of nursing. In J.J. Fitzpatrick & R.L. Taunton (Eds.), Annual review of nursing research (Vol. 5, pp. 229–246). New York: Springer.

Skidmore, W. (1975). Theoretical thinking in sociology. New York: Cambridge University Press.

Stevens, B.J. (1984). Nursing theory. Analysis, application, evaluation (2nd ed.). Boston: Little, Brown & Co.

Thomae, H. (1979). The concept of development and life-span developmental psychology. In P.B. Baltes & O.G. Brim, Jr. (Eds.), Life-span development and behavior (Vol. 2, pp. 281–312). New York: Academic Press.

Travelbee, J. (1966). Interpersonal aspects of nursing. Philadelphia: FA Davis.

Walker, L.O., & Avant, K. (in press). Strategies for theory construction in nursing (2nd ed.). Norwalk, CT: Appleton and Lange.

Waltz, C., & Bausell, R.B. (1981). Nursing research: Design, statistics and computer analysis. Philadelphia: FA Davis.

Watson, J. (1981). Nursing's scientific quest. Nursing Outlook, 29, 413–416.

Whall, A.L. (1980). Congruence between existing theories of family functioning and nursing theories. Advances in Nursing Science, 3(1), 59–67.

Whall, A.L. (1986). Family therapy theory for nursing. Four approaches. Norwalk, CT: Appleton-Century-Crofts.

Williams, C.A. (1979). The nature and development of conceptual frameworks. In F.S. Downs & J.W. Fleming, Issues in nursing research (pp. 89–106). New York: Appleton-Century-Crofts.

ANNOTATED BIBLIOGRAPHY

Adam, E. (1983). Frontiers of nursing in the 21st century: Development of models and theories on the concept of nursing. Journal of Advanced Nursing, 8, 41–45.
  The author maintains that nursing must have a conceptual base if it is to be recognized as a profession. Examples are given of the works of Roy, Orem, Johnson, and Henderson.

Adam, E. (1985). Toward more clarity in terminology: Frameworks, theories and models. Journal of Nursing Education, 24, 151–155.
  This article gives some of the varied meanings that are conveyed by terms such as conceptual model, conceptual framework, theory, and frame of reference.

Aggleton, P., & Chalmers, H. (1985). Critical examination. Nursing Times, 81(14), 38–39.
  This article describes how the medical model approaches aspects of patient care, including the nature of the person receiving care, the causes of problems experienced by the person, the nature of assessment, planning, and goal setting processes, the focus of intervention, and the nature of the evaluation process.

Aggleton, P., & Chalmers, H. (1986). Nursing research, nursing theory, and the nursing process. Journal of Advanced Nursing, 11, 197–202.
  The methods of inductive and deductive development of nursing theories are discussed and examples of such nursing theories are given. The authors advocate the use of the nursing process to facilitate nursing theory development.

Aggleton, P., & Chalmers, H. (1987). Models of nursing, nursing practice and nursing education. Journal of Advanced Nursing, 12, 573–581.
  The article identifies the distinctive features of developmental, systems, and interactionist conceptual models of nursing and explores the implications of each type for contemporary approaches to nursing practice and nursing education.

Battista, J.R. (1977). The holistic paradigm and general system theory. General Systems, 22, 65–71.
  The author discusses the concept of paradigm and compares the characteristics of vitalistic, mechanistic, and holistic views of the world. The relationship between the holistic world view and general system theory is discussed.

Benoliel, J.Q. (1977). The interaction between theory and research. Nursing Outlook, 25, 108–113.
  This article describes the influence of theory on the design and conduct of nursing research. Symbolic interactionism is described and its influence on the author's research program is outlined.

Bertalanffy, L. von (1968). General system theory. New York: George Braziller.
  This book defines and describes the elements of general system theory.

Chin, R. (1980). The utility of systems models and developmental models for practitioners. In J.P. Riehl and C. Roy, Conceptual models for nursing practice (2nd ed., pp. 21–37). New York: Appleton-Century-Crofts.
  This chapter identifies and describes the elements of developmental and systems models.

Chinn, P.L., & Jacobs, M.K. (1987). Theory and nursing. A systematic approach (2nd ed.). St. Louis: CV Mosby.
  This book presents a comprehensive discussion of a systematic manner of developing middle-range nursing theory. Chapter 1 includes a seminal discussion of empirical, esthetic, ethical, and personal knowledge and the methods to establish credibility of each of these types of nursing knowledge.

DeBeck, V. (1981). The relationship between senior nursing students' ability to formulate nursing diagnoses and the curriculum model. Advances in Nursing Science, 3(3), 51–66.

This article reports the findings of study that revealed that type of nursing curriculum (developmental, systems, mixed) did not influence students' abilities to make nursing diagnoses.

Donaldson, S.K., & Crowley, D.M. (1978). The discipline of nursing. Nursing Outlook, 26, 113–120.
This article identifies the characteristics of academic and professional disciplines. Nursing is described as a professional discipline. Recurring themes found in the nursing literature are outlined.

Duldt, B.W., & Giffin, K. (1985). Theoretical perspectives for nursing. Boston: Little, Brown & Co.
This book presents a discussion of theory, a framework for theory analysis, and Weaver's theory of humanistic nursing communication.

Eckberg, D.L., & Hill, L. Jr. (1979). The paradigm concept and sociology: A critical review. American Sociological Review, 44, 925–937.
This article reviews the multiple definitions of a paradigm and distinguishes among metaparadigms, paradigms or disciplinary matrices, and exemplars.

Ellis, R. (1982). Conceptual issues in nursing. Nursing Outlook, 32, 406–410.
The author discusses several different conceptualizations of nursing. The history of nursing, the disease model, and definitions of health were identified as factors that have affected the development of the discipline of nursing.

Erickson, H.C., Tomlin, E.M., & Swain, M.A.P. (1983). Modeling and role-modeling. A theory and paradigm for nursing. Englewood Cliffs, NJ: Prentice-Hall.
This book presents the theory of modeling and role-modeling developed by the authors. A description of application of the concepts of modeling and role-modeling in the nursing process is given. The authors include their philosophy and definition of nursing.

Faculty-curriculum development. Part III. Conceptual framework—its meaning and function. (1975). New York: National League for Nursing.
This book presents discussions of the influence of philosophies, conceptual models, and theories on curriculum development.

Fawcett, J. (1984). The metaparadigm of nursing. Current status and future refinements. Image. The Journal of Nursing Scholarship, 16, 84–87.

Brodie, J.M. (1984). A response to Dr. J. Fawcett's paper: "The metaparadigm of nursing: Present status and future refinements." Image. The Journal of Nursing Scholarship, 16, 87–89.

Conway, M.E. (1985). Toward greater specificity in defining nursing's metaparadigm. Advances in Nursing Science, 7(4), 73–81.
The article by Fawcett defines metaparadigm and describes the metaparadigm of nursing, including central concepts and major themes. Further refinement of the metaparadigm is suggested at the levels of disciplinary matrix or paradigm and exemplars.
Brodie's response to Fawcett's paper points out that relationships between central concepts and themes were not addressed nor were suggestions made for reconciling disparate orientations evident in various conceptual models of nursing.
Conway maintains that inclusion of the concept of nursing as a concept of nursing's metaparadigm is inappropriate.

Fawcett, J. (1986). Guest Editorial: Conceptual models of nursing, nursing diagnosis, and nursing theory development. Western Journal of Nursing Research, 8, 397–399.
This editorial focuses on the relationship of the North American Nursing Diagnosis Association's list of nursing diagnoses to conceptual models of nursing. The claim is made that the nursing diagnosis list is a middle-range descriptive theory that has no connection to an existing conceptual model of nursing. It is recommended that the implicit conceptual model from which nursing diagnoses were derived be identified and that theories of nursing diagnosis be derived from existing conceptual models of nursing.

Fawcett, J., & Downs, F.S. (1986). The relationship of theory and research. Norwalk, CT: Appleton-Century-Crofts.
This book includes definitions of conceptual model, theory, and research. The con-

struction of conceptual-theoretical-empirical structures is explained. Techniques for analysis of theory, called theory formalization, are a focal point of the book.

Field, L., & Winslow, E. H. (1985). Moving to a nursing model. American Journal of Nursing, 85, 1100–1101.
This book reviews the conceptual models of King, Orem, Rogers, and Roy and dis- The authors encourage the use of nursing conceptual models to define nursing practice and to systematically assess patients and administer nursing care.

Field, P.A. (1987). The impact of nursing theory on the clinical decision making process. Journal of Advanced Nursing, 12, 563–571.
This article explains the relationship of the nursing process and nursing diagnosis to nursing conceptual models. Included is a brief discussion of the use of nursing diagnosis in relation to Orem's, Neuman's, and Roy's models.

Fitzpatrick, J.J., Whall, A.L. Johnston, R.L., & Floyd, J.A. (1982). Nursing models and their psychiatric mental health applications. Bowie, MD: Brady.
This book reviews the conceptual models of King, Orem, Rogers, and Roy and discusses the changes, or reformulations, needed to link theories borrowed from other disciplines with these models in a logically congruent manner.

Flaskerud, J.H. (1983). Utilizing a nursing conceptual model in basic level curriculum development. Journal of Nursing Education, 22, 224–227.
This article identifies the assumptions that must be made when adopting a conceptual model as a framework for a curriculum and the steps to be followed to develop such a curriculum.

Flaskerud, J.H. (1984). Nursing models as conceptual frameworks for research. Western Journal of Nursing Research, 6, 153–155, 197–199.
The author identifies both advantages and problems inherent in using conceptual models to guide nursing research.

Flaskerud, J.H., & Halloran, E.J. (1980). Areas of agreement in nursing theory development. Advances in Nursing Science, 3(1), 1–7.
This article identifies and discusses areas of agreement in nursing theory development. The central concepts of nursing are identified as person, environment, health, and nursing.

Hall, B.A. (1981). The change paradigm in nursing: Growth versus persistence. Advances in Nursing Science, 3(4), 1–6.

Hall, B.A. (1983). Toward an understanding of stability in nursing phenomena. Advances in Nursing Science, 5(3), 15–20.
These articles identify the elements of the world views of change and persistence.

Hall, A.D., & Fagen, R.E. (1968). Definition of system. In W. Buckley (Ed.), Modern systems research for the behavioral scientist (pp. 81–92). Chicago: Aldine.
This chapter defines and describes a system.

Hardy, L.K. (1986). Identifying the place of theoretical frameworks in an evolving discipline. Journal of Advanced Nursing, 11, 103–107.
Some negative aspects of nursing conceptual frameworks are discussed by the author, including the gap between theory and practice, the fact that a given framework can stifle thinking and creativity, and the jargon that is used in some frameworks.

Heiss, J. (1981). The social psychology of interaction. Englewood Cliffs, NJ: Prentice-Hall.
This book represents a comprehensive discussion of the elements of interactionism.

Hinshaw, A.S. (1979). Theoretical substruction: An assessment process. Western Journal of Nursing Research, 1, 319–324.
Hinshaw presents a brief discussion of the technique of theoretical substruction, which facilitates identification of the components of a theory.

Johnson, D.E. (1987). Guest Editorial: Evaluating conceptual models for use in critical care nursing practice. Dimensions of Critical Care Nursing, 6, 195–197.
This editorial presents a discussion of the use of conceptual models of nursing and the importance of using an explicit nursing model for nursing practice.

Kim, H.S. (1983). The nature of theoretical thinking in nursing. Norwalk, CT: Appleton-Century-Crofts.

Kim, H.S. (1987). Structuring the nursing knowledge system: A typology of four domains. Scholarly Inquiry for Nursing Practice. 1, 99–110.

Hinshaw, A.S. (1987). Response to "Structuring the nursing knowledge system: A typology of four domains." Scholarly Inquiry for Nursing Practice: An International Journal, 1, 111–114.
    In her 1983 book, Kim defines and discusses the elements that form theories and discusses these elements in reference to three domains: client, environment, and nursing action. Examples from current conceptual models are used, but the models are not systematically analyzed or evaluated.
    In her 1987 publication, Kim presents a revised typology of the domains of nursing knowledge, including client, client-nurse, practice, and environment.
    Hinshaw's response focuses on the relevance of Kim's typology for practice, when to apply or utilize a typology in practice, and diversity versus standardization in adopting a typology for the discipline. She points out that Kim does not include health in her typology, although other typologies of nursing knowledge do so.

King, I.M. (1984). Philosophy of nursing education: A national survey. Western Journal of Nursing Research, 6, 387–406.
    The study reported in this article compared and contrasted concepts such as man, health, environment, social systems, role, perception, interpersonal relations, nursing, and God as used in philosophies of schools of nursing throughout the United States. Significant differences were found among diploma, associate degree, and baccalaureate programs but no differences were found between different regions of the country or between private and public schools.

Leininger, M. (1985). Transcultural care diversity and universality: A theory for nursing. Thorofare, NJ: CB Slack.
    Leininger presents her theory of transcultural nursing care in this book.

Looft, W.R. (1973). Socialization and personality throughout the life span: An examination of contemporary psychological approaches. In P.B. Baltes & K.W. Schaie (Eds.), Life span developmental psychology. Personality and socialization (pp. 25–52). New York: Academic Press.
    This chapter presents a detailed discussion of the mechanistic and organismic world views.

Marriner, A. (1986). Nursing theorists and their work. St. Louis: CV Mosby.
    The purpose of this book was to identify major thinkers in nursing and to provide the reader with a review of some of their ideas, lists of their publications, and major sources used for development of their ideas. Theorists are clustered into four categories according to major themes—the art and science of humanistic nursing, interpersonal relationships, systems, and energy fields. No distinctions were made between conceptual models and theories.

Meleis, A.I. (1985). Theoretical nursing: Development and progress. Philadelphia: JB Lippincott.
    This book presents a definition of theory and a comprehensive historical review of the development of nursing knowledge. Works are categorized as needs, outcomes, and interaction theories and reviewed using a schema that does not distinguish conceptual models from theories. Indeed, Meleis claims that calling a work a conceptual model lessens its value. Extensive bibliographies are included.

Newman, M.A. (1979). Theory development in nursing. Philadelphia: FA Davis.

Newman, M.A. (1986). Health as expanding consciousness. St. Louis: CV Mosby.
    Newman presents the rudiments of her grand theory of health, whose origins lie with Rogers's conceptual model, in her 1979 book. The theory is refined and further discussion is presented in the 1986 book. An application of the theory to individuals, families, and communities is included in the 1986 book. The 1979 book includes discussion of techniques of theory analysis.

Nye, F.I., & Berardo, F.N. (Eds.). (1966). Emerging conceptual frameworks in family analysis. New York: Macmillan.

Nye, F.I. & Berardo, F.N. (Eds.). (1981). Emerging conceptual frameworks in family analysis. New York: Macmillan.
    This book defines the term conceptual framework. The 1966 edition presents de-

tailed discussions of 11 conceptual frameworks related to family functioning found in the sociological literature, and the 1981 edition presents 16 conceptual frameworks.

Orlando, I.J. (1961). The dynamic nurse-patient relationship. New York: GP Putnam's Sons.

Orlando, I.J. (1972). The discipline and teaching of nursing process. New York: GP Putnam's Sons.
Orlando presents her theory of the interpersonal process between nurse and patient and a systematic approach to nursing process in her 1961 book. The 1972 book explains the findings of several years of research focused on testing the theory.

Pagana, K.D. (1986). Consider this. Journal of Nursing Administration, 16(2), 4.
The author presents a brief discussion of the value of using conceptual models to the nurse administrator.

Parse, R.R. (1981). Man-living-health. A theory of nursing. New York: John Wiley & Sons.
Parse presents her grand theory of nursing, which is derived from Rogers's conceptual model and existential-phenomenological thinking.

Parse, R.R. (1987). Nursing science. Major paradigms, theories, and critiques. Philadelphia: WB Saunders.
This book presents the papers read at the Nurse Theorist Conference held in Pittsburgh, Pennsylvania in May 1985. A presentation of two world views, called paradigms by Parse, is included. These are the totality and the simultaneity paradigms. Presentations of their works are by King, Orem, Parse, Rogers, and Roy. A critique of each work is included, using an evaluation scheme that does not distinguish between conceptual models and theories.

Peplau, H.E. (1952). Interpersonal relations in nursing. New York: GP Putnam's Sons.
Peplau presents her theory of the interpersonal relationship between nurse and patient.

Reese, H.W., & Overton, W.F. (1970). Models of development and theories of development. In L.R. Goulet & P.B. Baltes (Eds.), Life span developmental psychology. Research and theory (pp. 115–145). New York: Academic Press.
This chapter identifies the relationship between models and theories and discusses the characteristics of the mechanistic and organismic world views.

Reilly, D.E. (1975). Why a conceptual framework? Nursing Outlook, 23, 566–569.
This article differentiates between conceptual models and theories and discusses the development and uses of conceptual models.

Theory development. What, why, how? (1978). New York: National League for Nursing.
This book presents various papers dealing with development of nursing knowledge, including the relation of conceptual models to theories.

Stevens, B.J. (1979). Nursing theory. Analysis, application, evaluation. Boston: Little, Brown & Co.

Stevens, B.J. (1984). Nursing theory. Analysis, application, evaluation (2nd ed.). Boston: Little, Brown & Co.
This book presents a review of nursing theory. A classification scheme is offered with the following categories: intervention, substitution, conservation, sustenance, and enhancement. Stevens does not make any clear distinction between conceptual models and theories, although she does regard more abstract works as grand theories.

Thomae, H. (1979). The concept of development and life-span developmental psychology. In P.B. Baltes & O.G. Brim, Jr. (Eds.), Life-span development and behavior (Vol. 2, pp. 281–312). New York: Academic Press.
This chapter presents a discussion of the elements of the change and persistence world views.

Travelbee, J. (1966). Interpersonal aspects of nursing. Philadelphia: FA Davis.
Travelbee presents her theory of the interpersonal relationship between nurse and patient.

Walker, L.O., & Avant, K.C. (1983). Strategies for theory construction in nursing. Norwalk, CT: Appleton-Century-Crofts.

Walker, L.O., & Avant, K.C. (in press). Strategies for theory construction in nursing (2nd ed.). Norwalk, CT: Appleton and Lange.
These landmark books present various strategies for the analysis, evaluation, and synthesis of concepts and propositions of middle-range theories.

Watson, J. (1979). Nursing: The philosophy and science of caring. Boston: Little, Brown & Co. (Reissued by National League for Nursing, 1988.)

Watson, J. (1985). Nursing: Human science and human care. A theory of nursing. Norwalk, CT: Appleton-Century-Crofts.
Watson's 1979 book presents her ideas about nursing and rudimentary elements of her theory of caring. The 1985 book extends her earlier work on caring and presents her theory of human care.

Whall, A.L. (1986). Family therapy theory for nursing. Four approaches. Norwalk, CT: Appleton-Century-Crofts.
This book describes four approaches to development of family therapy theory for nursing. A deductive approach is taken using King's and Rogers's models to derive family treatment protocols. Two approaches to family therapy are deductively reformulated: Modane's theory is reformulated in light of Roy's model and developmental theories of family therapy are reformulated within the context of Rogers's model. Nursing theory is inductively derived using Jackson's family therapy approach, and a nursing approach to family therapy is derived inductively.

White, M.B. (Ed.). (1983). Curriculum development from a nursing model. The crisis theory framework. New York: Springer.
This book explains how a curriculum for nursing education can be guided by a conceptual framework of nursing. The crisis theory framework developed at the University of Connecticut School of Nursing is used.

Williams, C.A. (1979). The nature and development of conceptual frameworks. In F.S. Downs & J.W. Fleming, Issues in nursing research (pp. 89–106). New York: Appleton-Century-Crofts.
This chapter presents definitions of concept, hypothesis, theory, and conceptual framework. The differences between conceptual models and theories are identified.

Wright, S.C. (1986). Building and using a model of nursing. Baltimore: Edward Arnold & Co.
This book, written by a British nurse, discusses some of the problems with current nursing models developed by United States nurses and the difficulty in using them within the British health care system. A step-by-step approach to development of a nursing model is given, outlining the development of the author's nursing model. Examples are given from practice, management, education, and research.

CHAPTER

2

Analysis and Evaluation of Conceptual Models of Nursing_____

This chapter presents a framework for analysis and evaluation of conceptual models of nursing. The chapter also presents a discussion of the comparison of various models, as well as an outline of points to consider when selecting one to use for nursing activities.

The major components of analysis and evaluation of conceptual models of nursing are identified in the following key terms. Each component is discussed in detail in this chapter.

KEY TERMS_____

Analysis	Evaluation—*Cont.*
Development of the	World Views
Conceptual Model	Category of the Model
Content: Concepts and	Generation and Testing of
Propositions	Theory
Areas of Concern	Social Considerations
Evaluation	Social Congruence
Explication of Assumptions	Social Significance
Comprehensiveness of	Social Utility
Content	Contributions to Nursing
Logical Congruence	Knowledge

A FRAMEWORK FOR ANALYSIS AND EVALUATION OF NURSING MODELS

The analysis and evaluation framework presented here highlights the most important features of conceptual models of nursing and is appropriate to their level of abstraction. The framework was first published several years ago (Fawcett, 1980) and has undergone some revision since then. Initial and continued development of the framework has been motivated by dissatisfaction with other evaluation schemes.

Previously published evaluative schemes reflect the confusion between conceptual models and theories. The one proposed by Riehl and Roy in the 1974 edition of their book used the Dickoff, James, and Wiedenbach (1968) survey list for situation-producing theory. Therefore, this scheme is too concrete for conceptual models. Conversely, the authors of two other review systems claimed that their schemes were designed for theory evaluation but used them to evaluate conceptual models. Both the Duffey and Muhlenkamp (1974) and the Stevens (1979, 1984) schemes include some questions appropriate to a model's level of abstraction, but like the Riehl and Roy (1974) scheme, offer other items more germane to concrete theories. Three additional schemes are appropriate for conceptual model review but seem too limited for a comprehensive analysis and evaluation. Johnson's (1974) criteria are focused solely on social decisions, and Peterson's (1977) questions lack necessary scope and detail. Similarly, Johnson's unpublished lecture notes, cited by Riehl and Roy in the 1980 edition of their book, are limited in scope. Further, some more recently published evaluative schemes do not distinguish clearly between conceptual models and theories, in that they include some items appropriate for conceptual models, but other items are directed toward evaluation of middle range theories. (Fitzpatrick & Whall, 1983; Marriner, 1986; Meleis, 1985; Nursing Theories Conference Group, 1985). Parse (1987) presented a scheme similar to the one described in this chapter, but referred to conceptual models as theories. Finally, Thibodeau (1983) used an early version of the framework presented here. Some of these schemes, however, provided a few building blocks for construction of the analytic and evaluative framework presented in Figure 2–1.

This framework separates questions dealing with analysis from those more appropriate to evaluation. Analysis is an objective breakdown of content into component elements. This is done to explicitly identify concepts, propositions, and any relative hierarchy of ideas contained in the conceptual model. The intent of analysis, then, is to clarify the content of the conceptual model and to indicate its organization. In particular, analysis of elements requires identification of the conceptual model concepts and its propositions, including assumptions, definitions, and relationships between concepts. This facilitates

QUESTIONS FOR ANALYSIS

- What is the historical evolution of the conceptual model?
- What approach to development of nursing knowledge does the model exemplify?
- Upon what assumptions was the conceptual model based?
- How are nursing's four metaparadigm concepts explicated in the model?
    How is person defined and described?
    How is environment defined and described?
    How is health defined? How are wellness and illness differentiated?
    How is nursing defined? What is the goal of nursing? How is the nursing process described?
- What statements are made about the relationships among the four metaparadigm concepts?
- What areas of concern are identified by the conceptual model?
- What is the source of these concerns?

QUESTIONS FOR EVALUATION

- Are the assumptions upon which the conceptual model was based made explicit?
- Does the conceptual model provide complete descriptions of all four concepts of nursing's metaparadigm?
- Do the relational propositions of the conceptual model completely link the four metaparadigm concepts?
- Is the internal structure of the conceptual model logically congruent?
    Does the model reflect more than one contrasting world view?
    Does the model reflect characteristics of more than one category of models?
    Do the components of the model reflect logical translation of diverse perspectives?
- Does the conceptual model generate empirically testable theories?
- Do tests of derived theories yield evidence in support of the model?
- Is the conceptual model socially congruent?
    Does the conceptual model, when linked with relevant theories, lead to nursing activities that meet society's expectations or do the expectations created by the conceptual model require societal changes?
- Is the conceptual model socially significant?
    Does the conceptual model, when linked with relevant theories, lead to nursing actions that make important differences in the person's health status?
- Is the conceptual model socially useful?
    Does the conceptual model include explicit rules for research, practice, education, and administration?
    Is the conceptual model comprehensive enough to provide direction for research, practice, education, and administration when linked with relevant theories?

Figure 2–1.   Framework for analysis and evaluation of conceptual models of nursing. (*Figure continues on next page.*)

Is the investigator given sufficient direction about what to study and what questions to ask?

Is the practitioner able to make pertinent observations, decide that a nursing problem exists, and prescribe and execute a course of action that achieves the goal specified?

Does the educator have sufficient guidelines to construct a curriculum, and a reasonable understanding of what knowledge and skills are needed?

Does the administrator have sufficient guidelines to organize and deliver nursing services?

- What is the overall contribution of the conceptual model to nursing knowledge?

Figure 2–1.   *Continued*

recognition of stated and unstated assumptions, identification of motives, and comprehension of the interrelationships between concepts and propositions of the model. This also facilitates detection of logical fallacies in the model. The analysis of organizational principles requires examination of the overall arrangement or structure of the conceptual model, permitting a view of its gestalt (Bloom, 1956).

Analysis of a conceptual model of nursing is accomplished by examining exactly what its author has presented, rather than by making inferences about what might have been meant by any statement or by referring to others' interpretations of the author's work. When the author has not been clear about a point, or has failed to present certain information, it may be necessary to make inferences or to turn to other reviews of the author's work. This, however, must be noted explicitly, so that the distinction between the author's words and those of others is clear.

In summary, analysis requires a nonjudgmental, detailed examination of the conceptual model. Evaluation, in contrast, involves judgments about the value and logical structure of the conceptual model. Such judgments are made by determining the extent to which the model satisfies certain external criteria and meets certain standards (Bloom, 1956). Thus, evaluation of a conceptual model allows one to draw conclusions about its credibility.

QUESTIONS FOR ANALYSIS

Analysis of conceptual models of nursing may be accomplished by answering a series of questions about the development of the model, its content, and its areas of concern.

Development of the Conceptual Model

A conceptual model is formulated from an author's personal views of and assumptions about the world and nursing. Formulation of a conception model is a more intellectual than empirical endeavor, although empirical observations certainly may influence the work. The content of the model evolves as the author engages in inductive and/or deductive reasoning. Because it is not unusual to find that the content of a model has undergone revisions as the author refines concepts and propositions and formulates new ideas about nursing, it is important to trace the model from its initial version to the present one. The first aspect of the analysis, then, asks the following questions:

- What is the historical evolution of the conceptual model?
- What approach to development of nursing knowledge does the model exemplify?
- Upon what assumptions was the conceptual model based?

This part of the analysis of a conceptual model of nursing requires a review of all available publications and presentations by the author of the model. This is especially important because the historical evolution of the model, including revisions in content and influences on the author's thinking, often is revealed in early writings. The author's use of either or both inductive and deductive reasoning reflects a certain orientation to science in general and to development of knowledge in particular. This orientation often can be traced to the author's educational experiences as well as to exposure to the thinking of other scholars. Accordingly, analysis of the evolution of the model should include the author's link with earlier nurse educators and other authors, as well as the general climate of science at the time the model was formulated.

Following the extensive literature review, a description of the evolution of the model can be articulated. Furthermore, the review of the author's writings will provide clues or explicit descriptions of the underlying assumptions as well as the inductive and/or deductive strategies used to transform an implicit private image of nursing into a formal conceptual model.

Content of the Conceptual Model

The content of a conceptual model is presented in the form of abstract and general concepts and propositions. These ideas and statements reflect a distinctive perspective of the four concepts of nursing's metaparadigm—person, environment, health, and nursing. The second aspect of analysis therefore asks the following questions:

- How are nursing's four metaparadigm concepts expli-
  cated in the model?
  How is person defined and described?
  How is environment defined and described?
  How is health defined? How are wellness and illness dif-
  ferentiated?
  How is nursing defined? What is the goal of nursing?
  How is the nursing process described?
- What statements are made about the relationships among
  the four metaparadigm concepts?

Most authors of nursing models have not presented their ideas in
the form of explicit statements about each of the metaparadigm concepts. Therefore, this part of the analysis is most readily accomplished
first by categorizing the content of the model into definitions and descriptions of person, environment, health, and nursing. Then, in the
language of the conceptual model, statements reflecting the linkage of
these metaparadigm concepts are to be extracted.

This aspect of the analysis of a conceptual model will yield information about its elements and their relationships. An understanding
of the organizational principles of the model will emerge when the
propositions are arranged in a hierarchical manner. This may be done
by clearly differentiating between the assumptions upon which the
conceptual model was based and other propositions that describe and
link the concepts of the model.

Areas of Concern

The final aspect of analysis derives from the fact that each conceptual model presents a distinctive perspective of nursing. Although
most authors start with the same view of the general purpose of nursing, in final form the nursing models present different views of the
metaparadigm concepts (Johnson, 1974). Each conceptual model focuses on different areas of concern. In other words, different models
are concerned with different problems in nurse-patient situations or
different problems in person-environment interactions (Duffey &
Muhlenkamp, 1974). They also may be concerned with different actual and potential deviations from desired health states and with different modes of nursing intervention (Johnson, cited in Riehl & Roy,
1980; Johnson, 1987). The source of problems, deviations, and interventions also may vary from model to model. Different conceptual
models may identify different factors that are thought to influence the
development of problems or deviations or direct types of nursing interventions. Paraphrasing Duffey and Muhlenkamp (1974), the questions to be raised are

- What areas of concern are identified by the conceptual model?
- What is the source of these concerns?

The author's presentation of the conceptual model content will provide the answers to these questions. Coupled with the information obtained from the first two aspects of analysis, the identification of areas of concern and their sources will yield a comprehensive picture of the author's distinctive view of nursing.

QUESTIONS FOR EVALUATION

Evaluation of conceptual models of nursing is accomplished by comparing their content to criteria focusing on explication of assumptions, comprehensiveness of content, logical congruence, theory generating and testing capabilities, social considerations, and contributions to nursing knowledge.

Explication of Assumptions

The first aspect of evaluation concerns the assumptions upon which the conceptual model was based. The question is
- Are the assumptions upon which the conceptual model was based made explicit?

Identification of assumptions about the person, the environment, health, and nursing yields information about the author's values and about special points of emphasis in the view of nursing put forth by the conceptual model. The expectation is that these assumptions have been made explicit by the author. Indeed, "a statement of one's value system is an essential accompaniment to a model" (Johnson, 1987, p. 197).

Comprehensiveness of Content

The next aspect of evaluation deals with the content of the model. Here, the questions are
- Does the conceptual model provide complete descriptions of all four concepts of nursing's metaparadigm?
- Do the relational propositions of the conceptual model completely link the four metaparadigm concepts?

No well-accepted criterion for completeness of descriptions of the metaparadigm concepts has been established. It seems reasonable to expect, however, that the content of the model encompasses the four metaparadigm concepts and that this content is relatively unambiguous. Thus, we should expect the conceptual model to present a description of the person, an identification of the person's environment, a discussion of the author's meaning of health, a definition of nursing, a statement of nursing goals, and an outline of the nursing process.

Evaluation of the nursing process component of conceptual models may be expanded by employing the criteria proposed by Walker and Nicholson (1980). They maintained that the nursing process should

1. Incorporate an underlying knowledge base in making the judgment inherent in the nursing process.
2. Be as dynamic as practice itself, that is, the [process] should permit dynamic movement back and forth between steps.
3. Be applicable to nursing in general and not only to specific clinical settings.
4. Be compatible with ethical standards for nursing practice.
5. Be consistent with scientific findings on human behavior in health and illness. (p. 9)

The criterion for the linkage of concepts requires that the relational propositions of the conceptual model link all four metaparadigm concepts. This may be done in a series of statements linking two or more concepts, or it may be accomplished by one summary statement encompassing all four concepts. These statements will, of course, use the vocabulary of the particular conceptual model.

Logical Congruence

Evaluation of conceptual models must consider the logic of their internal structures. The criterion of logical congruence is based, in part, on the agreement between world views reflected by the model. The contrasting world views of mechanism and organicism and of change and persistence, discussed in Chapter 1, are appropriate here.

Logical congruence also must take into account the classification of models. As explained in Chapter 1, nursing models may be categorized as developmental, systems, or interaction models; needs or outcomes models; humanistic or energy field models; and intervention, substitution, conservation, sustenance, or enhancement models.

Evaluation of logical congruence is accomplished by comparing both implicit and explicit aspects of the conceptual model to the elements of the world views and the characteristics of categories of models. In other words, the content of the model is examined for its stands on mechanism versus organicism and on change versus persistence. The content of the model also is examined to determine to what extent it reflects the characteristics of various categories of models.

Consideration of logical congruence is especially important if the conceptual model incorporates more than one contrasting world view or category of models. This is because different schools of thought cannot be combined easily, if at all. However, viewpoints sometimes may be merged or translated by redefining all concepts in a consistent manner.

The questions to be asked when evaluating logical congruence are

- Is the internal structure of the conceptual model logically congruent?

  Does the model reflect more than one contrasting world view?

  Does the model reflect characteristics of more than one category of models?

  Do the components of the model reflect logical translation of diverse perspectives?

Contrasting world views obviously are not logically congruent. Moreover, various categories of conceptual models of nursing focus on different phenomena and, therefore, are not necessarily congruent. Conceptual models of nursing that strive to combine concepts and propositions derived from different world views and/or different categories of models must first translate the concepts and propositions to ensure just one congruent frame of reference. Translation, according to Reese and Overton (1970), is accomplished by redefining concepts and restating propositions that do not reflect the preferred world view or category type, so that all ideas presented in the conceptual model are consistent.

Generation and Testing of Theory

The next part of the evaluation of a conceptual model of nursing reflects the relationship between models and theories. As explained in Chapter 1, relatively specific and concrete theories can be derived from the abstract and general conceptual models of nursing. Thus, the theory generating contributions of the model should be judged, as well as the result of empirical tests of any such theories. These judgments can be made only after examination of the research literature related to the model.

The questions to be posed here are

- Does the conceptual model generate empirically testable theories?
- Do tests of derived theories yield evidence in support of the model?

The need for logically congruent conceptual-theoretical systems of nursing knowledge for nursing activities mandates that at least some theories be derived from each conceptual model. The expectation, therefore, is that the concepts and propositions of the model be sufficiently clear so that specific and concrete concepts and propositions can be deduced, and so that testable hypotheses can be formulated. Furthermore, it is expected that the tests of these theories will yield supporting evidence for the more abstract model. If not, the credibility of the model must be questioned seriously.

Social Considerations

The next aspect of evaluation takes into account the fact that conceptual models cannot be applied directly in real world situations. Rather, as explained in Chapter 1, they are linked with theories to form conceptual-theoretical systems of knowledge that then are used to guide and direct nursing research, practice, education, and administration. The results of use of a conceptual-theoretical system of nursing knowledge may be evaluated by means of criteria that contribute to determination of the credibility of conceptual models of nursing. The criteria have been adapted from the social decisions identified by Johnson (1974, 1987).

This portion of the evaluation is accomplished by reviewing not only all publications and presentations by the author of the conceptual model but also those by other nurses who have used the model.

The first social decision is social congruence, and the question is

- Does the conceptual model, when linked with relevant theories, lead to nursing activities that meet society's expectations, or do the expectations created by the conceptual model require societal changes?

Johnson (1987) maintained that social congruence is the most difficult social decision to satisfy and that its evaluation "requires both time and research" (p. 197). She noted that a conceptual model might lead to nursing actions that are not currently congruent with societal expectations, and, thus, society might have to be helped to develop new expectations. She explained that "current nursing practice is not entirely what it might become and that society might come to expect a different form of practice, given the opportunity to experience it" (Johnson, 1974, p. 376). The answer to this question, then, does not have to be an affirmation of current societal expectations. If, however, the answer is that changes in expectations are needed, nurses who want to use the model must recognize that they will have to help people to expect a different mode of nursing care. This is especially important, for without an affirmative answer to the question of social congruence, "nursing will not continue to be sanctioned as a profession or an occupation, and in a nursing shortage situation, . . . the nurse may be replaced with other health professionals" (Johnson, 1987, p. 197).

The second social decision is that of social significance, and here the question is

- Does the conceptual model, when linked with relevant

theories, lead to nursing actions that make important differences in the person's health status?

Johnson (1974) commented, "This criterion recognizes that a professional service is a highly valued one because it is critical to people in some way" (p. 376). The expectation, therefore, is that the use of the conceptual model has a significant, positive impact on the persons's well-being. Johnson (1987) pointed out that although the question of social significance "may be answered initially on the basis of reason, the ultimate answer will depend at least partially on research" (p. 197).

The third social decision is social utility, and one question takes into account the extent to which rules for research, practice, education, and administration are made explicit. As discussed in Chapter 1, a fully developed conceptual model represents a paradigm that guides the activities of its advocates. The professional discipline of nursing, with its mission of practice, requires paradigms that provide direction not only for research, but also for clinical practice, as well as for the education of clinicians and the administration of nursing services. The question is

- Does the conceptual model include explicit rules for research, practice, education, and administration?

The rules for various activities in nursing were identified in Chapter 1. The expectation is that these rules are explicit in the conceptual model.

A second question regarding social utility is

- Is the conceptual model comprehensive enough to provide direction for research, practice, education, and administration when linked with relevant theories?

This question may be phrased in more specific terms for each type of nursing activity. For research, the question is

- Is the investigator given sufficient direction about what to study and what questions to ask? (Johnson, 1987, p. 197)

For practice, the question is

- Is the practitioner able to make pertinent observations, decide that a nursing problem exists, and prescribe and execute a course of action that achieves the goal specified? (Johnson, 1987, p. 197)

For education, the question is

- Does the educator have sufficient guidelines to construct a curriculum, and a reasonable understanding of what knowledge and skills are needed? (Johnson, 1987, p. 197)

For administration, the question is

- Does the administrator have sufficient guidelines to organize and deliver nursing services?

The expectation here is that the conceptual model is a useful frame of reference for many nursing activities. Moreover, it is expected that when the conceptual model is linked with relevant theories it has utility in a variety of clinical situations. However, although the utility of the conceptual model in various settings certainly is a measure of its value, it is possible that the focus of the model precludes certain situations. In such a case, we must decide if the limitations are sufficient to warrant elimination of the model as a viable one for nursing.

Contributions to Nursing Knowledge

The final aspect of evaluation of nursing models is as general as the models themselves, and requires review of all of the literature dealing with a given conceptual model. This question judges the contribution of the model to the discipline of nursing, asking
- What is the overall contribution of the conceptual model to nursing knowledge?

Lippitt (1973) pointed out that "any model is valuable when it improves our understanding of obscure behavioral characteristics more than would be possible by observing the real system [without guidelines]" (p. 30). The expectation, therefore, is that use of a conceptual model of nursing will lead to more systematic observations of phenomena and hence to more systematic building of nursing knowledge through programs of nursing research. Given this, it seems reasonable to expect that use of a conceptual model will foster a higher quality of nursing practice and more organized nursing curricula and systems of nursing care delivery than is evident when an explicit model is not used to guide activities.

COMPARISON OF CONCEPTUAL MODELS

The framework for analysis and evaluation of nursing models presented above will assist nurses to examine and compare various conceptual models prior to selecting one to guide their endeavors. It is, however, imperative that the reader understand on what level conceptual models may be compared.

Analysis and evaluation allows one to draw conclusions about the internal validity of each model but does not extend to external comparisons among different models. This important distinction implies "that any conceptual model is valid insofar as it is reasonably sound with regard to the particular anthropology employed (i.e., man as developing, adapting, interacting)" (Zbilut, 1978, p. 128).

Thus, because each conceptual model presents a distinctive view of metaparadigm phenomena, direct external comparisons should not be made. As Reese and Overton (1970) explained, "because of basic lack of communication, the partial overlap in subject matter, and the difference in truth criteria, [each model] must be evaluated separately, and in obedience to its own ground rules" (p. 122). Thus, one should not, for example, criticize a given conceptual model for failing to consider problems in patients' self-care abilities when the model emphasizes the nurse's management of stimuli to promote the patient's adaptation.

Some external comparisons of conceptual models of nursing have appeared in the literature. Most of these are discussions of the qualitative differences among models and presentations of differences in approaches to nursing care. Stanton (1985), for example, presented a brief overview of different views of the nursing process steps of assessment, nursing diagnosis, planning, implementation, and evaluation. Similarly, Fitzpatrick and Whall (1983) developed a chart that compares various conceptual models with regard to the definition of nursing, derivation of nursing activity, and conceptualization of the person, health, and environment. Because such comparisons do not fault one model for excluding content that is encompassed by another model, they are appropriate approaches to exploring similarities and differences in various perspectives of nursing.

Jacobson (1984) has argued that certain quantitative external comparisons of conceptual models of nursing also are appropriate. She maintained that global appraisal of the total impact of a conceptual model is appropriate, using parameters that apply to all nursing models, regardless of the content of each. Using a questionnaire that measures the meaning of each model to the user, Jacobson found that conceptual models of nursing are regarded as worthwhile and consistent with the values of the discipline. Comparisons of the meaning profiles of various models revealed "a satisfying blend of similarities and differences" (p. 67). Jacobson explained, "The basic similarity of profiles is logical because all models deal with the same phenomenon; yet there is enough variation to indicate obvious differences among the models" (p. 67).

Suppe (1982) also supported external comparisons of conceptual models. He did not, however, present any technique or criteria for the comparisons.

SELECTING A CONCEPTUAL MODEL FOR CLINICAL PRACTICE

Once a nurse decides to structure her activities according to a conceptual model, it becomes necessary to select one from among the several models now in the literature. The following steps are offered as a guide for selection of that conceptual model:

1. The nurse should first state his or her beliefs and values about the metaparadigm concepts person, environment, health, and nursing, that is, his or her philosophy of nursing. Because the choice of a particular model to guide nursing activities ultimately is a value judgment (Hodgman, 1973), and because the author of each conceptual model based the model on certain personal beliefs and values, the nurse's own philosophical statement of beliefs and values about the metaparadigm concepts will facilitate the search for a model congruent with these ideas. Similarly, the nurse's private image of nursing should be articulated, as should theoretical notions about the metaparadigm concepts. Then, a model that is congruent with the nurse's philosophy and private image of nursing, as well as with his or her theoretical understanding can be located. Finally, the nurse should identify his or her usual way of practicing nursing, so that model choice can reflect congruence with pragmatics of practice.
2. Thoroughly analyze and evaluate several conceptual models of nursing in detail.
3. Compare the content of the model with the philosophical statements, private image of nursing, and theoretical notions, as well as usual ways of practicing nursing.
4. Select the conceptual model that most closely matches these beliefs, thoughts, and practices.
5. Use the conceptual model in a variety of nursing situations to determine its utility.

Additional points to consider when selecting a conceptual model for use in a clinical agency were offered by Capers (1986). She noted that it is important to determine if the nursing practice environment is conducive to using an explicit conceptual model, what outcomes are anticipated from use of the conceptual model, which nursing personnel will use the model, how the staff will be prepared to use the model, how and when use of the model will be evaluated, and the financial resources that are needed and those that are available.

The novice user of a conceptual model should not become discouraged if initial experiences with the model seem forced or awkward. Adoption of a model does require restructuring of the nurse's way of thinking about nursing situations and use of a new vocabulary. However, repeated use of the model should lead to more systematic and organized endeavors. Broncatello's (1980) words underscore these points.

> The nurse's consistent use of any model for the interpretation of observable client data is most definitely not an easy task. Much like the

development of any habitual behavior, it initially requires thought, discipline and the gradual evolvement of a mind set of what is important to observe within the guidelines of the model. As is true of most habits, however, it makes decision making less complicated. (p. 23)

CONCLUSION

In this chapter, a framework for analysis and evaluation of conceptual models was presented, along with a detailed discussion of each criterion. The framework will be applied in the next seven chapters, each of which will present a comprehensive examination of a conceptual model of nursing.

REFERENCES

Bloom, B.S. (Ed.). (1956). Taxonomy of educational objectives. The classification of educational goals. Handbook I. Cognitive domain. New York: McKay.

Broncatello, K.F. (1980). Auger in action: Application of the model. Advances in Nursing Science 2(2), 13–23.

Capers, C.F. (1986). Using nursing models to guide nursing practice: Key questions. Journal of Nursing Administration, 16(11), 40–43.

Dickoff, J., James, P., & Wiedenbach, E. (1968). Theory in a practice discipline: Part 1. Practice oriented theory. Nursing Research, 17, 415–435.

Duffey, M., & Muhlenkamp, A.F. (1974). A framework for theory analysis. Nursing Outlook, 22, 570–574.

Fawcett, J. (1980). A framework for analysis and evaluation of conceptual models of nursing. Nurse Educator, 5(6), 10–14.

Fitzpatrick, J.J., & Whall, A.L. (1983). Conceptual models of nursing. Analysis and application. Bowie, MD: Brady.

Hodgman, E.C. (1973). A conceptual framework to guide nursing curriculum. Nursing Forum, 12, 110–131.

Jacobson, S.F. (1984). A semantic differential for external comparison of conceptual nursing models. Advances in Nursing Science, 6(2), 58–70.

Johnson, D.E. (1974). Development of theory. A requisite for nursing as a primary health profession. Nursing Research, 23, 372–377.

Johnson, D.E. (1987). Guest Editorial: Evaluating conceptual models for use in critical care nursing practice. Dimensions of Critical Care Nursing, 6, 195–197.

Lippitt, G.L. (1973). Visualizing change. Model building and the change process. Fairfax, VA: NTL Learning Resources.

Marriner, A. (1986). Nursing theorists and their work. St. Louis: CV Mosby.

Meleis, A.I. (1985). Theoretical nursing: Development and progress. Philadelphia: JB Lippincott.

Nursing Theories Conference Group. (1985). Nursing theories. The base for professional nursing practice (2nd ed.). Englewood Cliffs, NJ: Prentice-Hall.

Parse, R.R. (1987). Nursing science. Major paradigms, theories, and critiques. Philadelphia: WB Saunders.

Peterson, C.J. (1977). Questions frequently asked about the development of a conceptual framework. Journal of Nursing Education, 16(4), 22–32.

Reese, H.W., & Overton, W.F. (1970). Models of development and theories of development. In L.R. Goulet & P.B. Baltes (Eds.), Life span development psychology. Research and theory (pp. 116–145). New York: Academic Press.

Riehl, J.P., & Roy, C. (1974). Conceptual models for nursing practice. New York: Appleton-Century-Crofts.

Riehl, J.P., & Roy, C. (1980). Conceptual models for nursing practice (2nd ed.). New York: Appleton-Century-Crofts.

Stanton, M. (1985). Nursing theories and the nursing process. In Nursing Theories Conference Group, Nursing theories. The base for professional nursing practice (2nd ed., pp. 319–337). Englewood Cliffs, NJ: Prentice-Hall.

Stevens, B.J. (1979). Nursing theory. Analysis, application, evaluation. Boston: Little, Brown and Co.

Stevens, B.J. (1984). Nursing theory. Analysis, application, evaluation (2nd ed.). Boston: Little, Brown and Co.

Suppe, F. (1982, April). Implications of recent developments in philosophy of science for nursing theory. Paper presented at the Fifth Biennial Eastern Conference on Nursing Research, Baltimore, MD.

Thibodeau, J.A. (1983). Nursing models: Analysis and evaluation. Monterey, CA: Wadsworth.

Walker, L.O., & Nicholson, R. (1980). Criteria for evaluating nursing process models. Nurse Educator, 5(5), 8–9.

Zbilut, J.P. (1978). Epistemologic constraints to the development of a theory of nursing. (Letter to the editor). Nursing Research, 27, 128–129.

ANNOTATED BIBLIOGRAPHY

Adam, E.T. (1975). A conceptual model for nursing. Canadian Nurse, 7(9), 40–41.
Positive aspects of using a conceptual model are given in this article. Criteria for choosing a particular conceptual model are presented.

Aggleton, P., & Chalmers, H. (1986). Model choice. Senior Nurse, 5(5/6), 18–20.
This article presents guidelines to help nurses evaluate and choose from among different nursing models. Stated as questions, the guidelines are:
What assumptions does the model make about people and their health-related needs? Do they match your own understandings of people and how they operate?
What values does the model work with? Do they match the values that you find socially desirable?
What are the key concepts a model uses? Are they useful in nursing and caring for people? Have they been derived from work in other disciplines or have they emerged from the research and concerns of nurses?
What relationships are suggested between these concepts? Do they seem reasonable in the light of your own nursing experience? Is there nursing research that supports the existence of these relationships?
How does the model see the role of the nurse? Is this a conception you can find acceptable?
Is the model parsimonious? Does it present things in a clear-cut and understandable way without being too simplistic in its claims?
Does the model have something of generality to say about nursing in the context for which its use is being considered?
Is the use of the model likely to lead to better care?
Did the nursing model provide adequate guidelines on assessment so that the patient's problems could easily be identified?
Did the planning of care and the setting of goals match the patient's own expectations?
Did the model suggest a range of nursing interventions that were practical in that particular care setting?
Did the nursing interventions enable the nurse to provide a standard of care acceptable both to her/himself and to the patient?

Buchanan, B.F. (1987). Conceptual models: An assessment framework. Journal of Nursing Administration, 17(10), 22–16.
This article presents a framework for assessing the adequacy, completeness, and appropriateness of nursing models. The context, form, and process of the model are analyzed, and consideration is given to the implications of the model for professional and legal standards. Roy's and King's models are reviewed.

Capers, C.F. (1986). Using nursing models to guide nursing practice: Key questions. Journal of Nursing Administration, 16(11), 40–43.

This article presents the following questions to be asked of a conceptual model when considering its adoption as a guide for nursing practice in a clinical agency. Is the nursing practice environment conducive to using a nursing conceptual model?
Which nursing conceptual model will serve as the guide for nursing practice?
What outcomes are anticipated from using the nursing conceptual model?
Who uses the model?
How will nurses be prepared for using the model?
How and when will goal attainment be evaluated?
What financial resources are available to support the project?

Cessario, L. (1987). Utilization of board gaming for conceptual models of nursing. Journal of Nursing Education, 26, 167–169.

The author describes a board game she developed to teach students about conceptual models of nursing.

Chinn, P.L., & Jacobs, M.K. (1987). Theory and nursing. A systematic approach. (2nd ed.). St. Louis: CV Mosby.

This book includes a scheme for analyzing and evaluating theories. Evaluation criteria include semantic clarity and consistency, structural clarity and consistency, simplicity, generality, empirical applicability, and consequences.

Dickoff, J., James, P., & Wiedenbach, E. (1968). Theory in a practice discipline: Part 1. Practice oriented theory. Nursing Research, 17, 415–435.

The authors discuss the relation of theory to practice and the structure of nursing practice theory. They maintain that any practice discipline requires a four-level hierarchy of theory, including factor-isolating theories, factor-relating or situation-depicting theories, situation-relating theories, including predictive and promoting or inhibiting theories, and situation-producing or prescriptive theories. The authors identify the essential ingredients of prescriptive theory as goal content, prescriptions for activity to achieve the goal, and specification of the following survey list items: who or what performs the activity, who or what is the recipient of the activity, the context in which the activity is performed, the end point of the activity, the guiding procedure for the activity, and the energy source of the activity.

Duffey, M., & Muhlenkamp, A.F. (1974). A framework for theory analysis. Nursing Outlook, 22, 570–574.

The authors identify four questions to be used in analyzing nursing theory:
What is the origin of the problems with which the theory is concerned?
What are the methods used?
What is the character of the subject matter dealt with by the theory?
What kind of outcomes of testing propositions generated by this theory would you expect to get?
The use of this framework for theory analysis was illustrated by examination of Peplau's and Rogers's work.

Ellis, R. (1968). Characteristics of significant theories. Nursing Research, 17, 217–222.

This article presents criteria for evaluation of theories, including scope, complexity, testability, usefulness, values, hypotheses, and terminology.

Fawcett, J. (1980). A framework for analysis and evaluation of conceptual models of nursing. Nurse Educator, 5(6), 10–14.

Fawcett, J. (1984). Analysis and evaluation of conceptual models of nursing. Philadelphia: FA Davis.

The article defines, describes, and differentiates conceptual models of nursing and nursing theories. A framework for analysis and evaluation appropriate for nursing models is identified. Chapters 1 and 2 of the 1984 book represent an expansion of the article, and include some modifications in the framework. Chapters 1, 2, and 10 of the present book present the most recent refinements in the discussion of conceptual models and theories and the most recent modifications in the analysis and evaluation framework.

Fawcett, J., & Downs, F.S. (1986). The relationship of theory and research. Norwalk, CT: Appleton-Century-Crofts.

This book presents definitions of theory and research and describes the relationship between theory and research in considerable detail. Techniques for analysis of theory are a focal point of the book. Criteria for the evaluation of theory are given, including significance, internal consistency, parsimony, testability, operational adequacy, empirical adequacy, and pragmatic adequacy.

Fitzpatrick, J.J., & Whall, A.L. (1983). Conceptual models of nursing. Analysis and application. Bowie, MD: Brady.

This book presents a scheme for analysis and evaluation of conceptual models of nursing. The scheme includes the following questions:

What are the definitions of person, environment, health, and nursing given by the model?

What is the understanding of these concepts basic to the model?

What are the relationships among these concepts?

How are nursing activities explicated?

What are the implicit and explicit assumptions of the model?

How do the implicit and explicit assumptions relate to each other?

What are the central components of the model?

What is the relative importance of the components?

What types of concepts are used?

What are the definitions of these components and what are the relationships among components?

What is the internal consistency of the model?

What is the meaning and logical adequacy of the model?

Are there operational definitions for the concepts, are these adequate, and may hypotheses be drawn from the model?

What is the scope of the model?

What is the complexity of the model?

What is the usefulness of the model?

Does the model generate new information?

What is the relationship of the model to nursing research, nursing education, and professional practice?

Works reviewed in the book are those of Nightingale, Peplau, Orlando, Wiedenbach, Henderson, Levine, Johnson, Orem, Roy, Paterson and Zderad, Neuman, King, Rogers, Newman, Parse, and Fitzpatrick. No clear distinctions between conceptual models and theories are made.

Hardy, M.E. (1978). Perspectives on nursing theory. Advances in Nursing Science, 1(1), 37–48.

This article presents a discussion of the stages of scientific development, the nature of theory, and criteria for evaluation of a theory, including logical adequacy, empirical adequacy, usefulness, and significance.

Hils-Williams, J. (1985). Conceptual models—A framework for nursing practice. Emphasis: Nursing, 1(2), 77–83.

A discussion of the use of conceptual models as guides for nursing practice is presented by the author. Questions to be answered prior to selecting a conceptual model for practice include:

Who is the patient?

What is the patient's role in the health care system?

What are the patient's rights?

What is the role of the family?

Who is responsible for patient outcomes?

What is the patient's relationship to the environment?

Can the environment affect health/illness? How?

Is the patient a part of or separate from the environment?

How does the environment affect the nurse?

Can the nurse affect the environment?

Is health and illness a dichotomy or a continuum?

What is health? Illness?

How is illness cured? How is health restored?

What is the relationship between a patient and illness?

Who defines "illness" in a patient?
How is "health" defined for a particular patient?
What relationship does the mind and body have to health/illness?
What is the nurse's role?
What is the nurse's responsibility to the patient?
What effect does the nurse have on the environment and health/illness?
What is the goal of nursing?
What does the nurse do to, for, or with the patient?
What is nursing's contribution to the health care team?

Hoon, E. (1986). Game playing: A way to look at nursing models. Journal of Advanced Nursing, 11, 421–427.
This article explains how conceptual models can be analyzed through the use of a board game.

Jacobson, S.F. (1984). A semantic differential for external comparison of conceptual models. Advances in Nursing Science, 6(2), 58–70.

Nicoll, L., Myer, P., & Abraham, I. (1985). Critique: External comparison of conceptual nursing models. Advances in Nursing Science, 7(4), 1–9.
Jacobson presents the findings of an exploratory study of the meaning of several conceptual models to student and faculty raters. A semantic differential instrument was used to measure meaning and the resultant profile for each model served as a basis for comparisons. The models included in the study were the works of King, Orem, Rogers, Roy, and Wiedenbach.
Nicoll, Myer, and Abraham critique Jacobson's philosophical stance and research using the semantic differential. They contend that Jacobson's rationale for external comparison of nursing models is invalid, citing Fawcett's statement in the first edition of this book that comparisons are not appropriate. However, Fawcett's statement was taken out of context.

Johnson, D.E. (1974). Development of theory: A requisite for nursing as a primary health profession. Nursing Research, 23, 372–377.
The author discusses the status of nursing science and the evolution of scientific disciplines, and differentiates the scientific and social functions of a profession. Alternative routes to theory development identified are the laissez-faire, following medicine's path, or acceptance of nursing as a distinctive profession. Contributions to the development of nursing's conceptual system are identified and conceptual models of nursing are discussed briefly. Criteria for evaluation of nursing models put forth by the author include social congruence, social significance, and social utility.

Johnson, D.E. (1980). Unpublished lecture notes and class handouts. University of California at Los Angeles, Fall 1975. In J.P. Riehl & C. Roy, Conceptual models for nursing practice (2nd ed., p. 7). New York: Appleton-Century-Crofts.
Johnson identifies the essential units of a conceptual model of nursing as: clear statements of assumptions and values; clear definitions of concepts; identification of a goal of action; description of patiency and of the nurse's role; and identification of the source of difficulty, the focus of intervention, and the intended and unintended consequences.

Johnson, D.E. (1987). Guest Editorial: Evaluating conceptual models for use in critical care nursing practice. Dimensions of Critical Care Nursing, 6, 195–197.
This editorial presents a discussion of the use of conceptual models of nursing and the importance of using an explicit nursing model for nursing practice. Johnson maintains that a nursing model must include a goal of action, a descriptive term for patiency, a source of difficulty, and the types of interventions that are appropriate and useful. She also presents the following three questions, affirmative answers to which demonstrate the utility of the conceptual model.
Is the practitioner able to make pertinent observations, decide that a nursing problem(s) exists, and prescribe and execute a course of action which achieves the goal specified?
Does the educator have sufficient guidelines to construct a curriculum, and does she have reasonable understanding of what knowledge and skills are needed?

Is the investigator given sufficient direction about what to study and what questions to ask?

Marriner, A. (1986). Nursing theories and their work. St. Louis: CV Mosby.

This book identifies major thinkers in nursing and provides a review of some of their ideas, lists of their publications, and major sources used for development of their ideas. No distinctions are made between conceptual models and theories and no explicit format for analysis and evaluation of the works is given. Works by Nightingale; Henderson; Abdellah; Hall; Orem; Adam; Leininger; Watson; Parse; Peplau; Travelbee; Orlando; Wiedenbach; King; Riehl-Sisca; Erickson, Tomlin, and Swain; Barnard; Johnson; Roy; Neuman; Levine; Rogers; Fitzpatrick; and Newman are reviewed. Marriner noted that the work of Paterson and Zderad was not included at their request.

Meleis, A.I. (1985). Theoretical nursing: Development and progress. Philadelphia: JB Lippincott.

This book reviews major works in nursing using a schema that does not distinguish conceptual models from theories. Indeed, Meleis claims that calling a work a conceptual model lessens its value. The works of Johnson, Roy, Rogers, King, Orlando, Paterson and Zderad, Travelbee, Wiedenbach, Levine, and Orem are reviewed. Extensive bibliographies are included.

Mooney, M.M. (1980). The ethical component of nursing theory. An analysis of ethical components of four nursing theories. Image. The Journal of Nursing Scholarship, 12, 7–9.

An analysis of ethical components of works by Travelbee, Rogers, Orem, and an adaptation model is presented in this article. Consideration is given to their stances on personhood, rights of person, consent, rights of society, distributive justice, and personal justice.

Nursing Theories Conference Group. (1980). Nursing theories. The base for professional nursing practice. Englewood Cliffs, NJ: Prentice-Hall.

Nursing Theories Conference Group. (1985). Nursing Theories. The base for professional nursing practice (2nd ed.). Englewood Cliffs. NJ: Prentice-Hall.

The 1980 edition of this book reviews the works of Abdellah, Hall, Henderson, King, Levine, Nightingale, Orem, Orlando, Peplau, Rogers, Roy, and Wiedenbach. Each review includes discussion of the historical setting of the nurse and the components of the work. The components are then interpreted and discussed by the chapter author(s) in relation to man, health, society, and nursing and to their use in the nursing process. The 1985 edition follows a similar format and includes all works in the 1980 edition as well as those of Johnson, Neuman, and Patterson and Zderad. Neither edition makes any distinction between conceptual models and theories.

Parse, R.R. (1987). Nursing science. Major paradigms, theories, and critiques. Philadelphia: WB Saunders.

This book presents the papers read at the Nurse Theorist Conference held in Pittsburgh, Pennsylvania in May 1985. Presentations of their works are by King, Orem, Parse, Rogers, and Roy. A critique of each work is included, using an evaluation scheme that does not distinguish between conceptual models and theories.

Peterson, C.J. (1977). Questions frequently asked about the development of a conceptual framework. Journal of Nursing Education, 16(4), 22–32.

The author defines the terms concept, proposition, hypothesis, theory, law, and conceptual framework. The latter is differentiated from a theoretical framework. The author maintains that the following questions must be answered by a conceptual framework if it is to be an adequate guide for curriculum development:

What is the nature of the service being provided to the client (consumer, patient)—that is, how is nursing described?

What is the goal or outcome to which the service is directed—that is, how is health or well-being viewed?

Why does the client need the services nursing provides?

How is the giver of the service—the nurse—described?

Riehl, J.P., & Roy, C. (1974). Conceptual models for nursing practice. New York: Appleton-Century-Crofts.

Riehl, J.P., & Roy, C. (1980). Conceptual models for nursing practice (2nd ed.). New York: Appleton-Century-Crofts.

In the 1974 edition, the authors maintain that the elements of nursing models are those of prescriptive theory, as defined and described by Dickoff, James, and Wiedenbach. The 1974 edition includes reviews and applications of the works of Chrisman and Riehl, Johnson, Neuman, Pierce, Preisner, Riehl, Rogers, Roy, and Travelbee. In the 1980 edition, the authors maintain that the elements of a nursing model are those put forth by Johnson in her 1975 lecture notes (see Johnson, 1980). The book includes reviews and applications of the works of Abbey, Brink, Chrisman and Fowler, Johnson, Neuman, Orem, Peplau, Preisner, Riehl, Rogers, and Roy. Neither edition makes clear distinctions between conceptual models and theories.

Stevens, B.J. (1979). Nursing theory. Analysis, application, evaluation. Boston: Little, Brown and Co.

Stevens, B.J. (1984). Nursing theory. Analysis, application, evaluation (2nd ed.). Boston: Little, Brown and Co.

In the 1979 edition, the author identifies and describes the following criteria for evaluation of nursing theories:

Internal Criticism: clarity, consistency, logical development, and level of theory development

External Criticism: adequacy, utility, significance, discrimination, scope of theory, and complexity

These criteria are used to examine the works of several nurse scholars, including Hall, Johnson, King, Levine, Neuman, Orem, Peplau, Rogers, and Roy. The 1984 edition presents slight modifications in the criteria for theory evaluation, including placement of adequacy under internal criticism and the addition of the criterion of reality convergence to external criticism. Distinctions are not made between conceptual models and theories.

Thibodeau, J.A. (1983). Nursing models: Analysis and evaluation. Monterey, CA: Wadsworth.

This book represents a scheme for analysis and evaluation of conceptual models of nursing that draws heavily from Fawcett's 1980 framework. The works reviewed include the crisis model and those by Travelbee, Neuman, and Orem. No clear distinction is made between conceptual models and theories.

Torres, G. (1986). Theoretical foundations of nursing. Norwalk, CT: Appleton-Century-Crofts.

This book presents brief overviews of some of the main concepts of works by Nightingale, Henderson, Abdellah, Orlando, Wiedenbach, Orem, Kinlein, Johnson, Rogers, King, Neuman, Roy, Peplau, Hall, Levine, Travelbee, and Watson. Works by the non-nurses Murray, Maslow, and Carl Rogers also are reviewed. No distinctions are made between conceptual models and theories.

Uys, L.R. (1987). Foundation studies in nursing. Journal of Advanced Nursing, 12, 275–280.

Three approaches to review of the content of conceptual models are presented in this article. Foundationalism focuses on questions about the primary foundations on which assertions about the truth of knowledge are based. Language critique emphasizes the language in which propositions and theories are expressed. Philosophical analysis focuses on the philosophical premises from which a particular model was developed.

Walker, L.O., & Nicholson, R. (1980). Criteria for evaluating nursing process models. Nurse Educator, 5(5), 8–9.

The authors identify and discuss the following criteria for evaluation of nursing process models. They maintain that a nursing process model should:

1. Incorporate an underlying knowledge base in making the judgment inherent in the nursing process.
2. Be as dynamic as practice itself, that is, the model should permit dynamic movement back and forth between steps in the process.
3. Be applicable to nursing in general and not only to specific clinical settings.
4. Be compatible with ethical standards for nursing practice.

5. Be consistent with scientific findings on human behavior in health and illness.

Winstead-Fry, P. (Ed.). (1986). Case studies in nursing theory. New York: National League for Nursing.

This book presents reviews of the works of Orlando, Orem, Rogers, Roy, Neuman, Paterson and Zderad, King, and Newman. King and Orem wrote the chapters dealing with their works. An attempt is made to distinguish between conceptual models and theories.

Winter, E.J.S., Bender, A.W., Hertz, J.E., & Reider, J.A. (1987). Analyzing and evaluating a baccalaureate nursing curriculum framework. Nurse Educator, 12(4), 10–13.

The authors used the framework for analysis and evaluation of conceptual models of nursing published in the first edition of this book to review the nursing curriculum framework at York College of Pennsylvania.

CHAPTER

3

Johnson's Behavioral System Model_____

This chapter presents an analysis and evaluation of Dorothy Johnson's conceptual model of nursing. This formulation clearly fits the definition of conceptual model used in this book and always has been classified as such by its author.

The key terms of Johnson's conceptual model are listed below. These terms were taken from the only published presentation of the model by Johnson (1980), entitled "The Behavioral System Model for Nursing."

KEY TERMS_____

Behavioral System	Subsystem Functional
Subsystems	Requirements—*Cont.*
Attachment or Affiliative	Stimulation
Dependency	Subsystem Structural Elements
Ingestive	Drive or Goal
Eliminative	Set
Sexual	Choice
Aggressive	Action or Behavior
Achievement	Behavioral System Balance and
Subsystem Functional	Stability
Requirements	Efficient and Effective Behavioral
Protection	System Functioning
Nurturance	

Behavioral System Imbalance and Instability	Nursing as an External Regulatory Force
Goals of Nursing Restore, Maintain, or Attain Behavioral System Balance and Stability	Impose External Regulatory or Control Mechanisms Change Structural Units Fulfill Functional Requirements

ANALYSIS OF JOHNSON'S BEHAVIORAL SYSTEM MODEL

This section presents an analysis of Johnson's conceptual model. The analysis relies heavily on Johnson's 1980 publication. "The behavioral system model for nursing."

Development of the Model

The rudimentary ideas of Johnson's conceptual model were evident in her 1959 article. "A philosophy of nursing," and in her 1961 article, "The significance of nursing care." However, Johnson did not present her entire conceptual model in the literature until she prepared a chapter for the second edition of Riehl and Roy's (1980) book, *Conceptual models for nursing practice*. Prior to this publication, the only public records of the model were a widely cited paper of Johnson's 1968 presentation at Vanderbilt University in Nashville, Tennessee and her 1978a presentation at the Second Annual Nurse Educator Conference. Versions of the model, however, had been available to interested nurses since Grubbs published her interpretation of Johnson's conceptual model in 1974 and Auger published her interpretation in 1976. Johnson has not presented any revisions in her conceptual model since the 1980 publication.

Johnson's various publications indicate her continuous interest in the development of nursing as a science and a profession. In particular, she has been interested in identifying the nature of the service offered by nursing and in delineating the knowledge needed to provide that service (Johnson, 1974). She certainly may be considered a pioneer in this endeavor, despite the fact that she did not publish her model until recently. In fact, Johnson (1978a) stated that she has been developing her model since the early 1940s, when she began to teach nursing. Her educational activities led her to ask: What content is properly included in a nursing course? This question led to two others: (1) Knowledge for what purpose? and (2) Knowledge to what end?

Johnson (1978a) stated that she based the answers to those questions on the following two premises:

1. Nursing is a profession that makes a distinctive contribution to the welfare of society.
2. Nursing has an explicit goal of action in patient welfare that is different from but complementary to that of other health professions.

Given these premises, the task then was delineated as the need to clarify nursing's social mission from the perspective of a theoretically sound view of the person served by nursing. This task was approached historically, empirically, and analytically. The historical approach led Johnson to accept from Nightingale nursing's traditional concern with the person who is ill, rather than with the person's disease, per se. The empirical approach led to a review of studies of nursing tasks. Johnson noted that this approach, which defines nursing as what nurses do, was not fruitful. However, it kept the focus on people who are ill or who might be prevented from becoming ill. Finally, the analytical approach led Johnson to consider what reason suggests. This turned out to be the most useful approach.

Through reasoning, Johnson (1980) finally came to conceive of nursing's specific contribution to patient welfare as "the fostering of efficient and effective behavioral functioning in the patient to prevent illness and during and following illness" (p. 207). This focus led Johnson to accept a view of the patient as a behavioral system.

The basic idea of Johnson's conceptual model, then, is the behavioral system. The acceptance of this idea, according to Johnson (1980), "is made possible by the relatively recent development and rapid expansion of . . . an interdisciplinary literature . . . focused on the behavior of the individual as a whole—on what he does, why, and on the consequences of that behavior—not on why or how he has changed over time in an intraorganismic sense" (p. 207). More specifically, this literature focuses on observable features and actions that comprise social behavior, and in particular, on behavior that has major adaptive significance.

Johnson (1980) acknowledged the limitations of current knowledge in supporting the idea of the behavioral system as a whole. However, she noted the contributions of the developing knowledge of "systems in general and the laws that govern the operation of all systems" (p. 208) to an understanding of the behavioral system and of the integration of the specific response systems comprising the whole system. Johnson's discussion of the systems literature included references to works by Buckley (1968), Chin (1961), and Rapoport (1968). Furthermore, she commented that this interdisciplinary literature is being developed by behavioral and biologic scientists, animal and human ethologists, and some nurses, although she did not cite specific authors.

Johnson (1980) identified the following 12 assumptions about the nature and operation of the behavioral system:

1. A system is a whole which functions as a whole.
2. Parts or elements of a system are organized, interactive, interdependent, and integrated.
3. The system tends to achieve a balance among various forces acting within and upon it.
4. Man strives continually to maintain behavioral system balance and a steady state by more or less automatic adjustments and adaptations to the natural forces impinging upon him.
5. Man actively seeks new experiences that may disturb balance and may require small or large behavioral system modification to reestablish balance.
6. Observed regularities and constancies in human behavior that result from behavioral system balance and stability are functionally significant for the individual and for social life.
7. When behavioral regularities are disturbed, integrity of the person is threatened and functions served by such order are less than adequately fulfilled.
8. Behavioral system balance represents adjustments and adaptations that are successful to some degree and in some way, even though observed behavior may not match cultural or biologic norms for acceptable or healthy behavior.
9. Living systems can and do operate at varying levels of efficiency and effectiveness, but in order for a system to operate at all, it must maintain a certain level of balance and stability internally and in its environmental interactions.
10. Behavioral systems have sufficient flexibility to take account of the usual fluctuations in the impinging forces and enough stress tolerance for adjustment to many common, but extreme, fluctuations.
11. During their lives, most individuals probably experience a psychologic or social crisis or physical illness grave enough to disturb system balance and require external assistance.
12. Nursing is, or could be, the force that supplies assistance both when disturbances in system balance occur and at other times to prevent such disturbances. (pp. 208–209)

Johnson (1980) stated "the conception of man as a behavioral system, or the idea that man's specific response patterns form an organized and integrated whole is original with me, so far as I know" (p. 208). She further noted that the literature indicates that others support her idea. Indeed, Ackoff used the term behavioral system in 1960.

Johnson's description of the development of her conceptual model suggests that she used a deductive approach. Her conception of the person as a behavioral system reflects a synthesis of knowledge, primarily from the systems literature but also from nursing's historical past. Further documentation of the deductive method used in the development of the model is provided by Johnson's reference to many authors when discussing the subsystems of the behavioral system. These authors include Ainsworth (1964, 1972); Atkinson and Feather (1966); Crandal (1963); Feshbach (1970); Gewirtz (1972); Heathers (1955); Kagan (1964); Lorenz (1966); Mead (1953); Resnik (1972); Robson (1967); Rosenthal (1967); Sears, Maccoby, and Levin (1954); and Walike, Jordan, and Stellar (1969). There are indications that Johnson also may have used induction to develop her conceptual model. The evidence for an inductive approach comes from the following statement: "Over a period of some twenty years and in the light of my clinical experiences, thinking, reading, and conversations with colleagues, I evolved the notion that one potentially useful way of viewing man is as a behavioral system" (Johnson, 1978b, pp. 7–8).

Content of the Model: Concepts

Person

The person of interest in Johnson's conceptual model is the individual behavioral system. The model focuses on the whole individual, defined as a behavioral system. "All patterned, repetitive, and purposeful ways of behaving that characterize each man's life are considered to comprise his behavioral system" (Johnson, 1980, p. 209). The parts of the behavioral system are called subsystems. They carry out specialized tasks or functions needed to maintain the integrity of the whole behavioral system and manage its relationship to the environment.

Johnson (1980) identified seven subsystems. These subsystems and their specialized functions are listed below.

1. Attachment or affiliative subsystem: Functions are attainment of the security needed for survival as well as social inclusion, intimacy, and the formation and maintenance of social bonds.
2. Dependency subsystem: Functions are succoring behavior that calls for a response of nurturance as well as approval, attention, or recognition, and physical assistance.
3. Ingestive subsystem: Function is appetite satisfaction, with regard to when, how, what, how much, and under what conditions the individual eats, which is governed by social and psychological considerations as well as biologic requirements for food and fluids.
4. Eliminative subsystem: Function is elimination, with regard to when, how, and under what conditions the individual eliminates wastes.
5. Sexual subsystem: Functions are procreation and gratification, with regard to behaviors dependent upon the

individual's biologic sex, including but not limited to courting and mating.

6. Aggressive subsystem: Function is protection and preservation of self and society.
7. Achievement subsystem: Function is mastery or control of some aspect of self or environment, with regard to intellectual, physical, creative, mechanical, social, and care-taking (of children, spouse, home) skills.

Johnson (1980) commented that the subsystems are found cross-culturally and across a broad range of the phylogenetic scale, suggesting that they are genetically programmed. She also noted the significance of social and cultural factors involved in the development of the subsystems. The seven subsystems are not to be regarded as a complete set, because "the ultimate group of response systems to be identified in the behavioral system will undoubtedly change as research reveals new systems or indicates changes in the structure, functions, or behavior pattern groupings in the original set" (Johnson, 1980, p. 212).

Johnson (1980) explained that the subsystems "are linked and open, . . . and a disturbance in one subsystem is likely to have an effect on others" (p. 210). She further explained that "although each subsystem has a specialized task or function, the system as a whole depends on an integrated performance" (p. 210).

The ability of the subsystems to fulfill their functions depends upon certain requirements "that must be met through the individual's own efforts, or through outside assistance" (Johnson, 1980, p. 212). The functional requirements are (1) protection from noxious influences with which the system cannot cope, (2) nurturance through the input of appropriate supplies from the environment, and (3) stimulation to enhance growth and prevent stagnation.

In addition to function, each subsystem has structure. The four structural elements of each are drive or goal, set, choice, and action or behavior. The drive or goal of a subsystem refers to motivation for behavior. In general, the drive of each subsystem is the same for all people, "but there are variations among individuals in the specific objects or events that are drive-fulfilling, in the value placed on goal attainment, and in drive strength" (Johnson, 1980, p. 210). The specific drive of each subsystem cannot be observed directly but must be inferred from the individual's actual behavior and from the consequences of that behavior.

Set, which also is inferred from observed behavior, refers to the individual's predisposition to act in certain ways, rather than in other ways, to fulfill the function of the subsystem. Johnson (1980) explained that "through maturation, experience, and learning, the individual comes to develop and use preferred ways of behaving under particular circumstances and with selected individuals" (p. 211).

Choice refers to the individual's total behavior repertoire for fulfilling subsystem functions. The behavioral repertoire encompasses the scope of action alternatives from which the person can choose. Johnson (1980) pointed out that the individual rarely uses all these alternatives but, rather, chooses certain preferred behaviors. However, the other behaviors are available should the preferred ones not work in a certain situation.

Action refers to the actual behavior in a situation and is the only structural element that can be observed directly. Johnson (1980) commented that behavior is instigated, inhibited, shaped, continued, or terminated by the complex biological, psychological, sociological, and physical factors that constitute the other structural elements. She described behavior as "a set of behavioral responses, responsive tendencies, or actions systems" (p. 209). She went on to say,

> these responses are developed and modified over time through maturation, experience, and learning. They are determined developmentally and are continuously governed by a multitude of physical, biologic, psychologic, and social factors operating in a complex and interlocking fashion. These responses are reasonably stable, though modifiable, and regularly recurrent, and their action pattern is observable. (p. 209)

Environment

Johnson (1980) referred to the internal and external environment of the system, as well as to "the interaction between the person and his environment and . . . to the objects, events and situations in his environment" (p. 209). She also referred to forces that impinge on the person and to which the person adjusts and adapts. However, Johnson gave no specific definition for environment, nor did she identify what she considered internal versus external environment. Her discussion suggests that objects, events, situations, and forces are part of the environment. This was not, however, made explicit.

Health

Johnson (1978b) commented that health in its most global sense is a concern of the members of all health professions, political scientists, agronomists, and others. Her particular focus, however, and one that she considered appropriate for nursing, is the behavioral system. This focus is reflected in Johnson's (1968) statement, "One or more of [the behavioral system] subsystems is likely to be involved in any episode of illness, whether in an antecedent or a consequence way, or simply in association, directly or indirectly, with the disorder or its treatment" (p. 3). In various presentations and publications, Johnson has mentioned behavioral system balance and stability, efficient and effective behavioral functioning, behavioral system imbalance and instability, and the person who is ill.

Johnson (1978a) stated that behavioral system balance and stability is demonstrated by observed behavior that is purposeful, orderly, and predictable. Purposeful behavior is goal directed; that is, actions reveal a plan and cease at an identifiable point. Orderly behavior is methodical and systematic, as opposed to diffuse and erratic. Further, orderly behavior encompasses actions that build sequentially toward a goal and form a recognizable pattern. Predictable behavior is that which is repetitive under particular circumstances.

Purposeful, orderly, and predictable behavior is maintained when it is efficient and effective in managing the person's relationship to the environment. Behavior changes when efficiency and effectiveness are no longer evident or when a more optimal level of functioning is perceived (Johnson, 1978a). Individuals are said to achieve efficient and effective behavioral functioning when their behavior is commensurate with social demands, when they are able to modify their behavior in ways that support biologic imperatives, when they are able to benefit to the fullest extent during illness from the physician's knowledge and skill, and when their behavior does not reveal unnecessary trauma as a consequence of illness (Johnson, 1978a, 1980).

Behavioral system imbalance and instability is not described explicitly but can be inferred to be a malfunction of the behavioral system from the following statement:

> The subsystems and the system as a whole tend to be self-maintaining and self-perpetuating so long as conditions in the internal and external environment of the system remain orderly and predictable, the conditions and resources necessary to their functional requirements are met, and the interrelationships among the subsystems are harmonious. If these conditions are not met, malfunction becomes apparent in behavior that is in part disorganized, erratic, and dysfunctional. Illness or other sudden internal or external environmental change is most frequently responsible for such malfunctions. (Johnson, 1980, p. 212)

Johnson did not define illness. She mentioned psychological and social crisis and physical illness (Johnson, 1978a, 1980), but did not describe manifestations of these conditions. Though it may be inferred that behavioral system imbalance and instability are equated with illness, the quotation above suggests that Johnson may view illness as separate from behavioral system functioning.

Furthermore, although Johnson (1980) referred to physical and social health, she did not explicitly define wellness. Just as an inference about illness may be made, it may be inferred that wellness is behavioral system balance and stability, as well as efficient and effective behavioral functioning. These inferences suggest that Johnson views health as a dichotomy, rather than a continuum. Caution must be observed, however, when assessing the validity of these inferences.

Nursing

Johnson (1980) viewed nursing as "a service that is complementary to that of medicine and other health professions, but which makes its own distinctive contribution to the health and well-being of people" (p. 207). More specifically, she described nursing "as an external regulatory force which acts to preserve the organization and integration of the patient's behavior at an optimal level under those conditions in which the behavior constitutes a threat to physical or social health, or in which illness is found" (Johnson, 1980, p. 214). Johnson clearly distinguished nursing from medicine by stating that nursing views the patient as a behavioral system and medicine views the patient as a biologic system.

The goal of nursing action is "to restore, maintain, or attain behavioral system balance and stability at the highest possible level for the individual" (Johnson, 1980, p. 214). This goal may be expanded to include helping the person to achieve a more optimum level of balance and functioning when this is possible and desired (Johnson, 1978a). The goal of nursing is based on the following propositions:

1. If extraordinarily strong impinging forces, or a lowered resistance to or capacity to adjust to more moderate forces, disturb behavioral system balance, the integrity of the person is threatened.
2. The attempt by man to preserve or re-establish behavioral system balance in the face of continuing excessive forces making for imbalance requires an extraordinary expenditure of energy.
3. Insofar as behavioral system balance requires a minimum (for the moment at least and in reference to a particular individual) expenditure of energy, a larger supply of energy is available in the service of biologic processes and recovery. (Johnson, 1968, p. 4)

Johnson did not identify a specific nursing process, although she mentioned analysis of system functioning and measures through which nursing operates as an external regulatory force in her presentations and publications. Questions to be asked when analyzing system functioning include

- Is the behavior succeeding or failing to achieve the consequences sought?
- Are more skillful motor, expressive, or social skills needed?
- Are the choices appropriate?
- Is the sequence of action purposeful and orderly; does it demonstrate economy of action; is the action socially and biologically appropriate? (Johnson, 1968, 1978a)

Measures encompassed by the external regulatory force that is nursing include

- imposition of external regulatory or control mechanisms
- attempts to change structural units in desirable directions
- the fulfillment of the functional requirements of the subsystem. (Johnson, 1980, p. 214)

Further specification of these elements was extracted from Johnson's (1968, 1978a) discussions of use of her conceptual model and is presented in Table 3–1.

TABLE 3–1. Using Johnson's Behavioral System Model

I. Analysis of system functioning
  A. Study man as a behavioral system
    1. Collect data to describe the structure and function of the system as a whole and the subsystems
      a. Observe system input, output, feedback, and regulatory and control mechanisms
      b. Obtain measures of
        (1) Expenditure of energy required for behavioral functioning
        (2) Compliance of behavior with biological and social imperatives
        (3) Degree of personal satisfaction expressed about the behavior
    2. Analyze data to determine degree of efficiency and effectiveness of the behavioral system
      a. Ask questions such as:
        (1) Is the behavior succeeding or failing to achieve the consequences sought?
        (2) Are more skillful motor, expressive, or social skills needed?
        (3) Is the sequence of action purposeful and orderly; does it demonstrate economy of action; is the action socially and biologically appropriate?
      b. Compare behavior to indices of behavioral system and subsystem balance
        (1) Is the observed behavior purposeful? That is, is the behavior goal directed? Do actions reveal a plan and cease at an identifiable point?
        (2) Is the observed behavior orderly? That is, is the behavior methodological and systematic? Do actions build sequentially toward a goal and form a recognizable pattern?
        (3) Is the observed behavior predictable? That is, is the behavior repetitive under particular circumstances?
      c. Compare behavior to indices of efficient and effective behavioral functioning
        (1) Is energy expenditure acceptable?
        (2) Does behavior comply with biological and social imperatives?
        (3) Is behavior satisfying to the patient?

TABLE 3–1.   *Continued*

      3. Identify origin and nature of structural or functional problems of the behavioral system and subsystems
 II. Identification of goal of nursing action
   A. General goal of action
      1. Restore, maintain, or attain the patient's behavioral system balance and stability
      2. Help the patient achieve a more optimum level of balance and functioning when this is possible and desired
   B. Determine what nursing is to accomplish on behalf of the behavioral system
      1. Determine what level of behavioral system balance and stability is acceptable
      2. Determine who makes the judgment regarding acceptable level of behavioral system balance and stability
         a. Identify value system of nursing profession
         b. Identify own explicit value system
III. Identification of nursing intervention
   A. Modes of intervention
      1. Temporarily impose external regulatory or control measures
         a. Modify behavior; for example
            (1) Set limits for behavior by either permissive or inhibitory means
            (2) Inhibit ineffective behavioral responses
            (3) Assist patient to acquire new responses
      2. Change structural units in desirable direction
         a. Repair damaged structural units; for example
            (1) Alter set by instruction or counselling
            (2) Add choices by teaching new skills
      3. Fulfill functional requirements of the subsystems
         a. Supply essential environmental conditions or resources (or help patient to find own supplies); for example
            (1) Protect patient from overwhelming noxious influences
            (2) Supply adequate nurturance through an appropriate input of essential supplies
            (3) Provide stimulation to enhance growth and to inhibit stagnation
   B. Negotiate treatment modality with patient
      1. Establish a contract with the patient
      2. Help patient understand meaning of nursing diagnosis and proposed treatment
      3. If diagnosis and/or proposed treatment are rejected, continue to negotiate with the patient until agreement is reached
IV. Evaluation of goal achievement
   A. Compare behavior after intervention to indices of behavioral system and subsystem balance (c.f. I.A.2.b.)
   B. Compare behavior to indices of efficient and effective behavioral system functioning (c.f. I.A.2.c.)

Adapted from Johnson, D.E. (1968, April). One conceptual model of nursing. Paper presented at Vanderbilt University, Nashville, TN; and Johnson, D.E. (1978a, December). Behavioral System Model for Nursing. Paper presented at Second Annual Nurse Educator Conference, New York. (Cassette recording)

As noted in Table 3–1, Johnson expects the nurse to base judgments about behavioral system balance and stability on an explicit value system. She set forth her own value system, which is capsulized in the following quotation:

> There is a wide range of behavior which is tolerated in this society or any other, and only the middle section of the continuum can be said to represent the cultural norms. So long as behavior does not threaten the survival of society, either directly through the death or lack of productivity of individuals or indirectly through the creation of massive disorder or deviance from established social values, it appears to be acceptable. The outer limits of acceptable, and therefore tolerated, behavior are thus set for the professions by society, but in fact, the limits of acceptable behavior set by the health professions, including nursing, probably tend to be narrower in some areas and in some respects than those set by the larger society.
>
> Since the professions have an obligation which goes beyond accepting the current state of affairs to shaping the reality of the future, an additional facet of this problem of values is that of determining what is desirable, rather than simply acceptable behavior. At least two closely related facts must be remembered in this connection. In the first place, forced change in behavior in one area of life may and often does require other behavioral modifications. The consequences may be unforeseen, unintended, and undesirable. Secondly, the current status of knowledge about man and his universe does not allow us to predict, with reasonable certainty, a configuration of behavioral responses which measured against some established standards could be said to be of a "better" or "higher" level in an absolute way.
>
> Applying these considerations to the establishment of a value system for the use of this model leads us to certain conclusions. First of all nursing must not, in our opinion, purposefully support, certainly over a prolonged period or in the absence of other counteractive measures, behavioral responses which are so deviant that they are intolerant to society or constitute a threat to the survival of the individual, either socially or biologically, and thus ultimately are a threat to society. We believe further that while nursing has an obligation to [help the person] seek the highest possible level of behavioral functioning, and to contribute, through research, to the specification of what that level might be, we cannot afford to go very far beyond what is known. Quite specifically, we do not think that nursing can presume to transform the values, beliefs, and norms of the individuals we serve to those in accordance with the culture of middle-class, urban, American society which we generally represent. We cannot, and must not, substitute our judgments at any given point in time for those of the individual or of the larger society. (Johnson, 1968, pp. 4–5)

In her 1978a presentation, Johnson added to her value system by stating that the final judgment of the desired level of functioning is the right of the individual, given that this level is within survival limits and that the individual has been provided with adequate understanding of the potential for and the means to obtain a more optimal level of behavioral functioning than is evident at the present time.

Johnson's value system also emphasized the need for a contract between nurse and patient for treatment, as noted in Table 3–1. Johnson (1978a) maintained that continuous negotiation between nurse and patient is necessary if the initial diagnosis or proposed treatment is rejected by the patient.

Content of the Model: Propositions

The linkage of the metaparadigm concepts, person and environment, is reflected in the following statements:

> All the patterned, repetitive, and purposeful ways of behaving that characterize each man's life are considered to comprise his behavioral system. These ways of behaving form an organized and integrated functional unit that determines and limits the interaction between the person and his environment and establishes the relationship of the person to the objects, events, and situations in his environment. (Johnson, 1980, p. 209)

> The behavioral system has many tasks or missions to perform in maintaining its own integrity and in managing the system's relationship to its environment. (Johnson, 1980, p. 209)

The concepts, person, environment, and health, are linked in the following statement:

> The subsystems and the system as a whole tend to be self-maintaining and self-perpetuating so long as conditions in the internal and external environment of the system remain orderly and predictable, the conditions and resources necessary to their functional requirements are met, and the interrelationships among the subsystems are harmonious. If these conditions are not met, malfunction becomes apparent in behavior that is in part disorganized, erratic, and dysfunctional. Illness or other sudden internal or external environmental change is most frequently responsible for such malfunctions. (Johnson, 1980, p. 212)

The linkages among the metaparadigm concepts, person, health, and nursing, are evident in these statements:

> Most individuals probably experience at one or more times during their lives a psychologic crisis or a physical illness grave enough to disturb the system balance and to require external assistance. Nursing is (or could be) the force that supplies assistance both at the time of occurrence and at other times to prevent such occurrences. (Johnson, 1980, p. 209)

> Nursing is thus seen as an external regulatory force which acts to preserve the organization and integration of the patient's behavior at an

optimal level under those conditions in which the behavior constitutes a threat to physical or social health, or in which illness is found. (Johnson 1980, p. 214)

Areas of Concern

The areas of concern, or problems, that Johnson's conceptual model addresses are structural or functional problems in the behavioral system as a whole and in the various subsystems. In addition, the model is concerned with behavioral functioning that is at a less than desired or optimal level. In particular, this model is concerned with behavioral system disorders of two types.

Those that are related tangentially or peripherally to disorder in the biological system; that is, they are precipitated simply by the fact of illness or the situational context of treatment.

Those that are an integral part of a biological system disorder in that they are either directly associated with or a direct consequence of a particular kind of biological system disorder or its treatment. (Johnson, 1968)

All of these problems present actual or potential imbalances in the behavioral system. The sources of these problems are inadequate or inappropriate development of the system and its parts, a breakdown in internal regulatory and control mechanisms of the system, the system's exposure to noxious influences, its failure to be adequately stimulated, or lack of adequate environmental input (Johnson, 1980).

EVALUATION OF JOHNSON'S BEHAVIORAL SYSTEM MODEL

This section presents an evaluation of Johnson's conceptual model. The evaluation is based on the findings of the analysis of the model as well as on publications and presentations by others who have used or commented on Johnson's work.

Explication of Assumptions

Johnson presented the assumptions underlying her conceptual model explicitly and concisely. She clearly stated the premises regarding nursing and her assumptions regarding the nature and operation of the behavioral system.

Johnson's presentation of her conceptual model indicates that she values a focus on the person's behavior and views that behavior as a manifestation of the momentary condition of the whole behavioral system as well as the subsystems. Johnson also values nursing intervention before, during, and following illness. Moreover, she values the patient's contributions to his or her care, as indicated by her insistence on establishment of a contract for nursing intervention.

Johnson stated that the use of her conceptual model is based on values of the nursing profession, as well as those of the individual nurse. She explicitly set forth her own value system for use of the model, which was outlined in the analysis section.

Comprehensiveness of Content

Johnson addressed all four concepts of nursing's metaparadigm—person, environment, health, and nursing. Person is clearly defined and described. Although the description of the ingestive and eliminative subsystems seems to emphasize biologic processes, behaviors related to ingestion and elimination are highlighted.

All other metaparadigm concepts are described, although in some instances this is done so globally that clarity needs to be enhanced. For one thing, environment is not defined explicitly. Thus, what constitutes the environment is not clear, nor are the parameters of the relevant environment known. Moreover, Johnson did not make a clear distinction between what she called the internal environment and the external environment.

Health also is not defined explicitly. As a consequence, inferences must be made about what Johnson meant by wellness and illness, as well as how these are distinguished. In particular, the relation of health to behavioral system balance and stability versus imbalance and instability needs to be clarified. Further, although behavioral system balance and stability is clearly and comprehensively described, the description of behavioral system imbalance and instability is not explicit. It must be inferred that this is the converse of behavioral system balance and stability.

Other aspects of Johnson's discussion of health also require clarification. Although the model clearly focuses on behavior, Johnson uses the terms psychologic and social crises and physical illness. The meaning of these terms in relation to the various subsystems of the behavioral system is not clear. One interpretation of Johnson's statements about illness is that this condition is separate from behavioral system functioning. Thus, it is not clear if illness (physical, psychologic, or social) is an external condition that affects certain subsystems, or if it is manifested when these subsystems are not functioning efficiently and effectively. Similarly, the meaning of the terms physical and social health and their relation to the condition of the behavioral system require specification.

It must be pointed out, however, that Johnson (1978b) regarded health as "an extremely elusive state" (p. 6). It is not surprising, then, that the conceptual model does not include an explicit definition of health and that there is some lack of clarity about aspects of this concept.

Nursing is defined and described adequately, as is the goal of nursing. The description of the nursing process, however, lacks specificity. The nursing process format presented in Table 3–1 had to be extracted from Johnson's discussions of the use of the model. The application of Walker and Nicholson's (1980) criteria for nursing process is based on the content of Table 3–1.

Johnson's model emphasizes that judgments regarding behavioral system functioning are to be based on theoretical and empirical knowledge of systems, as well as that related to each subsystem. Johnson (1980) underscored this aspect of her model by outlining the various sciences that must be studied prior to using her model. These are discussed in the section on social utility.

In Johnson's model, the nursing process is not presented as a particularly dynamic activity, although some dynamism is evident in the negotiation of proposed treatment between patient and nurse. Johnson (1978a) claimed that her model provides clear direction for practice, education, and research. This is documented in the section on social utility. It may be concluded, then, that the nursing process is useful in a variety of settings.

Johnson's explication of her own value system, her statement that the use of the model should be based on the values of the nursing profession as well as the individual nurse, and the inclusion of negotiation of treatment between patient and nurse all attest to her concern for ethical standards for nursing practice. Furthermore, this conceptual model is clearly and explicitly based on scientific findings in nursing and other disciplines.

The propositions of Johnson's conceptual model link the person and the environment; the person, the environment, and health; and the person, health, and nursing. No one statement links all four metaparadigm concepts, and there is no direct link between environment and nursing. This linkage is implied, however, when Johnson (1980) stated that nursing is "an external regulatory force . . . that operates through the imposition of external regulatory or control mechanisms" (p. 214). It may be inferred that nursing is part of the environment.

Some limitations of Johnson's model, especially those related to the lack of comprehensive descriptions of the metaparadigm concepts, have been overcome by others who have extended the model. Auger (1976) provided an interpretation of the model that focused on the person as a personality system (Johnson, personal communication, October 17, 1977), thus extending the model further into the psychological realm. Grubbs (1974, 1980) presented an interpretation of the model that expanded each of the metaparadigm concepts considerably. She also presented a comprehensive description of a nursing process that is in keeping with Johnson's major ideas.

Logical Congruence

World Views

Johnson's conceptual model primarily reflects the organismic world view, but includes a mechanistic element as well. The focus on the behavioral system as a whole and emphasis on behavior, per se, indicates a holistic view of the person. The subsystems are explicitly identified as parts of the whole behavioral system, rather than as discrete entities.

The organismic view of the world also is reflected in Johnson's (1980) description of the person as actively seeking new experiences. The active organism view is underscored by the ideas that each subsystem strives to achieve a particular goal and that each person makes certain behavioral choices. This viewpoint is further documented by Johnson's (1980) statement that the behavioral system "determines and limits the interaction between the person and his environment" (p. 209). In fact, Johnson (cited in Conner & Watt, 1986) views the behavioral system as active, not reactive. Furthermore, she believes that individuals are active beings who adjust environments to ensure better functioning for themselves.

However, Johnson (1980) at least implied a mechanistic, reactive organism viewpoint when she noted that forces operate upon the system and that nursing is an external regulatory force. An attempt to reconcile the logically incompatible world views of mechanism and organicism may be inferred from the following quotation:

> Man strives continually to maintain a behavioral system balance and steady states by more or less automatic adjustments and adaptations to the "natural" forces impinging upon him. At the same time, . . . man also actively seeks new experiences that may disturb his balance. (Johnson, 1980, p. 208)

Johnson's emphasis on behavioral system balance and stability indicates a persistence view of the world. Hall's (1981) comments support this judgment. She stated:

> Interestingly, one of the first of the current nursing theorists, Dorothy Johnson, tried to head the profession in the direction of persistence. She takes equilibrium as a starting point in her original conception. The goal of nursing care, in her model, emphasizes balance, order, stability, and maintenance of the integrity of the patient. (p. 5)

Change, in Johnson's model, is postulated to occur only when necessary for survival. As Johnson (1980) noted, the behavioral system "both requires and results in some degree of regularity and constancy in behavior. . . . Behavioral system balance reflects adjustments and adaptations that are successful in some way and to some degree" (p. 208).

Classification of the Model

Johnson's conceptual model was classified as a systems model by Marriner (1986), Riehl and Roy (1980), and Stevens (1984). The appropriateness of this categorization is evident in the following comparison of the concepts and propositions of Johnson's model with the characteristics of systems models.

Johnson's conceptual model addresses system in the definition of the person as a behavioral system. The integration of the parts, called subsystems, is evident in the comment that they are "linked and open, as is true in all systems, and a disturbance in one subsystem is likely to have an effect on others" (Johnson, 1980, p. 210).

Environment is addressed throughout the presentation of the model, although its parameters are never identified beyond the comment that it is both internal and external. Boundary is not addressed explicitly in Johnson's conceptual model. Boundary permeability is alluded to in this statement: "There appears to be built into the system sufficient flexibility to take account of the usual fluctuations in the impinging forces and enough stress tolerance for the system to adjust to many common, but extreme, fluctuations" (Johnson, 1980, p. 209).

The systems model characteristic of tension, stress, strain, and conflict is addressed through the discussion of the "natural" forces impinging upon the behavioral system. These forces lead to "more or less automatic adjustments and adaptations" required for continuing behavioral system balance and stability (Johnson, 1980, p. 208).

Johnson (1980) used the term steady state in conjunction with behavioral system balance. Although the concept of behavioral system balance and stability implies that the system is at a fixed point or achieves an equilibrium when stable, Johnson apparently regarded stability as a dynamic equilibrium. This aspect of the conceptual model requires clarification.

The characteristic of feedback is addressed only briefly in this conceptual model, when Johnson (1978a) commented that it is necessary to understand input, output, feedback, and regulatory control mechanisms to analyze behavioral system functioning. However, the nature of these system operations was not described.

Meleis (1985) regarded Johnson's conceptual model as a prominent example of the outcome category of models, although she commented that the model incorporates the needs category view of the human being. Although Stevens (1984) classified Johnson's conceptual model as a systems model, she also placed the model within the intervention category of her classification scheme.

Generation and Testing of Theory

The formation of conceptual-theoretical systems of nursing knowledge is evident in many of the applications of Johnson's Behavioral System Model, as can be seen in the section on social utility. In several instances, selected concepts of the model were linked with theories borrowed from other disciplines. The outcomes of these applications, especially the findings of the studies, provide evidence that supports the credibility of the conceptual model. For example, Holaday (1981) found that "patterns of maternal response provided information related to the . . . behavioral set, that is, the degree of proximity and speed of maternal response. Crying behavior in the ill infant provided an illustration of a type of signal in which the mother had to make the discrimination of when and when not to respond. Mothers with chronically ill infants rarely did not respond to a cry" (p. 347).

Holaday (personal communication, August 26, 1987) has begun to develop a theory dealing with the structural elements and functional requirements (sustenal imperatives) of Johnson's conceptual model. This theory development work is part of an ongoing study of what chronically ill 10- to 12-year-old children do with their time out-of-school. Holaday commented that she and a colleague "are interested in identifying the important sustenal imperatives for each subsystem and how they influence choice and action. We will attempt to see if there is a hierarchy of sustenal imperatives for each subsystem."

Although some theory development work has been done, no theories of the behavioral system as a whole have been formulated yet. Commenting on this, Johnson (1980) stated,

> At this point, research and theoretical attention have been directed primarily toward specific response systems within the total complex of the whole behavioral system; an empirical literature supporting the notion of the behavioral system as a whole is largely yet to be developed. This is not unlike the case of the growth of knowledge about the biologic system, in which knowledge of the parts preceded knowledge of the whole. Fortunately, there is also developing concurrently a body of knowledge about systems in general and the laws that govern the operation of all systems, on which we can rely in a tentative way until further knowledge of the behavioral system is developed. (p. 208)

Social Considerations

Social Congruence

Johnson's conceptual model is generally congruent with contemporary social expectations regarding nursing practice. Commenting on this criterion, Johnson (1980) stated, "Insofar as it has been tried in practice, the resulting nursing decisions and actions have generally been judged acceptable and satisfactory by patients, families, nursing staff, and physicians" (p. 215). Furthermore, Grubbs (1980) maintained that the role of the nurse, as described in this model, "is congruent with society's expectations of nursing and that nursing's contribution to health care is a socially valued service" (p. 218). However, neither Johnson nor Grubbs provided empirical evidence to support their contentions.

Johnson (1968) deliberately attempted to structure nursing practice so that it would be congruent with societal expectations. She maintained, "The value of the model does not lie so much in the fact that it leads to very different forms of action—if it did depart markedly from currently accepted practice, it would perhaps be open to greater question than it otherwise might be" (p. 6).

In contrast to her 1968 comment, 10 years later Johnson (1978a) indicated that in some situations, the nurse and/or the patient may accept a wider range of behavior than prescribed by cultural norms. In such cases, society would have to be helped to accept variances from the average. Additionally, society may have to be helped to accept the role of nursing in assisting people to maintain efficient and effective behavioral functioning when the threat of illness exists. This is because some people still do not expect nursing care prior to the onset of illness. Indeed, Johnson (cited in Conner & Watt, 1986) maintained that preventive nursing, whether aimed at prevention of behavioral system disorder or some other goal, needs to be developed.

Social Significance

Johnson (1980) claimed that her conceptual model leads to nursing actions that are socially significant, stating "resulting [nursing] actions have been thought to make a significant difference in the lives of the persons involved" (p. 215). Grubbs (1980) agreed with Johnson, noting that the model "provides the framework for categorizing all aspects of the nursing process so that the science of nursing, the personal satisfaction of the nurse, and ultimately the welfare of the patient will improve" (p. 249). Again, however, neither Johnson nor Grubbs supported her claim with empirical evidence.

Johnson's insistence on continued negotiation with the patient until agreement is reached on treatment strategies may contribute to improved health status for the patient. This is because there may be a greater likelihood of patient adherence to a prescribed treatment in a climate of negotiation than when treatment is established solely by the nurse. This thesis is supported by Swain and Steckel's (1981) findings of improved health status for hypertensive patients when the treatment was established through a contract between nurse and patient.

Social Utility

Johnson (1980) claimed that her conceptual model "has already proved its utility in providing clear direction for practice, education, and research" (p. 215). Articles by advocates of Johnson's model indicate that it also has provided useful guidelines for administration. The following examples, as well as the annotated bibliography at the end of this chapter, support Johnson's claim of social utility.

The utility of Johnson's Behavioral System Model for nursing research is documented by the several studies that have been conducted within this paradigm. Although several rules for research have not yet been developed for this conceptual model, the rules dealing with the nature of problems and phenomena to be studied are explicit. In particular, Johnson (1968) maintained that within the context of her conceptual model, the research task "is to identify and explain the behavioral system disorders which arise in connection with illness, and to develop the rationale for and the means of management" (p. 6).

The focus on the behavioral system is evident in several master's theses and doctoral dissertations known to have been based on Johnson's conceptual model. Holaday (personal communication, August 26, 1987) identified several master's theses that were based on the Behavioral System Model. These studies were conducted by Broering (1985), Dawson (1984), Kizpolski (1985), Miller (1987), Moran (1986), and Wilkie (1985). Doctoral dissertation research includes Carino's (1976) comparison of differences in behavioral system responses of disoriented and oriented intensive care unit patients, Kosten's (1977) exploration of professional nurses' assessment of practice in psychiatric settings, Lovejoy's (1982) development of a family assessment tool derived from Johnson's model, and Dee's (1987) study of the validation of a patient classification instrument based on Johnson's model (Holaday, personal communication, August 26, 1987; Silva & Sorrell, 1987). Nishimoto's (1987) doctoral dissertation also was derived from Johnson's conceptual model. She explored the perceived sexuality of men who had experienced prostate surgery.

Investigation of the behavioral system also is evident in several published research reports. One of the earliest reports of research based on Johnson's conceptual model was Stamler and Palmer's (1971) investigation of dependency behaviors in children who made repetitive visits to an elementary school nurse. Other reports include Holaday's (1974, 1981, 1982, 1987) four studies derived from Johnson's conceptual model. For one investigation, Holaday (1974) used the concepts of the achievement subsystem, behavioral system balance, drive, and set to study the differences in achievement behavior between chronically ill and well children. These concepts were linked with theoretical knowledge about children's achievement behavior, social learning theory, and attribution theory. In another study, Holaday (1981) used the concept of behavioral set to guide her investigation of the effects of degree of illness, infant's sex, and ordinal position on maternal response to infants' crying. Theories of attachment behavior provided the rationale for the study hypotheses. In her third and fourth studies, Holaday (1982, 1987) again used the concept of behavioral set to continue her examination of mothers' responses to the crying behaviors of their chronically ill infants. Holaday (personal communication, August 26, 1987) explained that her 1987 study was "a 'second check' on the structural component of conceptual set" and that the data from this study led to identification of "the general characteristics of the stages of conceptual set."

Damus (1980) also used Johnson's model for her study of patients who had post-transfusion hepatitis. She investigated "the relationship between selected physiologic disequilibria and behavioral disequilibria as well as the correlation of particular nursing diagnoses with effective nursing interventions" (p. 275). Damus used the behavioral subsystems as the classification scheme for nursing diagnoses and the functional requirements to classify nursing interventions. Theoretical knowledge was drawn from literature dealing with serum hepatitis.

Furthermore, Small (1980) discussed the findings of her investigation in the context of Johnson's conceptual model. Her study compared perceived body image and spatial awareness of visually handicapped preschool children with that of normally sighted preschoolers. The study was based on theoretical knowledge of visual handicaps.

Other research based on Johnson's conceptual model includes Derdiarian's (1983, 1984; Derdiarian & Forsythe, 1983) innovative work on development of an instrument to measure perceived behavioral changes in cancer patients, and Lovejoy's (1983) futher work on development of a family assessment tool. Derdiarian's and Lovejoy's studies are noteworthy in that their instruments encompass several subsystems of the behavioral system.

Lovejoy (1985) also has conducted a study of the needs of visitors of patients with cancer. Additional research, which deals with quality assurance, is discussed in the section on utility for administration.

The utility of the Behavioral System Model for nursing practice also is documented in the literature. Rules for practice are not explicit, but some can be extracted from the content of the conceptual model.

Clearly, nursing practice is directed toward restoration, maintenance, or attainment of behavioral system balance and stability, and clinical problems encompass conditions in which behavior is a threat to health or in which illness is found. The nursing process, although not explicated completely by Johnson, is inherent in the model. These rules and the utility of the model in various clinical settings are reflected in several publications.

Holaday (1980) used the model to assess health status and to derive nursing interventions for a 6-year-old child scheduled for surgery, for a 12-year-old with meningomyelocele and multiple urinary tract problems, and for a 15-year-old retarded child with a discrepancy of the eliminative subsystem. In each of these situations, Holaday linked concepts of Johnson's model with theories of development. Skolny and Riehl (1974) used the model to guide their actions to promote development of hope for the mother of a dying brain-injured 22-year-old man. They used theories of grief and mourning and of hope to direct their nursing actions. Rawls (1980) used the model to guide nursing care of an adult amputee with a problem in body image. She linked Johnson's model with theoretical notions about body image. McCauley and her colleagues (1984) used the model to guide assessment and nursing intervention for family-centered nursing care of the patient with ventricular tachycardia. They linked the model with theoretical knowledge of physiologic, psychologic, and sociologic responses to cardiac arrhythmias.

Another use of Johnson's model in nursing practice was reported by Hackley (1987), who redesigned nursing care processes within the context of this conceptual model for the psychiatric unit at the U.S. Naval Hospital in Philadelphia, Pennsylvania. Furthermore, B. Sanchez, J. de Uriza, and M. Orjuela (personal communication, March 18, 1986) reported the progress they had made in using Johnson's model to guide nursing care of elderly patients in Colombia, South America.

Johnson's model emphasizes and focuses explicitly on the individual behavioral system. However, for those nurses who are interested in the care of families and other groups, Johnson (1978a) suggested the use of Chin's (1961) intersystem model. This approach permits consideration of each individual behavioral system and the interaction of these systems. Furthermore, Conner and Watt (1986) explained how the model could be used in community health nursing. Thus, the model may be readily extended to a variety of clinical nursing situations.

Rawls (1980) summarized the utility of Johnson's model for nursing practice by stating:

> Use of the Model allowed me to systematically assess the patient and facilitated identification of specific factors which influenced the effectiveness of nursing care. The assessment data allowed identification of

interventions which had the desired effect and resulted in effective care for the patient. (p. 16)

Johnson claimed that her conceptual model has utility for nursing education and identified guidelines for curriculum development based on the model. She stated:

Adoption of this model for practice carries with it direct responsibilities in education. The user will need a thorough grounding in the underlying natural and social sciences. Emphasis should be placed in particular on the genetic, neurologic, and endocrine bases of behavior; psychologic and social mechanisms for the regulation and control of behavior; social learning theories; and motivational structures and processes. (Johnson, 1980, p. 214)

Johnson (1980) also stated that the user of the model must study the behavioral system as a whole and as a composite of subsystems, pathophysiology, medicine's and nursing's clinical sciences, and the health system.

Johnson's statements suggest some rules for nursing education. In particular, the focus of the curriculum is the behavioral system and subsystems, and content is drawn from the natural, social, and clinical sciences.

The utility of Johnson's conceptual model for nursing education is documented by its use as a guide for curriculum construction in nursing education programs. Hadley (1970) described the use of Johnson's conceptual model at the University of Colorado in Denver. Harris (1986) described the use of a modified version of the conceptual model at the University of California in Los Angeles. Asay and Ossler (1984) indicated that Johnson's model has been used by the Department of Nursing at California State University in Bakersfield. In addition, Meleis (1985) reported that Johnson's model has served as a basis for curriculum in schools of nursing in Hawaii and Tennessee. She did not, however, give the names of the schools. The utility of Johnson's conceptual model for nursing education also is documented by Derdiarian (1981), who discussed the application of the model to cancer nursing education.

The utility of Johnson's model for nursing service administration is evident, although specific rules for administration have not yet been formulated. Rogers (1973) proposed that the behavioral subsystems form areas for clinical specialization in nursing. Chance (1982) claimed that nursing models provide guidelines for professional accountability and quality of nursing care. Although she reviewed the major concepts of Johnson's model, she did not demonstrate their application to quality assurance programs.

Application of the conceptual model to quality assurance programs was demonstrated by Majesky, Brester, and Nishio (1978), who derived the Patient Indicators of Nursing Care instrument from Johnson's conceptual model. This instrument was designed "to measure quality of nursing care, defined as prevention of nursing care complications" (p. 365). More specifically, the tool assesses the "degree to which nursing intervention contributes to the deterioration or improvement of a patient's condition, based on selected physiological measures, over a seven- to nine-day (hospital or nursing home) stay" (p. 366). The specific items comprising the tool were drawn from theoretical knowledge of the effects of infection, immobility, and fluid imbalance.

Bruce and associates (1980) also used Johnson's model for a quality assurance program. Their work focused on the patient with end-stage renal disease. They designed a comprehensive program and developed a tool to measure outcome criteria for fluid and electrolyte balance. The tool was based on Johnson's ingestive, eliminative, and achievement subsystems and theoretical knowledge of renal physiology, end-stage renal disease, client education, fluid and electrolyte balance, and development and use of outcome criteria.

Glennin (1980) developed standards for nursing practice from Johnson's conceptual model. These were developed for hospitalized patients receiving acute care from professional registered nurses. Emphasis was placed on psychosocial, rather than physiological management. Glennin classified the standards according to the nursing process areas of data-gathering, assessment, diagnosis, prescription, implementation, and evaluation. In each area, specific standards were formulated for relevant concepts and propositions of Johnson's model.

Auger and Dee (1983) developed a patient classification system based on Johnson's model. Each behavioral subsystem was operationalized as critical behaviors. Overall level of behavior for each patient then was categorized as adaptive, in the process of being learned and/or minimally maladaptive, or maladaptive. Nursing interventions were linked to behaviors and also categorized. Dee and Auger (1983) described the application of the patient classification system within the Child Inpatient Service of the Mental Retardation and Child Psychiatry Division of the University of California Los Angeles-Neuropsychiatric Institute. The authors maintained that although the patient classification system was developed for use in psychiatric settings, it can be extended for use in various clinical settings by identifying relevant patient behaviors and nursing interventions for each setting. It is noteworthy that this patient classification system encompasses all subsystems and the entire nursing process. Indeed, Dee and Auger commented that use of the system led to many practical benefits and had a major impact on all phases of the nursing process. They explained,

> The assessment of patient behaviors . . . [is] now systematically and comprehensively reviewed within the framework of the behavioral

subsystems. . . . The correlated nursing care actions with patient behaviors has assisted in both the planning and the intervention phases
of the process by identifying a broad range of general areas of potential
nursing activity. . . . The use of a model also provides an objective
means for evaluating the quality of nursing care. . . . Instead of evaluating patient outcome for groups based on medical diagnoses, it becomes feasible to evaluate outcome for groups of patients based on
common behavioral problems or nursing treatment approaches. (p. 23)

Contributions to Nursing Knowledge

Johnson's conceptual model makes a substantial contribution to
nursing knowledge by focusing attention on the person's behavior,
rather than on his or her health state or disease condition. Johnson
used this distinction to clarify the different foci of nursing and medicine, a clarification that is especially important for continued development of nursing as a distinct discipline. However, she recognized the
boundary overlaps that are inevitable in all disciplines. This point is
elaborated in the following quotation:

This model attempts to specify [the goal of nursing] in keeping with
our historical concerns, and to reclarify nursing's mission and area of
responsibility. In doing so, no denial of nursing's old relationship with
medicine is intended. Nursing has, and undoubtedly always will play
an important role in assisting medicine to fulfill its mission. We do this
directly by taking on activities delegated by medicine, but also, and
perhaps more importantly, we may contribute to the achievement of
medicine's goals by fulfilling our own mission. (Johnson, 1968, p. 9)

Johnson (1968) identified the advantages she saw in her model.
This list adequately summarizes the many contributions her conceptual model makes to nursing knowledge.

1. The assumptions and values of the model are made explicit. This
   allows their examination and offers the possibility that those assumptions which have not been adequately verified can be logically and perhaps empirically tested.
2. The model offers a reasonably precise and limited ideal goal for
   nursing by stating the end product desired. Specification of this
   ideal state or condition is the first step in its operational definition
   in the concrete case. It thus offers promise for the establishment of
   standards against which to measure the effectiveness and significance of nursing actions.
3. The model directs our attention to those aspects of the patient, in
   all his complex reality, with which nursing is concerned, and provides a systematic way to approach the identification of nursing
   problems.
4. It provides us with clues as to the source of difficulty (i.e., either
   functional or structural stress).

5. It offers a focus for intervention and suggests the major modes of intervention which will be required.
6. It opens the door to focused research programs in nursing and the possibility that the findings of individual investigators will become cumulative and of theoretical as well as of practical significance. (pp. 7–8)

Johnson's Behavioral System Model is especially attractive to those nurses who are familiar with system theory and the attendant vocabulary. Although Rawls (1980) regarded the complex and unique terminology used to explain the model as a disadvantage, this limitation is readily overcome by studying the model's vocabulary.

In conclusion, Johnson's conceptual model of nursing has been enthusiastically adopted by many nurses interested in a systematic approach to nursing. It has documented utility in practice, administration, and research. And it provides direction for curriculum development. The credibility of the conceptual model is beginning to be established by means of studies directly derived from several of its components. This empirical work needs to be expanded and more systematic evaluations of the use of the model in various clinical situations and educational settings are needed.

REFERENCES

Ackoff, R.L. (1960). Systems, organizations, and interdisciplinary research. General Systems, 5, 1–8.

Ainsworth, M. (1964). Patterns of attachment behavior shown by the infant in interaction with mother. Merrill-Palmer Quarterly, 10(1), 51–58.

Ainsworth, M. (1972). Attachment and dependency: A comparison. In J. Gewirtz (Ed.), Attachment and dependency (pp. 97–137). Englewood Cliffs, NJ: Prentice-Hall.

Asay, M.K., & Ossler, C.C. (Eds.). (1984). Conceptual models of nursing. Applications in community health nursing. Proceedings of the Eighth Annual Community Health Nursing Conference. Chapel Hill, NC: Department of Public Health Nursing, School of Public Health, University of North Carolina.

Atkinson, J.W., & Feather, N.T. (1966). A theory of achievement maturation. New York: John Wiley & Sons.

Auger, J.R. (1976). Behavioral systems and nursing. Englewood Cliffs, NJ: Prentice-Hall.

Auger, J.R., & Dee, V. (1983). A patient classification system based on the Behavioral System Model of Nursing: Part I. Journal of Nursing Administration, 13(4), 38–43.

Broering, J. (1985). Adolescent juvenile status offenders' perceptions of stressful life events and self-perception of health status. Unpublished master's thesis, University of California, San Francisco.

Bruce, G.L., Hinds, P., Hudak, J., Mucha, A., Taylor, M.C., & Thompson, C.R. (1980). Implementation of ANA's quality assurance program for clients with end-stage renal disease. Advances in Nursing Science, 2(2), 79–95.

Buckley, W. (Ed.). (1968). Modern systems research for the behavioral scientist. Chicago: Aldine.

Carino, C. (1976). Behavioral responses of disoriented patients compared to oriented patients in intensive care units. Dissertation Abstracts International, 37, 162B.

Chance, K.S. (1982). Nursing models: A requisite for professional accountability. Advances in Nursing Science, 4(2), 57–65.

Chin, R. (1961). The utility of system models and developmental models for practitioners. In W.G. Bennis, K.D. Beene, & R. Chin (Eds.), The planning of change (pp. 201–214). New York: Holt, Rinehart and Winston.

Conner, S.S., & Watt, J.K. (1986). Dorothy E. Johnson. Behavioral System Model. In A. Marriner, Nursing theorists and their work (pp. 283–296). St. Louis: CV Mosby.

Crandal, V. (1963). Achievement. In H.W. Stevenson (Ed.), Child psychology (pp. 416–459). Chicago: University of Chicago Press.

Damus, K. (1980). An application of the Johnson behavioral system model for nursing practice. In J.P. Riehl & C. Roy, Conceptual models for nursing practice (2nd ed., pp. 274–289). New York: Appleton-Century-Crofts.

Dawson, D.L. (1984). Parenting behaviors of mothers with hospitalized children under two years of age. Unpublished master's thesis, University of California, San Francisco.

Dee, V. (1986). Validation of a patient classification instrument for psychiatric patients based on the Johnson model for nursing. Dissertation Abstracts International, 47, 4822B.

Dee, V., & Auger, J.A. (1983). A patient classification system based on the Behavioral System Model of Nursing: Part 2. Journal of Nursing Administration, 13(5), 18–23.

Derdiarian, A.K. (1981). Nursing conceptual frameworks: Implications for education, practice, and research. In D.L. Vredevoe, A.K. Derdiarian, L.P. Sarna, M. Eriel, & J.C. Shipacoff, Concepts of oncology nursing (pp. 369–385). Englewood Cliffs, NJ: Prentice-Hall.

Derdiarian, A.K. (1983). An instrument for theory and research using the Behavioral Systems Model for Nursing: The cancer patient (Part I). Nursing Research, 32, 196–201.

Derdiarian, A.K. (1984). An investigation of the variables and boundaries of cancer nursing: A pioneering approach using Johnson's Behavioral Systems Model for Nursing. In Proceedings of the 3rd International Conference on Cancer Nursing (pp. 96–102). Melbourne, Australia: The Cancer Institute/Peter MacCallum Hospital and the Royal Melbourne Hospital.

Derdiarian, A., & Forsythe, A.B. (1983). An instrument for theory and research using the Behavioral Systems Model for Nursing: The cancer patient (Part II). Nursing Research, 32, 260–266.

Feshbach, S. (1970). Aggression. In P. Mussen (Ed.), Carmichael's manual of child psychology (Vol. 2, 3rd ed., pp. 159–259). New York: John Wiley & Sons.

Gewirtz, J. (Ed.). (1972). Attachment and dependency. Englewood Cliffs, NJ: Prentice-Hall.

Glennin, C.G. (1980). Formulation of standards for nursing practice using a nursing model. In J.P. Riehl & C. Roy, Conceptual models for nursing practice (2nd ed., pp. 290–301). New York: Appleton-Century-Crofts.

Grubbs, J. (1974). An interpretation of the Johnson Behavioral System Model. In J.P. Riehl & C. Roy, Conceptual models for nursing practice (pp. 160–197). New York: Appleton-Century-Crofts.

Grubbs, J. (1980). An interpretation of the Johnson Behavioral System Model. In J.P. Riehl & C. Roy, Conceptual models for nursing practice (2nd ed., pp. 217–254). New York: Appleton-Century-Crofts.

Hackley, S. (1987, January). Application of Johnson's Behavioral System Model. Paper presented at the University of Pennsylvania School of Nursing. Philadelphia.

Hadley, B.J. (1970, March). The utility of theoretical frameworks for curriculum development in nursing: The happening at Colorado. Paper presented at WICHEN General Session, Honolulu, Hawaii.

Hall, B.A. (1981). The change paradigm in nursing: Growth versus persistence. Advances in Nursing Science, 3(4), 1–6.

Harris, R.B. (1986). Introduction of a conceptual nursing model into a fundamental baccalaureate course. Journal of Nursing Education, 25, 66–69.

Heathers, G. (1955). Acquiring dependence and independence: A theoretical orientation. Journal of Genetic Psychology, 87, 277–291.

Holaday, B. (1974). Achievement behavior in chronically ill children. Nursing Research, 23, 25–30.

Holaday, B. (1980). Implementing the Johnson model for nursing practice. In J.P. Riehl

& C. Roy, Conceptual models for nursing practice (2nd ed., pp. 255–263). New York: Appleton-Century-Crofts.

Holaday, B. (1981). Maternal response to their chronically ill infants' attachment behavior of crying. Nursing Research, 30, 343–348.

Holaday, B. (1982). Maternal conceptual set development: Identifying patterns of maternal response to chronically ill infant crying. Maternal-Child Nursing Journal, 11, 47–59.

Holaday, B. (1987). Patterns of interaction between mothers and their chronically ill infants. Maternal-Child Nursing Journal, 16, 29–45.

Johnson, D.E. (1959). A philosophy of nursing. Nursing Outlook, 7, 198–200.

Johnson, D.E. (1961). The significance of nursing care. American Journal of Nursing, 61(11), 63–66.

Johnson, D.E. (1968, April). One conceptual model of nursing. Paper presented at Vanderbilt University, Nashville, TN.

Johnson, D.E. (1974). Development of theory: A requisite for nursing as a primary health profession. Nursing Research, 23, 372–377.

Johnson, D.E. (1978a, December). Behavioral System Model for Nursing. Paper presented at the Second Annual Nurse Educator Conference, New York. (Cassette recording)

Johnson, D.E. (1978b). State of the art of theory development in nursing. In Theory development: What, why, how? (pp. 1–10). New York: National League for Nursing.

Johnson, D.E. (1980). The Behavioral System Model for Nursing. In J.P. Riehl & C. Roy, Conceptual models for nursing practice (2nd ed., pp. 207–216). New York: Appleton-Century-Crofts.

Kagan, J. (1964). Acquisition and significance of sex typing and sex role identity. In M. Hoffman & L. Hoffman (Eds.), Review of child development research, Vol. 1, pp. 137–167. New York: Russell Sage Foundation.

Kizpolski, P.A. (1985). Family adaptation during the midstage of cancer. Unpublished master's thesis, University of California, San Francisco.

Kosten, P.A. (1977). Professional nurses' assessment of practice in psychiatric settings. Dissertation Abstracts International, 38, 140B.

Lovejoy, N.C. (1982). An empirical verification of the Johnson Behavioral System Model for Nursing. Dissertation Abstracts International, 42, 2781B.

Lovejoy, N.C. (1983). The leukemic child's perceptions of family behaviors. Oncology Nursing Forum, 10(4), 20–25.

Lovejoy, N.C. (1985). Needs of vigil and nonvigil visitors in cancer research units. In Fourth Cancer Nursing Research Conference Proceedings (pp. 142–164). Honolulu: American Cancer Society.

Lorenz, K. (1966). On aggression. New York: Harcourt.

Majesky, S.J., Brester, M.H., & Nishio, K.T. (1978). Development of a research tool: Patient indicators of nursing care. Nursing Research, 27, 365–371.

Marriner, A. (1986). Nursing theorists and their work. St. Louis: CV Mosby.

McCauley, K., Choromanski, J.D., Wallinger, C., & Liu, K. (1984). Current management of ventricular tachycardia: Symposium from the Hospital of the University of Pennsylvania. Learning to live with controlled ventricular tachycardia: Utilizing the Johnson model. Heart and Lung, 13, 633–638.

Mead, M. (1953). Cultural patterns and technical change. World Federation for Mental Health: UNESCO.

Meleis, A.I. (1985). Theoretical nursing. Development and progress. Philadelphia: JB Lippincott.

Miller, M. (1987). Uncertainty, coping, social support and family functioning in parents of children with myelomeningocele. Unpublished master's thesis. University of California, San Francisco.

Moran, T.A. (1986). The effect of an AIDS diagnosis on the sexual practices of homosexual men. Unpublished master's thesis, University of California, San Francisco.

Nishimoto, P.W. (1987). Perceived impact of prostate surgery on sexual stability. Dissertation Abstracts International, 47, 4114B.

Rapoport, A. (1968). Forward. In W. Buckley (Ed.), Modern systems research for the behavioral scientist (pp. xiii–xxii). Chicago: Aldine.

Rawls, A.C. (1980). Evaluation of the Johnson Behavioral Model in clinical practice. Image, 12, 13–16.

Resnik, H.L.P. (1972). Sexual behaviors. Boston: Little, Brown and Co.

Riehl, J.P., & Roy, C. (1980). Conceptual models for nursing practice (2nd ed.). New York: Appleton-Century-Crofts.

Robson, K.K. (1967). Patterns and determinants of maternal attachment. Journal of Pediatrics, 77, 976–985.

Rogers, C.G. (1973). Conceptual models as guides to clinical nursing specialization. Journal of Nursing Education, 12(4), 2–6.

Rosenthal, M. (1967). The generalization of dependency from mother to a stranger. Journal of Child Psychology and Psychiatry, 8, 177–183.

Sears, R., Maccoby, E., & Levin, H. (1954). Patterns of child rearing. White Plains, NY: Row, Peterson.

Silva, M.C., & Sorrell, J.M. (1987, April). Doctoral dissertation research based on five nursing models: A select bibliography. January 1952 through February 1987. (Available from M.C. Silva, George Mason University School of Nursing, Fairfax, VA.)

Skolny, M.S., & Riehl, J.P. (1974). Hope: Solving patient and family problems by using a theoretical framework. In J.P. Riehl & C. Roy, Conceptual models for nursing practice (pp. 206–218). New York: Appleton-Century-Crofts.

Small, B. (1980). Nursing visually impaired children with Johnson's model as a conceptual framework. In J.P. Riehl & C. Roy, Conceptual models for nursing practice (2nd ed., pp. 264–273). New York: Appleton-Century-Crofts.

Stamler, C., & Palmer, J.O. (1971). Dependency and repetitive visits to the nurse's office in elementary school children. Nursing Research, 20, 254–255.

Stevens, B.J. (1984). Nursing theory. Analysis, application, evaluation (2nd ed.). Boston: Little, Brown and Co.

Swain, M.A., & Steckel, S.B. (1981). Influencing adherence among hypertensives. Research in Nursing and Health, 4, 213–222.

Walike, B., Jordan, H.A., & Stellar, E. (1969). Studies of eating behavior. Nursing Research, 18, 108–113.

Walker, L.O., & Nicholson, R. (1980). Criteria for evaluating nursing process models. Nurse Educator, 5(5), 8–9.

Wilkie, D. (1985). Pain intensity and observed behaviors of adult cancer patients experiencing pain. Unpublished master's thesis, University of California, San Francisco.

ANNOTATED BIBLIOGRAPHY

Aggleton, P., & Chalmers, H. (1984). Defining the terms. Nursing Times, 80(36), 24–28. This article includes a description of Johnson's conceptual model. The subsystems, set, action, choice, drive, and methods of nursing intervention are addressed and several brief examples of application are given.

Auger, J.R. (1976). Behavioral systems and nursing. Englewood Cliffs, NJ: Prentice-Hall. The Johnson model is presented and examined as it relates to general system theory. Each behavioral subsystem is discussed and potential regulators of behavioral systems are explicated. Behavioral subsystems are interpreted within physiological and psychosocial contexts. The concept of environment is elaborated more fully than in Johnson's original work. An assessment tool and two examples of its application in clinical situations are presented.

Auger, J.A., & Dee, V. (1983). A patient classification system based on the Behavioral System Model of Nursing: Part 1. Journal of Nursing Administration 13(4), 38–43.

Dee V., & Auger, J.A. (1983). A patient classification system based on the Behavioral System Model of Nursing: Part 2. Journal of Nursing Administration, 13(5), 18–23. Part 1 of the two-part article presents the development of a patient classification system using Johnson's Behavioral System Model. The classification system was developed for use at the Neuropsychiatric Institute at the University of California, Los Angeles. The authors contend, however, that the classification system can be adapted to various clinical settings.

Part 2 describes use of the classification system within an inpatient child psychiatric unit and includes staff education, use of an assessment tool, and use of a care plan based on Johnson's conceptual model.

Broncatello, K.F. (1980). Auger in action: Application of the model. Advances in Nursing Science, 2(2), 13–24.

Auger's interpretation of Johnson's conceptual model is described. The model is applied to patients receiving long-term hemodialysis. Theoretical knowledge of stressors confronting this population was combined with the conceptual model to form the conceptual-theoretical system of nursing knowledge for the application. The author concluded that the model is useful for nursing practice.

Bruce, G.L., Hinds, P., Hudak, J., Mucha, A., Taylor, M.C., & Thompson, C.R. (1980). Implementation of ANA's quality assurance program for clients with end-stage renal disease. Advances in Nursing Science, 2(2), 79–95.

Johnson's conceptual model was used to establish criteria for a quality assurance program for patients with end-stage renal disease. The ingestive, eliminative, and achievement subsystems were used to develop the audit tool, which was helpful in revealing deficiencies in the nursing care of patients.

Conner, S.S., & Watt, J.K. (1986). Dorothy E. Johnson. Behavioral System Model. In A. Marriner, Nursing theorists and their work (pp. 283–296). St. Louis: CV Mosby.

This chapter presents an overview of Johnson's conceptual model and a brief evaluation of the model.

Crawford, G. (1982). The concept of pattern in nursing: Conceptual development and measurement. Advances in Nursing Science 5(1), 1–6.

The concept of pattern is discussed from the perspectives of different conceptual models of nursing. Johnson's concept of set is identified as a view of pattern as repetition and regularity. Grubbs's extension of Johnson's model is noted, and her concept of perseverative set is mentioned.

Damus, K. (1974). An application of the Johnson Behavioral System Model for Nursing practice. In J.P. Riehl & C. Roy. Conceptual models for nursing practice (pp. 218–233). New York: Appleton-Century-Crofts. Reprinted in J.P. Riehl & C. Roy, (1980). Conceptual models for nursing practice (2nd ed., pp. 274–289). New York: Appleton-Century-Crofts.

An application of Johnson's conceptual model to a study of the nursing care of 10 post-transfusion hepatitis patients is presented. Reasons for selection of the patient population are discussed, along with a detailed account of methodology and limitations of the study. A relationship between behavioral disequilibrium and physiologic disequilibrium was found. The results indicated that Johnson's model is useful when applied to nursing practice and research.

Derdiarian, A.K. (1981). Nursing conceptual frameworks: Implications for education, practice, and research. In D.L. Vredevoe, A.K. Derdiarian, L.P. Sarna, M. Eriel, & J.C. Shipacoff, Concepts of oncology nursing (pp. 369–385). Englewood Cliffs, NJ: Prentice-Hall.

This chapter presents a brief overview of how a conceptual model can benefit nursing education, practice, and research. The application of Johnson's conceptual model to cancer nursing education, nursing service, and nursing research is discussed.

Derdiarian, A.K. (1983). An instrument for theory and research using the Behavioral Systems Model for Nursing: The cancer patient (Part I). Nursing Research, 32, 196–201.

Derdiarian, A.K., & Forsythe, A.B. (1983). An instrument for theory and research using the Behavioral Systems Model for Nursing: The cancer patient (Part II). Nursing Research, 32, 260–266.

Part I of this two-part article describes the use of Johnson's conceptual model to develop an instrument to measure perceived behavioral changes of the cancer patient. Theoretical development of the instrument and derivation of categories of behavioral change are discussed.

Part II describes data collection and procedures used to determine validity of the instrument.

Derdiarian, A.K. (1984). An investigation of the variables and boundaries of cancer nursing: A pioneering approach using Johnson's Behavioral Systems Model for Nursing. In Proceedings of the 3rd International Conference on Cancer Nursing (pp. 96–102). Melbourne, Australia: The Cancer Institute/Peter MacCallum Hospital and the Royal Melbourne Hospital.

The paper describes the development of an instrument derived from Johnson's conceptual model. The instrument was designed to determine whether changes due to illness can be measured by the subsystems of Johnson's model and whether the subsystems are inclusive of the problems experienced by cancer patients.

Glennin, C.G. (1974). Formulation of standards of nursing practice using a nursing model. In J.P. Riehl & C. Roy, Conceptual models for nursing practice (pp. 234–246). New York: Appleton-Century-Crofts. Reprinted in J.P. Riehl & C. Roy (1980). Conceptual models for nursing practice (2nd ed., pp. 290–301). New York: Appleton-Century-Crofts.

The nursing process component of Johnson's model is used as the basis for development of standards for nursing practice. Data-gathering, assessment, diagnostic, prescriptive, implementation, and evaluation standards are presented. The conclusion is that the model served as a useful framework for development of these standards.

Grubbs, J. (1974). An interpretation of the Johnson Behavioral System Model. In J.P. Riehl & C. Roy, Conceptual models for nursing practice (pp. 160–197). New York: Appleton-Century-Crofts. Reprinted in J.P. Riehl & C. Roy, (1980). Conceptual models for nursing practice (2nd ed. pp. 217–254). New York: Appleton-Century-Crofts.

The author presents her interpretation of Johnson's conceptual model. Basic assumptions and concepts of the model are discussed. Subsystems, goals, sustenal imperatives (functional requirements), and regulating and control mechanisms are presented in detail. The restorative subsystem is added to Johnson's list of behavioral subsystems. A nursing process compatible with Johnson's model is outlined and a first-level assessment tool is included.

Harris, R.B. (1986). Introduction of a conceptual nursing model into a fundamental baccalaureate course. Journal of Nursing Education, 25, 66–69.

This article presents a detailed discussion of the use of a modified version of Johnson's conceptual model in a beginning course in the baccalaureate program at the University of California, Los Angeles.

Holaday, B.J. (1974). Achievement behavior in chronically ill children. Nursing Research, 23, 25–30.

Johnson's conceptual model is used to guide a study of the comparison of achievement behavior in chronically ill and well children. Social learning theory and attribution theory serve as the theoretical framework for the study. Findings indicated the presence of disequilibrium in achievement behavior of chronically ill children.

Holaday, B.J. (1974). Implementing the Johnson model for nursing practice. In J.P. Riehl & C. Roy, Conceptual models for nursing practice (pp. 197–206). New York: Appleton-Century-Crofts. Reprinted in J.P. Riehl & C. Roy. (1980). Conceptual models for nursing practice (2nd ed., pp. 255–263). New York: Appleton-Century-Crofts.

The author facilitates readers' use of Johnson's conceptual model by defining its central terms. An assessment tool based on the model and theories of psychosocial and cognitive development is presented. Examples of assessment are described, with delineation of specific nursing interventions for a child with meningomyelocele, a child scheduled for surgery, and a child with a disturbance of the eliminative system. The author concluded that the model is beneficial for nursing practice.

Holaday, B.J. (1981). The Johnson Behavioral System Model for Nursing and the pursuit of quality health care. In G.E. Lasker (Ed.), Applied systems and cybernetics. Vol. 4. Systems research in health care, biocybernetics and ecology (pp. 1723–1728). New York: Pergamon.

The major elements of Johnson's conceptual model are reviewed. The model's potential for improving nursing care and thereby enhancing the quality of health care is identified, including its potential for providing more efficient judgments than the traditional nursing history approach, its potential for identification of relevant and significant behavioral responses to illness, and its ability to lend substantive insights, which are unavailable from the perspective of other conceptual models of nursing.

Holaday, B.J. (1981). Maternal response to their chronically ill infants' attachment behavior of crying. Nursing Research, 30, 343–348.

Johnson's model and attachment theory are combined to form the conceptual-theoretical framework for the study. The concept of behavioral set is examined in regard to the response patterns of mothers to their chronically ill children. Differences in the crying behavior of well and ill children are described. Study findings are compared with data from an investigation of maternal responses to well children.

Holaday, B. (1982). Maternal conceptual set development: Identifying patterns of maternal response to chronically ill infant crying. Maternal-Child Nursing Journal, 11, 47–69.

This article describes use of Johnson's conceptual model to guide a study of interaction between mothers and chronically ill infants. Six mother-infant pairs were studied by use of observation and interviews.

Holaday, B. (1987). Patterns of interaction between mothers and their chronically ill infants. Maternal-Child Nursing Journal, 16, 29–45.

This article describes a second check on the structural component of conceptual set used by mothers when responding to the crying of their chronically ill infants.

Johnson, D.E. (1959). A philosophy of nursing. Nursing Outlook, 7, 198–200.

The author clarifies the definition and nature of nursing. A discussion of nursing as a science and an art is included. The author puts forth her belief that there is a common core of nursing knowledge used by all nurses, regardless of their area of specialization.

Johnson, D.E. (1959). The nature of a science of nursing. Nursing Outlook, 7, 291–294.

The concept of nursing science is discussed. Attempts to clarify the goal of nursing and types of knowledge required by the profession are presented. Examples of nursing research questions are identified.

Johnson, D.E. (1961). The significance of nursing care. American Journal of Nursing, 61(11), 63–66.

Nursing care is defined and the need for a guiding framework is presented. The idea of promotion or maintenance of equilibrium as the primary role of nursing is set forth. Tension is offered as a possible indicator of disequilibrium. Potential nursing interventions related to reduction of stressors are presented.

Johnson, D.E. (1974). Development of theory: A requisite for nursing as a primary health profession. Nursing Research, 23, 372–377.

The need for nursing theory is discussed. The current status of nursing science is presented along with a discussion of other professions as sciences. Alternative directions for theory development are identified. Conceptual models of nursing are discussed and three criteria—social congruence, social significance, and social utility—are offered as appropriate standards for evaluation of nursing models.

Johnson, D.E. (1978). State of the art of theory development in nursing. In Theory development: What, why, how? (pp. 1–10). New York: National League for Nursing.

Johnson reports on the state of nursing research, concluding that little research basic to nursing is being conducted. The testing of conceptual models in practice is discussed. The possibility of agreement on one model for nursing is explored. The distinction is made between a theory of nursing and theory in nursing. The development of theory that identifies and explains patient care problems is advocated.

Johnson, D.E. (1980). The Behavioral System Model for Nursing. In J.P. Riehl & C. Roy, Conceptual models for nursing practice (2nd ed., pp. 207–216). New York: Appleton-Century-Crofts.

Johnson's behavioral system model is presented in detail, including assumptions upon which the concept of man as a behavioral system is based, subsystems of the behavioral system, structural elements of each subsystem, and functional requirements. The social utility of the model for education, practice, and research is discussed. This is the only publication of the Behavioral System Model by Johnson.

Lobo, M.L. (1985). Dorothy E. Johnson. In Nursing Theories Conference Group Nursing theories. The base for professional practice (2nd ed., pp. 195–213). Englewood Cliffs, NJ: Prentice-Hall.
This chapter presents a review of the content of Johnson's conceptual model and a brief evaluation of the model.

Lovejoy, N. (1983). The leukemic child's perception of family behaviors. Oncology Nursing Forum, 10(4), 20–25.
This article presents a report of a study designed to develop a projective assessment tool of family functioning based on Johnson's conceptual model. The tool was tested on 25 leukemic children. Study results indicated that the tool was helpful in assessing behavioral functioning.

Lovejoy, N. (1985). Needs of vigil and nonvigil visitors in cancer research units. In Fourth Cancer Nursing Research Conference Proceedings (pp. 142–164). Honolulu: American Cancer Society.
This report describes the needs of visitors of patients in cancer research units. Comparisons are made of the needs of visitors who maintain vigils at the patient's bedside and those who do not. Johnson's conceptual model was used as a base for the study.

Loveland-Cherry C., & Wilkerson, S.A. (1983). Dorothy Johnson's Behavioral System Model. In J.J. Fitzpatrick & A.L. Whall, Conceptual models of nursing. Analysis and application (pp. 117–135). Bowie, MD: Brady.
This chapter presents a review and evaluation of Johnson's conceptual model.

Majesky, S.J., Brester, M.H., & Nishio, K. T. (1978). Development of a research tool: Patient indicators of nursing care. Nursing Research, 27, 365–371.
Johnson's conceptual model is used to guide development of a tool designed to measure quality of nursing care. The concept of tensions causing disruptions in man's environment was operationalized as the presence of complications in the sample subjects. The tool is discussed and presented in the article. Study findings indicated the tool is an effective measure of the quality of nursing care.

McCauley, K., Choromanski, J.D., Wallinger, C., & Liu, K. (1984). Current management of ventricular tachycardia: Symposium from the Hospital of the University of Pennsylvania. Learning to live with controlled ventricular tachycardia: Utilizing the Johnson model. Heart and Lung, 13, 633–638.
This article describes how Johnson's behavioral subsystems were used to make assessments and plan nursing strategies for the patient suffering from ventricular tachycardia. A family-centered approach was used and examples are given for each subsystem.

Rawls, A.C. (1980). Evaluation of the Johnson Behavioral Model in clinical practice. Image, 12, 13–16.
Johnson's conceptual model is reviewed and applied to the nursing care of a patient with amputation of the left hand. First and second level assessments are reported. Theoretical knowledge of body image was combined with the Johnson model to form a guide for nursing practice. Advantages and disadvantages of the model in this clinical situation are discussed.

Rogers, C.G. (1973). Conceptual models as guides to clinical nursing specialization. Journal of Nursing Education, 12(4), 2–6.
Johnson's conceptual model is used to outline areas for clinical specialization in nursing. The behavioral subsystems are identified as appropriate specialty areas in nursing. The model is regarded as an effective way to avoid fragmentation of clinical specialties.

Skolny, M.A., & Riehl, J.P. (1974). Solving patient and family problems by using a theoretical framework. In J.P. Riehl & C. Roy, Conceptual models for nursing practice (pp. 206–218). New York: Appleton-Century-Crofts.
The concepts of hope and loss are discussed. Hope is operationalized in terms of Johnson's model. A case study of the nursing care of the mother of a dying brain-injured 22-year-old man is presented. The nursing care plan is included.

Small, B. (1980). Nursing visually impaired children with Johnson's model as a conceptual framework. In J.P. Riehl & C. Roy, Conceptual models for nursing practice (2nd ed., pp. 264–273). New York: Appleton-Century-Crofts.

Johnson's conceptual model guided a study of the body image and spatial awareness of visually impaired children. The theoretical framework for the study was
based on knowledge of visual handicaps. All behavioral subsystems are included
in plans of nursing care for visually impaired children and their families. The author concluded that the model is a useful guide to the nursing care of this patient
population.

Stamler, C., & Palmer, J.O. (1971). Dependency and repetitive visits to the nurse's office
in elementary school children. Nursing Research, 20, 254–255.

This article presents a report of a study derived from the dependency subsystem of
Johnson's conceptual model that was designed to test the hypothesis that the child
who frequently visits the nurse (the repeater) will have a higher dependency score
than the non-repeater. Results yielded support for the hypothesis and indicated
that girl repeaters had higher dependency scores than boy repeaters.

4

King's Interacting Systems Framework_____

This chapter presents an analysis and evaluation of Imogene M. King's conceptual framework of nursing and a discussion of the theory that she derived from the framework. In accordance with King's preference, the term conceptual framework, rather than conceptual model, with be used throughout this chapter.

King's work now can be separated into a conceptual framework and a theory. Her conceptual framework encompasses three interacting systems, and her theory focuses on goal attainment. Inasmuch as the purpose of this book is to analyze and evaluate conceptual models, emphasis will be placed on King's conceptual framework. Her pioneering work in theory generation and testing, however, is described in the evaluation section of this chapter.

The key terms of King's conceptual framework are listed below. These terms were taken primarily from King's (1981) book, *A theory for nursing. Systems, concepts, process.*

KEY TERMS_____

Personal System	Personal System—*Cont.*
Perception	Space
Self	Learning
Growth and Development	Interpersonal System
Body Image	Interaction
Time	Communication

Interpersonal System—*Cont.*	Environment—*Cont.*
Transaction	External
Role	Health
Stress	Dynamic Life Experiences
Coping	Ability to Function in Social
Social System	Roles
Organization	Goal of Nursing
Authority	Help Individuals Maintain
Power	Their Health So They Can
Status	Function in Their Roles
Decision Making	Nursing Process
Control	Action, Reaction, Interaction,
Environment	Transaction
Internal	Theory of Goal Attainment

ANALYSIS OF KING'S INTERACTING SYSTEMS FRAMEWORK

This section presents an analysis of King's conceptual framework. The analysis relies heavily on King's (1981) book, *A theory for nursing. Systems, concepts, process,* and attempts to deal only with that portion of King's work that is a conceptual model.

Development of the Model

King presented the foundation for her conceptual framework in the 1964 publication, "Nursing theory—Problems and prospect." She then identified several concepts of the framework in her 1968 article, "A conceptual frame of reference for nursing." In 1971, the entire conceptual framework was presented in her book, *Toward a theory for nursing.* King described refinements of the framework in her 1978 speech at the Second Annual Nurse Educator Conference. Further refinements were presented in her 1981 book, *A theory for nursing. Systems, concepts, process.* King (personal communication, July 18, 1987) recently stated that her conceptual framework "will not change but will continue to generate theories."

King began to develop her conceptual framework at a time when nursing was striving for status as a science and hence as a legitimate profession. She along with other writers of the 1960s (e.g., Moore, 1968, 1969), maintained that delineation of a theoretical body of knowledge was necessary for the advancement of nursing. Indeed, King voiced her concern that an existing "antitheoretical bias" in nursing had resulted in "nursing theory . . . based on practical techniques—the 'how' rather than the 'why'" (King, 1964, p. 395). She therefore deliberately set out to develop a conceptual frame of reference for nursing as a precursor to theory explicating the "why" of nursing actions. At that time, she offered two major and several minor propositions "not as a theory of nursing but rather another approach in thinking about fundamental concepts in nursing" (King, 1964, p. 401). These propositions are listed below.

> Major proposition: The nursing process is conducted within a social system. The dimensions include:
> 1. The nursing process
> 2. The individuals involved in the nursing process
> 3. The individuals involved in the environment within which the nursing process is activated
> 4. The social organization within which the process takes place
> 5. The community within which the social organization functions
>
> Minor propositions:
> The nursing process will differ, dependent upon the individual nurse and each recipient of nursing service.
> The nursing process will differ relative to all individuals in the environment.
> The nursing process will differ relative to the social organization in which the nursing process takes place.
> The relationships among the dimensions have an effect upon the nursing process.
>
> Major proposition: Nursing includes specific components.
> 1. Nursing judgment
> 2. Nurse action
> 3. Communication
> 4. Evaluation
> 5. Coordination
>
> Minor propositions:
> The nursing judgment will vary relative to each nursing action.
> The effectiveness of nursing action will vary with the extent to which it is communicated to those responsible for its implementation.
> Nursing action is more effectively assured if the goals are communicated and standards of nursing performance have been established.
> Nursing action is based on facts, which may change; thus, nursing judgments and action are evaluated and revised as the situation changes.
> Nursing action is one component of health care; thus health care is effected by the coordination of nursing with health services. (King, 1964, pp. 401–402)

King (1971) later stated that the particular concepts of her framework were formulated in response to several questions emanating from her "personal concern about the changes influencing nursing, a conscious awareness of the knowledge explosion, and a hunch that some of the essential components of nursing have persisted" (p. 19). The questions were:

1. What are some of the social and educational changes in the United States that have influenced changes in nursing?
2. What basic elements are continuous throughout these changes in nursing?
3. What is the scope of the practice of nursing, and in what kind of settings do nurses perform their functions?
4. Are the current goals of nursing similar to those of the past half century?
5. What are the dimensions of practice that have given the field of nursing unifying focus over time?

King (1971) then noted, "These questions established a framework for thinking about nursing today, for reading about nursing in society, for discussing ideas with nurses and other individuals" (p. 19). This led King to exploration of systems analysis and general system theory, and hence to another set of questions. These questions were:

1. What kind of decisions are nurses required to make in the course of their roles and responsibilities?
2. What kind of information is essential for them to make decisions?
3. What are the alternatives in nursing situations?
4. What alternative courses of action do nurses have in making critical decisions about another individual's care, recovery, and health?
5. What skills do nurses now perform and what knowledge is essential for nurses to make decisions about alternatives? (King, 1971, pp. 19–20)

Recently, King (1985a) commented that her perspective of nursing evolved in response to the questions, What is the essence of nursing? and What is the human act? She further commented that she believes the focus of nursing is the human being and human acts.

Elaborating on the origin of her conceptual framework, King (1971) explained, "concepts that consistently appeared in nursing literature, in research findings, in speeches by nurses, and were observable in the world of nursing practice were identified and synthesized into a conceptual framework" (pp. 20–21). This synthesis resulted in selection of four universal ideas—social systems, health, perception, and interpersonal relations. King (1971) maintained that these ideas formed a conceptual framework that "suggests that the essential characteristics of nursing are those properties that have persisted in spite of environmental changes" (p. ix). The four universal ideas then were used as a general frame of reference for identification of the other concepts of the framework.

In addition to delineating the thought processes underlying formation of her conceptual framework, King (1971) identified the following beliefs, upon which selection of the four ideas was based:

- Nurses, in the performance of their roles and responsibilities, assist individuals and groups in society to attain, maintain, and restore health.
- In the process of functioning in social institutions, nurses assist individuals to meet their basic needs at some point in time in the life cycle when they cannot do this for themselves.
- An understanding of basic human needs in the physical, social, emotional, and intellectual realm of the life process from conception to old age, within the context of social systems of the culture in which nurses live and work, is essential and basic content for learning the practice of nursing. (p. 22)

According to King (1981), her conceptual framework and her derived theory are based on the following overall assumption: "The focus of nursing is human beings interacting with their environment leading to a state of health for individuals, which is an ability to function in social roles" (p. 143).

King also identified more specific assumptions upon which her conceptual framework and theory are based.

Assumptions about human beings:
- Individuals are social beings.
- Individuals are sentient beings.
- Individuals are rational beings.
- Individuals are reacting beings.
- Individuals are perceiving beings.
- Individuals are controlling beings.
- Individuals are purposeful beings.
- Individuals are action-oriented beings.
- Individuals are time-oriented beings.

Assumptions about nurse-client interactions:
- Perceptions of nurse and of client influence the interaction process.
- The goals, needs, and values of nurse and client influence the interaction process.
- Individuals have a right to knowledge about themselves.
- Individuals have a right to participate in decisions that influence their life, their health, and community services.
- Health professionals have a responsibility to share information that can help individuals make informed decisions about their health care.
- Individuals have a right to accept or to reject health care.
- The goals of health professionals and of recipients of health care may be incongruent. (King, 1981, pp. 143–144; 1986b, pp. 199–200)

Still another assumption, with its extension to encompass family phenomena, is: "The assumption that individuals (nurse and client) are capable of interacting to set mutual goals and agree on means to achieve the goals has been extended to include mutual goal setting with family members in relation to clients and families" (King, 1986b, p. 200).

King used both inductive and deductive thought processes to formulate her conceptual framework. Explaining her approach, King (1975) commented:

> My personal approach to synthesizing knowledge for nursing was to use data and information available from research in nursing and related fields and from my 25 years in active practice, teaching, and research. . . . A search of the literature in nursing and other behavioral science fields, discussion with colleagues, attendance at numerous conferences, inductive and deductive reasoning, and some critical thinking about the information gathered, led me to formulate my own framework. (pp. 36–37)

Content of the Model: Concepts

Person

King (1981) stated, "human beings are the focus for nursing" (p.13). The primary concerns of nursing are human behavior, social interaction, and social movements (King, 1976). Thus, within the context of the metaparadigm concept of person, King included three dynamic interacting open systems—personal systems (individuals), interpersonal systems (groups), and social systems (society). Each system is described through a set of related concepts. King maintained that knowledge of these concepts is necessary for the nurse's thorough understanding of the systems.

King (1981) characterized individuals, or personal systems, as social beings who are rational and sentient. She conceptualized the individual as a personal system who processes selective inputs from the environment through the senses. Concepts related to the personal system were identified as perception, self, growth and development, body image, time, space, and learning (King, 1986a).

King (1981) defined perception as "a process of organizing, interpreting, and transforming information from sense data and memory. It is a process of human transactions with the environment. It gives meaning to one's experience, represents one's image of reality, and influences one's behavior" (p. 24).

In formulating this definition of perception, King drew upon the work of Bruner and Krech (1968), Gibson (1966), and Klein (1970), among others. The incorporation of the notion of transactions in the definition is based on the work of Ittleson and Cantril (1954).

King (1981) described the personal system as "a unified, complex whole, self who perceives, thinks, desires, imagines, decides, identifies goals and selects means to achieve them" (p. 27). She accepted as her definition of the self that proposed by Jersild (1952):

The self is a composite of thoughts and feelings which constitute a person's awareness of his individual existence, his conception of who and what he is. A person's self is the sum total of all he can call his. The self includes, among other things, a system of ideas, attitudes, values and commitments. The self is a person's total subjective environment. It is a distinctive center of experience and significance. The self constitutes a person's inner world as distinguished from the outer world consisting of all other people and things. The self is the individual as known to the individual. It is that to which we refer when we say "I." (pp. 9–10)

King's (1981) description of growth and development drew from the works of Erikson (1950), Freud (1966), Gesell (1952), Havighurst (1953), and Piaget (1969). She identified the following two characteristics of growth and development:

- Growth and development include cellular, molecular, and behavioral changes in human beings.
- Growth and development are a function of genetic endowment, meaningful and satisfying experiences, and an environment conducive to helping individuals move toward maturity. (pp. 30–31)

The concept of body image was defined by King (1981) as "a person's perceptions of his own body, others' reactions to his appearance, and is a result of others' reactions to self" (p. 33). This definition was derived from the writings of Fisher and Cleveland (1968), Schilder (1951), Shontz (1969), and Wapner and Werner (1965).

King (1981) defined time as "the duration between the occurrence of one event and the occurrence of another event" (p. 44). She noted that the term is used "to give order to events and to determine duration based on perceptions of each person's experiences" (King, 1981, p. 45). This definition was based on the writings of Fraser (1972) and Orme (1969), among others.

Space was defined by King (1981) as "existing in all directions and is the same everywhere. . . . as the physical area called territory and by the behavior of individuals occupying space" (pp. 37–38). She incorporated territory and the related idea of personal space into her discussion, citing the works of Hall (1959), Lyman and Scott (1967), and Sommer (1969).

King (1986a) added learning to the list of concepts related to the personal system in her discussion of use of her conceptual framework as a guide for curriculum development. She did not, however, define or describe this concept.

King (1981) linked all concepts except learning related to the personal system in the following statement:

An individual's perceptions of self, of body image, of time and space influence the way he or she responds to persons, objects, and events in his or her life. As individuals grow and develop through the life span, experiences with changes in structure and function of their bodies over time influence their perceptions of self. (p. 19).

The interpersonal system is composed of "two, three, or more individuals interacting in a given situation" (King, 1976, p. 54). The concepts associated with this system are interaction, communication, transaction, role, stress, and coping (King, 1987).

King (1981) defined interactions as:

> the acts of two or more persons in mutual presence. Interactions can reveal how one person thinks and feels about another person, how each perceives the other and what the other does to him, what his expectations are of the other, and how each reacts to the actions of the other. (p. 85)

According to King (1981), "The process of interactions between two or more individuals represents a sequence of verbal and nonverbal behaviors that are goal directed" (p. 60). Following a social psychological perspective, King (1971, 1981) explained that this process consists of each person's simultaneous perceptions and judgments about the other in the interaction, the taking of some mental actions based on the judgments, and reacting to the other's perceptions. Interaction follows these mental processes, and this is followed in turn by transaction. Moreover,

> In the interactive process, two individuals mutually identify goals and the means to achieve them. When they agree to the means to implement the goals, they move toward transactions. Transactions are defined as goal attainment. (King, 1981, p. 61)

King (1981) pointed out that the perceptions, judgments, actions, and reactions of the individuals cannot be directly observed, but must be inferred from the directly observable interaction. Elaborating, she stated:

> First, the informational component of interactions can be observed as communication. Second, the valuational component of interactions can be observed as transaction because one obviously values a goal, identifies means to achieve it, and takes action to attain it. (p. 62)

King (1981) viewed communication as "the vehicle by which human relations are developed and maintained" (p. 79). She went on to say, "all behavior is communication" (p. 80). This concept encompasses intrapersonal and interpersonal communication, as well as verbal and nonverbal communication. In formulating her view of communication, King drew primarily from works by Cherry (1966), Ruesch and Kees (1972), and Watzlawick, Beavin, and Jackson (1967).

Communication is involved in transactions, which is defined as "a process of interaction in which human beings communicate with environment to achieve goals that are valued. Transactions are goal-directed human behaviors" (King, 1981, p. 82).

In this conceptual framework, the concept of role was derived from the work of Benne and Bennis (1959), Haas (1964), and Parsons (1951). The three elements of role were identified as:

(1) role is a set of behaviors expected when occupying a position in a social system; (2) rules or procedures define rights and obligations in a position in an organization; (3) role is a relationship with one or more individuals interacting in specific situations for a purpose. (King, 1981, p. 93)

King (1981) developed her definition of stress from the writings of Janis (1958), Monat and Lazarus (1977), and Selye (1956). She stated:

Stress is a dynamic state whereby a human being interacts with the environment to maintain balance for growth, development, and performance, which involves an exchange of energy and information between the person and the environment for regulation and control of stressors. (p. 98)

Stress was viewed as negative and positive, as well as constructive and destructive. King (1981) explained that stress is reduced when transactions are made.

Coping, King (1987) maintained, is an essential area of knowledge related to the interpersonal system. However, she did not give a definition or description of this concept.

King (1981) defined a social system as "an organized boundary system of social roles, behaviors, and practices developed to maintain values and the mechanisms to regulate the practices and rules" (p. 115). She also stated, "Social systems describe units of analysis in a society in which individuals form groups to carry on activities of daily living to maintain life and health and, hopefully, happiness" (King, 1976, p. 54). The concepts related to social systems are organization, authority, power, status, decision making, and control (King, 1986a).

The definition of organization was based on the work of DiVincenti (1977) and Katz and Kahn (1966), and is as follows: "An organization is composed of human beings with prescribed roles and positions who use resources to accomplish personal and organizational goals" (King, 1981, p. 119).

King (1981) drew from Katz and Kahn (1966) and Simon (1962), among others, for her definition of authority. She stated:

Authority is a transactional process characterized by active, reciprocal relations in which members' values, background, and perception play a role in defining, validating, and accepting the authority of individuals within an organization. One person influences another, and he recognizes, accepts, and complies with the authority of that person. (p. 124)

The concept of power was defined as "the process whereby one or more persons influence other persons in a situation. Power defines a situation in a way that people will accept what is being done while they may not agree with it" (King, 1981, p. 127). This definition was based on the work of Etzioni (1975), Griffiths (1959), Katz and Kahn (1966), and Zald (1970).

King (1981) defined status as "the position of an individual in a group or a group in relation to other groups in an organization" (p. 129). She drew from Linton's (1963) work to characterize status as described or achieved.

The works of Bross (1953) and Simon (1957) were used to formulate the definition of decision making used in this conceptual framework. This definition is as follows:

> Decision making in organizations is a dynamic and systematic process by which goal-directed choice of perceived alternatives is made and acted upon by individuals or groups to answer a question and attain a goal. (King, 1981, p. 132)

King (1986a) added control to the list of concepts related to the social system in her discussion of the use of her conceptual framework as a guide for curriculum development. She did not, however, provide a definition or description of this concept.

The relationships among the personal, interpersonal, and social systems are illustrated in Figure 4–1. The figure depicts the three systems as "open systems in a dynamic interacting framework" (King, 1981, p. 10).

Environment

King used the terms environment, health care environment, internal environment, and external environment. She linked the latter two terms in the following statement: "The internal environment of human beings transforms energy to enable them to adjust to continuous external environmental changes" (King, 1981, p. 5). She also noted that the person continuously adjusts to stressors in the internal and external environment. It appears, then, that these environments are the source of stressors. No other discussion of environment was provided, nor were any definitions of these terms given.

Health

King (1981) defined health as "dynamic life experiences of a human being, which implies continuous adjustment to stressors in the internal and external environment through optimum use of one's resources to achieve maximum potential for daily living" (p. 5). She also

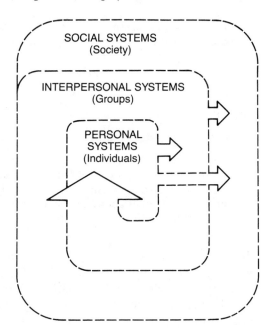

Figure 4–1. A conceptual framework for nursing: dynamic interacting systems. (From King, IM (1971). Toward a theory for nursing. New York: John Wiley & Sons, p. 20, with permission.)

defined health as "an ability to function in social roles" (p. 143). King (1985b) maintained that the idea of health as functional ability is the predominant view of this concept in her conceptual framework.

Although King did not use the term wellness, it may be inferred that her definitions of health refer to wellness. This interpretation is supported by her definition of illness:

Illness is defined as a deviation from normal, that is, an imbalance in a person's biological structure or in his psychological make-up, or a conflict in a person's social relationships. (King, 1981, p. 5)

She went on to say that one kind of illness is disease. Other kinds of illnesses were not identified.

King's discussion of health does not permit an unequivocal interpretation of wellness and illness as a continuum or a dichotomy. The continuum interpretation is supported by the following quotation:

The polarity between health and illness is almost a thing of the past. Individuals are viewing health as a functional state in the life cycle, and illness indicates some interference in the cycle. (King, 1981, p. 5)

Conversely, the following comments support an interpretation of health as a dichotomy:

It is reasonable to assume that the events and situations that prevent illness are not necessarily identical with those factors that promote health. (King, 1981, p. 6)

> As methods of measurement continue to be designed, validated, and used, the current arbitrary distinction between health and illness will be more pronounced. (King, 1981, p. 7)

Nursing

King (1981) stated that nursing is

> perceiving, thinking, relating, judging, and acting vis-a-vis the behavior of individuals who come to a nursing situation. A nursing situation is the immediate environment, spatial and temporal reality, in which nurse and client establish a relationship to cope with health states and adjust to changes in activities of daily living if the situation demands adjustment. (p. 2)

She went on to define nursing as "a process of action, reaction, and interaction whereby nurse and client share information about their perceptions in the nursing situation. Through purposeful communication they identify special goals, problems, or concerns. They explore means to achieve a goal and agree to means to the goal. When clients participate in goal setting with professionals, they interact with nurses to move toward goal attainment in most situations" (p. 2).

The domain of nursing "includes promotion of health, maintenance and restoration of health, care of the sick and injured, and care of the dying" (King, 1981, p. 4). Furthermore, King (1976) viewed nursing as a helping profession that "provides a service to meet a social need" (p. 52). This service extends to the care of individuals and groups who are ill and hospitalized, those who have chronic diseases and require rehabilitation, and those who require guidance for the maintenance of health.

According to King (1976), nurses are key figures in health care delivery. She viewed nurses as "partners with physicians, social workers, and allied health professionals in promoting health, in preventing disease, and in managing patient care. They cooperate with physicians, families, and others to coordinate plans of health care" (p. 52).

The person seeks help from the nurse when he or she cannot perform usual daily activities (Daubenmire & King, 1973). Accordingly, the goal of nursing "is to help individuals maintain their health so they can function in their roles" (King, 1981, pp. 3–4). In particular,

> The goal of nursing is to help individuals and groups attain, maintain, and restore health. If this is not possible, nurses help individuals die with dignity. (King, 1981, p. 13)

Nursing is practiced through the nursing process. Daubenmire and King (1973) defined the nursing process as "a dynamic, ongoing interpersonal process in which the nurse and the patient are viewed as a system with each affecting the behavior of the other and both being affected by factors within the situation" (p. 513).

King (1976) likened the nursing process to all human processes. She commented.

> The nursing act [is] as all other human acts, that is, a sequence of behaviors of interacting persons that occur in the following three phases: recognition of presenting conditions, operations or activities related to the conditions or situations, and motivation to exert some control over the events to achieve goals. (p. 54)

Thus, the process of interaction discussed in relation to the interpersonal system is applicable to the nurse-client situation.

As specified in the definition of nursing, the components of the nursing process were identified as action, reaction, interaction, and transaction. The process follows as sequence that encompasses two people who meet in some situation, perceive each other, make judgments about the other, take some mental action, react to each one's perceptions of the other, interact, and transact, or achieve a goal. King (1981) pointed out that although perception, judgment, action, and reaction cannot be observed, interaction can be observed directly and data about the interaction can be recorded. Transactions also can be observed, in the form of goal attainment measures (King, 1985b).

The nursing process component of King's conceptual framework is more fully specified in her theory of goal attainment. This theory is discussed in detail in the theory generation and testing section of this chapter. Suffice it to say now that the nursing process components of action, reaction, interaction, and transaction are operationalized through the Goal-Oriented Nursing Record (GONR). The components of the GONR are described in the social utility section of this chapter.

Content of the Model: Propositions

The propositions of King's conceptual framework encompass all four metaparadigm concepts. Person and environment are linked in the following statement:

> In open systems, such as human beings interacting with their environments, there is continuous and dynamic communication occurring. (King, 1981, p. 66)

The concepts of person, environment, and nursing are linked in the following quotation:

> The artificial boundaries of nursing are individuals and groups interacting with the environment. Nurses function in their roles in a variety of health care environments. (King, 1981, p. 1)

Person, health, and nursing are linked in this statement:

> As professionals, nurses deal with the behavior of individuals and groups in potentially stressful situations relative to health and illness and help people meet needs that are basic in performing activities of daily living. (King 1976, p. 51)

Finally, all four metaparadigm concepts are linked in the following quotation:

> The focus of nursing is human beings interacting with their environment leading to a state of health for individuals, which is an ability to function in social roles. (King, 1981, p. 143)

Areas of Concern

The major area of concern in King's conceptual framework is the continuing ability of individuals to meet their basic needs so they may function in their socially defined roles. Although King did not identify an explicit source of this problem, it may be inferred to be stressors in the internal and external environment. This interpretation is supported by the following statement:

> Health is defined as dynamic life experiences of a human being, which implies continuous adjustment to stressors in the internal and external environment through optimum use of one's resources to achieve maximum potential for daily living. (King, 1981, p. 5)

EVALUATION OF KING'S INTERACTING SYSTEMS FRAMEWORK

An evaluation of King's conceptual framework is presented below. The evaluation is based on the results of the analysis as well as publications and presentations by others who have used or commented on King's work.

Explication of Assumptions

King presented the assumptions upon which her conceptual framework was based in an explicit manner. Her statement of major and minor propositions constitutes assumptions underlying the content of the conceptual framework. Other assumptions are King's statements about human beings and nurse-client interactions. Taken together, the assumptions provide a clear and concise philosophical base for the concepts of the conceptual framework.

The assumptions indicate that King values the client's participation in his or her nursing care. They also indicate that King values the client's right to accept or reject the care offered by nurses and other health care professionals.

King's discussions of interaction and the nursing process indicate that she values equally the nurse's and the client's perceptions of any given situation. In particular, her definition of nursing as a process indicates that both nurse and client participate in setting goals and determining the means to achieve the goals.

Comprehensiveness of Content

King provided a comprehensive discussion of the metaparadigm concept, person. In fact, her descriptions of the several concepts associated with personal systems, interpersonal systems, and social systems provide more specification of individuals, groups, and society than usually is found in a conceptual model.

In contrast to the comprehensive consideration of the person, King's discussion of environment was vague. She failed to define this concept and to identify the particular parameters of the internal and external components. Further explication of this metaparadigm concept would provide much needed clarification.

Health was clearly defined in this conceptual framework. King did not, however, provide an explicit definition of wellness. As noted in the analysis section above, the definition of health appears to refer to wellness. Furthermore, although King defined illness, she did not relate it to her definition of health. Thus, it must be inferred that if health (wellness) is the ability to perform social roles, then illness must be, at least in part, the inability to perform these roles. This aspect of the conceptual framework requires further clarification, as does the conception of health as a continuum or a dichotomy.

King defined and described nursing in a relatively comprehensive manner. One point, however, requires clarification. King indicated that the "person" of her model encompasses individuals, groups, and society. However, her description of the nursing process is geared only to the individual. Thus, it is not clear whether the process also can be used with groups and society, and if so, how that might be accomplished. King (1983a, 1983b, 1983c) has begun to extend the nursing process to families, although explicit use of the process of action, reaction, interaction, and transaction was not evident in the examples given.

Furthermore, although King carefully delineated the concepts associated with the personal, interpersonal, and social systems and described the nursing process clearly, she failed to link these in any way in the conceptual framework. The linkages are, however, more obvious in the theory of goal attainment.

King's version of the nursing process, with its components of action, reaction, interaction, and transaction, meets most of the criteria proposed for nursing processes by Walker and Nicholson (1980). King (1971) stated emphatically, "Judgments made by nurses will be influenced by their knowledge of the physical, psychological, and social components of man, by their system of values, and by their selected perceptions in the nursing situation" (p. 92). In particular, interaction is based on the actions, perceptions, judgments, and reactions of the nurse and the client engaged in a nursing situation. Furthermore, as will be seen in the forthcoming discussion of the Goal-Oriented Nursing Record (GONR), the data base requires collection of considerable information about the person for the identification of nursing problems. Therefore, it may be concluded that this nursing process incorporates an underlying knowledge base that is used to make judgments regarding nursing problems and goals.

King conceptualized human interaction as a dynamic process. She explained:

> Perception of the nurse leads to judgments and to action by the nurse. Simultaneously, the perception of the patient leads to judgments and then to action by the patient. This is a continuous dynamic process rather than separate incidents in which the action of one person influences the perceptions of the other and vice versa. (King, 1971, p. 92)

Moreover, although King did not conceptualize the nursing process as the typical cycle of assessment, planning, intervention, and evaluation, the GONR suggests a dynamic nursing process. This nursing record involves continual monitoring of changes in status of nursing diagnoses and recording of the client's current health status. The nursing diagnoses and goal list are revised frequently on the basis of outcomes of nursing care.

There is little written documentation of the use of this conceptual framework in various nursing practice settings. However, King maintained that nursing extends to care of persons in acute and chronic care settings as well as in settings appropriate to delivery of care for the maintenance of health. And the use of the conceptual framework as a curriculum guide in basic nursing programs (Daubenmire, 1985; Fromen & Sanderson, 1985) suggests that it is appropriate in many different clinical practice settings.

King's concern for ethical standards for nursing practice is evident in her insistence on consideration of clients' perceptions of a situation and their participation in goal setting. Finally, King deliberately related the concepts of her conceptual framework to scientific findings about human behavior. This is evident in the strong scientific knowledge base used to describe each concept of the personal, interpersonal, and social systems.

The criterion stipulating the linkage of all four metaparadigm concepts was satisfied by the proposition linking person, environment, health, and nursing presented in the analysis section above.

Logical Congruence

World Views

In general, King's conceptual framework reflects an organismic world view. The holistic element of this viewpoint is indicated by the focus of the framework on the personal, interpersonal, and social systems as wholes. The concepts associated with each system in no way represent parts or subsystems. Rather, they may be construed as global characteristics of the system. In fact, no parts or subsystems are ever mentioned.

The organismic view of the world is further reflected by King's view of human beings as active participants in interaction with one another. Despite the use of terms such as action and reaction, the framework does not reflect a reactive, mechanistic view. King (1981) effectively translated these terms to conform with organicism by describing the process of interaction as a dynamic "sequence of verbal and nonverbal behaviors that are goal-directed" in which both individuals participate (p. 60).

Mechanistic elements are introduced into King's conceptual framework by her reference to reactive formulations such as those of Freud and Selye when describing concepts associated with the various systems of her framework. Mechanism also is reflected in King's (1981) comment that health "implies continuous adjustment to stressors in the internal and external environement" (p. 5). Perhaps it was these aspects of the conceptual framework that led Magan (1987) to regard it as mechanistic and consistent with the totality paradigm. But as explained in Chapter 1, Parse's (1987) description of the totality paradigm suggests a bridge between mechanism and organicism. Logical congruence of the conceptual framework certainly could be enhanced by selection of formulations of psychological development and stress that reflect an organismic world view.

King's Interacting Systems Framework reflects a change view of the world. This is attested to by King's (1981) statement that health is a dynamic life experience implying continuous adjustment to environmental stressors. This framework views change as continuous, natural, and desirable, as is documented by King's (1981) comment that normal changes in growth and development take place continuously. Realization of potential is addressed directly by King (1981) in the following statement:

> Growth and development describe the processes that take place in people's lives that help them move from potential capacity for achievement to self-actualization. (p. 31)

Classification of the Model

King has always maintained that her conceptual framework is a derivative of systems thinking, King (personal communication, May 12, 1980) also acknowledged the contributions of social psychology to her thinking, although she stated that she "never followed the symbolic interactionist school." Close examination of the content of the framework, however, revealed that characteristics of both systems and interaction models are represented.

King's conceptual framework addresses most of the characteristics of systems models. System is addressed through the personal, interpersonal, and social systems. King (1981) viewed these as open, dynamic, and interacting. Furthermore, the nurse and the patient were viewed as a system (Daubenmire & King, 1973).

This conceptual framework addresses environment in terms of internal and external components. The parameters of these environments, however, are not identified. King (1981) repeatedly referred to the interaction between open systems and environment and indicated that matter, energy, and information are exchanged. The dynamic quality of this interaction is explained in the following quotation from Daubenmire and King (1973):

> The nursing process is defined as a dynamic, ongoing interpersonal process in which the nurse and the patient are viewed as a system with each affecting the behavior of the other and both being affected by factors within the situation. (p. 513)

Boundary was addressed in King's framework in the following statement: "Open systems, such as man interacting with the environment, exhibit permeable boundaries permitting an exchange of matter, energy, and information" (King, 1981, p. 69). King (1981) also referred to the "artificial boundaries of nursing," which she identified as "individuals and groups interacting with the environment" (p. 1). She did not, however, explain the meaning of "artificial."

King (1981) addressed the systems model characteristic of tension, stress, strain, and conflict in her discussion of stress and transaction as they relate to the interpersonal system. She commented, "When transactions are made, tension or stress is reduced in a situation" (p. 82).

King (1981) did not address the characteristic of equilibrium or steady state in her framework. She did, however, refer to the dynamic life experience of health and stated that this involves continuous adjustment to environmental stressors. This statement suggests that King would accept the idea of a steady state, rather than a fixed point equilibrium.

King dealt with the characteristic of feedback in a dynamic manner in her discussion of nurse-patient interaction. She stated:

> Perception of the nurse leads to judgments and to action by the nurse. Simultaneously, the perception of the patient leads to judgments and then to actions by the patient. This is a continuous dynamic process rather than separate incidents in which the action of one person influences the perceptions of the other and vice versa. (King, 1971, p. 92)

King's conceptual framework also addresses each of the characteristics of interaction models. A major feature of the framework is the social act of human interaction that occurs in the relationship between nurse and patient. In fact, King (1981) indicated that a social psychological perspective is reflected in her description of human interaction.

The characteristic of perception is considered in detail as a major concept of the personal system. Moreover, perception is a central aspect of the process of human interaction described in this conceptual framework.

Communication is a major concept associated with the interpersonal system. According to King (1981), communication is used to establish and maintain relationships between human beings. Furthermore, nurses and patients communicate to establish mutual goals and decide on the means to achieve these goals.

Similarly, role is a concept related to the interpersonal system. The emphasis on role is seen in King's (1981) definition of health as "an ability to function in social roles" (p. 143).

The interaction model characteristic of self-concept is addressed in King's conceptual framework through the concept of self, which is associated with the personal system. In fact, King's use of Jersild's (1952) definition of the self as "a composite of thoughts and feelings which constitute a person's awareness of his individual existence, his conception of who and what he is" (p. 9), coincides with Heiss's (1981) definition of self-concept as "the individual's thoughts and feelings about himself" (p. 83) given in Chapter 1 of this book.

Meleis (1985) classified King's conceptual framework as an interaction model, and Marriner (1986) stated that it reflects a focus on interpersonal relationships. Stevens (1984) commented that King's conceptual framework cannot be categorized in her classification scheme. She explained that King's work "seems to desire interaction for its own sake rather than for the sake of a determined change (intervention), for conservation, for substitution, for sustenance, or for enhancement" (p. 259).

Although King's conceptual framework reflects the characteristics of both systems and interaction models, there is no evidence of logical incompatibility. The development of a framework combining all these characteristics was accomplished by using an open systems view along with a perspective of active participation of individuals in human interactions.

Generation and Testing of Theory

King derived a theory of goal attainment from the interpersonal system component of her conceptual framework, as well as from certain concepts included in the personal system component. The theory encompasses the concepts of self, perception, communication, interaction, transaction, role, stress, growth and development, time, and space. The following constitutive definitions of these concepts were given by King (1986b), who cited pages in her 1981 book:

Self is defined as a personal system synonymous with the terms I, me and person. Self is "a unified, complex whole [person] who perceives, thinks, desires, imagines, decides, identifies goals and selects means to achieve them" (p. 27).

Perception is each person's representation of a subjective world of experience (p. 146).

Communication is a process whereby information is given from one person to another either directly in face-to-face meetings or indirectly through telephone, television, or the written word (p. 146).

Interaction is a process of perception and communication between person and person and person and environment, represented by verbal and nonverbal behaviors that are goal-directed (p. 145).

Transaction is defined as observable behavior of human beings interacting with their environment that leads to goal attainment (p. 147).

Role is a set of behaviors expected of persons occupying a position in a social system; rules that define rights and obligations in a position; a relationship with one or more individuals interacting in specific situations for a purpose (p. 147).

Stress is a dynamic state whereby a human being interacts with the environment to maintain balance for growth, development, and performance (p. 147).

Growth and development are defined as "continuous changes in individuals at the cellular, molecular and behavioral levels of activities" (p. 148).

Time is a sequence of events moving onward to the future; a continuous flow of events in successive order that implies change; a past and a future (p. 148).

Space is that element that "exists in all directions and is the same everywhere. . . . a physical area called territory, and is defined by the behavior of individuals occupying space; such as, gestures, postures, and visible boundaries erected to mark off personal space" (p. 148).

King (1987) stated that she plans to substitute the concept of coping for stress as she refines the theory of goal attainment.

Drawing from Dewey's (1963) theory of knowledge, King (1987) commented that communication is the information component of the

theory of goal attainment, and transaction is the valuational component. Furthermore, King (1986b) considered transaction as "a critical
dependent variable in nurse-client interactions that lead to goal attainment" (p. 202) and has developed an operational definition of the concept. The following operations, or behaviors, comprise the operational
definition of transaction.

1. One member of the nurse-client dyad initiates behavior: asks questions, make statements, reaches out with arms, walks toward the
   other, looks at the other, gives something to the other.
2. The opposite member of the nurse-client dyad responds with behavior: answers questions, makes statements, reaches out with
   arms, walks toward the other, returns a look, gives or accepts
   something from the other.
3. Disturbance (or problem) is noted in the dyadic situation if a state
   or condition is identified.
4. Some goal is mutually agreed upon by both members of dyad; the
   goal may be implicit in behavior that is observed or verbalized, and
   each member shows or states agreement.
5. Exploration of means to achieve goals is iniated by one member of
   the dyad, or one member exhibits behavior that moves toward a
   goal.
6. The other member agrees to the means to achieve goal, and both
   move toward goal.
7. Transactions are made and the goal is attained. (King, 1981, pp.
   150–151; 1986b, p. 202)

Although King has never identified health as a concept in the theory, she views health as an outcome variable. She explained, "The
outcome is a state of health for individuals. A state of health is an ability to function in social roles" (King, 1986b, p. 200). Health is constitutively defined as "dynamic life experiences of a human being,
which implies continuous adjustment to stressors in the internal and
external environment through optimum use of one's resources to
achieve maximum potential for daily living" (King, 1981, p. 5; 1986b,
p. 200).

King (1985b, 1986b) has developed a criterion-referenced instrument for assessment of physical and behavioral functional abilities,
goal setting with clients and families, and measurement of goal attainment. The instrument has predictive and content validity and is reliable.

The theory of goal attainment proposes that

nurse and client interactions are characterized by verbal and nonverbal
communication, in which information is exchanged and interpreted;
by transactions, in which values, needs, and wants of each member of
the dyad are shared; by perceptions of nurse and client and the situation; by self in role of client and self in role of nurse; and by stressors

influencing each person and the situation in time and space. (King, 1981, p. 144)

King has continually refined the statements that link the concepts of the theory of goal attainment. The most recently available list of specific propositions is as follows:

1. If perceptual accuracy is present in nurse-client interactions, transactions will occur.
2. If nurse and client make transactions, goals will be attained.
3. If goals are attained, effective nursing care will occur.
4. If transactions are made in nurse-client interactions, growth and development will be enhanced for both.
5. If nurses with special knowledge and skills communicate appropriate information to clients, mutual goal setting will occur.
6. When mutual goals have been identified, means have been explored, and nurse and client agree on means to achieve goals, transactions will be made and goals achieved.
7. If role expectations and role performance as perceived by nurse and client are congruent, transactions will occur.
8. If role conflict is experienced by nurse, client, or both, stress in nurse-client interactions will occur.
9. Accurate perception of time and space dimensions in nurse-client interactions leads to transactions.
10. Knowledge of one's concept of self will help bring about a helping relationship with clients. (King, 1986b, p. 203)

King (1986b) derived the following hypotheses from the theory propositions:

1. Functional abilities will be greater in patients who participate in mutual goal setting than in those who do not participate.
2. Goal attainment will be greater in patients who participate in mutual goal setting than in patients who do not participate.
3. There is a positive relationship between functional abilities and goal attainment.
4. Mutual goal setting will increase functional abilities in performance of activities of daily living.
5. Mutual goal setting will increase the morale of elderly patients.
6. Mutual goal setting decreases stress in planning and implementing decisions about goals to be attained.
7. Mutual goal setting increases transactions, which increases goal attainment, which leads to effective nursing care.
8. Goal attainment in nursing situations leads to growth and development in nurse and client.
9. Transactions increase nurses' and patients' self-awareness in goal attainment.
10. Accurate perceptions of time-space relations in nurse-client interactions increase transactions and goal attainment.
11. Goal attainment decreases stress and anxiety.

12. Goal attainment increases patients' learning and coping abilities in nursing situations. (King, 1986b, p. 206)

The theory of goal attainment was developed to describe the nature of the nurse-client encounter. This middle-range theory is broad in scope but does have certain boundaries. King (1981) delineated the interior and exterior boundaries of the theory as follows:

Interior Boundaries
1. Nurse and client do not know each other.
2. Nurse is licensed to practice professional nursing.
3. Client is in need of the services provided by the nurse.
4. Nurse and client are in a reciprocal relationship in that the nurse has special knowledge and skills to communicate appropriate information to help client set goals; client has information about self and perceptions of problems or concerns that when communicated to nurse will help in mutual goal setting.

Exterior Boundaries
1. Interactions are in a two-person group.
2. Interactions are limited to licensed professional nurse and to client in need of nursing care.
3. Interactions are taking place in natural environments. (p. 150)

King (1987) identified another boundary of the theory when she noted that the client's locus of control must be taken into account because it is difficult to set mutual goals with a client who has an external locus of control.

Research designed to test the theory of goal attainment is being conducted by King and others. The findings from King's (1981) descriptive study provided initial support for the theory and facilitated development of a classification system to analyze nurse-patient interactions that lead to transactions and goal attainment. Other studies currently are being conducted by King and her colleagues as well as by several graduate students (King, 1986b). Research based on King's conceptual framework is discussed in the section on social utility.

Social Considerations

Social Congruence

The social congruence of this conceptual framework and the theory of goal attainment is based, in part, on the fact that King (1975) deliberately constructed the framework from "recurring ideas or . . . concepts that were undergoing verification through systematic investigation" (p. 37). Thus, the conceptual-theoretical system of knowledge emphasizes nursing care based on valid scientific findings and enduring traditions deemed acceptable by society.

Moreover, with its emphasis on mutual goal setting, this conceptual-theoretical knowledge system is especially appropriate for those health care consumers who wish to participate actively in their nursing care. Those members of society who do not subscribe to such an approach to nursing care would have to be helped to see its value. This is especially so when caring for clients with external locus of control. In fact, this conceptual framework may not be appropriate for such clients.

Furthermore, Meleis (1985) pointed out that although the emphasis on mutual goal setting is congruent with values espoused by western societies, including the United States, it may not be appropriate for patients in some cultures. She commented,

> Many other societies that consider patients helpless, that espouse the sick role as abandonment of social roles and responsibilities, and that support the rights of patients to be sheltered from prognosis and health care goals (such as some middle-eastern cultures) would consider this theory culturally limited. Patients in these societies prefer to relinquish all decisions and goal setting to the expertise of the health care professionals. (p. 238)

Meleis's comments indicate that the patient's cultural background certainly should be considered prior to using King's conceptual-theoretical knowledge system.

Social Significance

Systematic empirical evidence is not yet available to support the contention that use of King's conceptual framework and theory leads to improvements in individuals' health status. However, her focus on helping individuals to function in their social roles should lead to such improvements. Furthermore, the emphasis on mutual goal setting and determination of means to achieve goals might enhance clients' willingness to adhere to the prescribed nursing regimen. In fact, the findings of the descriptive study conducted by King (1981) indicated that goals were attained when both nurse and patient explored the situation, shared information, mutually set goals, explored means to resolve the problem and achieve the goal, and moved forward to implement the plan of care.

Social Utility

Documentation of the utility of King's conceptual framework and her theory of goal attainment is beginning to appear in the literature, and much work that should provide additional documentation is in progress. The examples given here, as well as the annotated bibliography at the end of this chapter, support the social utility of King's work.

The concepts of King's conceptual framework have begun to provide guidelines for research. Some rules for research are evident. King (1986b) identified transaction as "a critical dependent variable in nurse-client interactions that lead to goal attainment" (p. 202) and health, or the ability to function in social roles, as "an outcome variable" (p. 200) in her theory of goal attainment. King's criterion-referenced instrument was designed especially for research that will test the theory of goal attainment. Byers (1985) indicated that the theory of goal attainment leads to both qualitative and quantitative research. She described experimental designs that are consistent with the theory and identified three approaches to measuring goal attainment. One approach is to view goal attainment as a dichotomy—the goal is attained or not attained. Another approach is to use King's criterion-referenced instrument, which yields ordinal scores. Still another approach is to adapt the technique of goal attainment scaling developed in psychology.

Moreover, King's (1968, 1971) typology of variables that could generate research hypotheses identifies phenomena that could be studied within the context of her conceptual framework. One set of variables could serve as predictors of nurse behaviors. These include the nurse's education and experience, which could be used to predict effectiveness of nursing care. Another set of variables influences the whole complex of behaviors entering into the nursing process, such as patient perceptions and expectations as well as the structure of the clinical agency. Still another set focuses on situational behaviors related to nurse-patient interaction, including communication and interpersonal relationships, among others. A final set of variables encompasses criteria of effectiveness of nursing care, such as the patient's performance of activities of daily living and knowledge about health maintenance. King's (1981) descriptive study and planned future research that will test the goal attainment theory are discussed in the section on generation and testing of theory. The hypotheses recently formulated by King (1986b), which also are presented in the section on theory generation and testing, identify phenomena for research with even greater specificity.

Research based on King's conceptual framework and theory includes a descriptive study designed to identify the elements of transactions (King, 1981), Brower's (1981) study of nurses' attitudes toward older persons, and Rosendahl and Ross's (1982) study of the effect of attending behavior on mental status measurements. King (1986b) outlined planned future studies designed to test hypotheses derived from the theory of goal attainment and indicated that other studies are being conducted. A mark of the growing body of research focused on King's work is the research conference, held in February 1988 at the University of South Florida College of Nursing, that was devoted exclusively to presentation of studies that tested the goal attainment theory.

King (1968) stated that her framework provides a useful approach for nursing practice. Rules for practice are not explicit, but some can be extracted from the content of the conceptual framework and theory. Nursing practice clearly is directed toward helping people function in their social roles. Legitimate recipients of nursing care are patients who can actively participate in decisions that influence their care as well as patients who have family members with whom nurses can make transactions until the patients can participate (King, 1986b). The nursing process is clearly and explicitly identified as a process of action, reaction, interaction, and transaction and is implemented through the Goal-Oriented Nursing Record (GONR). Behaviors required for transactions are specified clearly and precisely in the operational definition of this concept given in the theory generating and testing section of this chapter.

King (1981) adapted Weed's (1969) Problem-Oriented Medical Record to develop the GONR. This nursing record represents an information system that encompasses collection of data, generation of a list of nursing diagnoses and a goal list, development of a plan of nursing care, and documentation of progress. Furthermore, although King included use of the SOAP format in her 1981 presentation of the GONR, she has since indicated that this format "is not logical" (King, 1985b). Furthermore, she has stated that nursing diagnoses taken from the North American Nursing Diagnosis Association list have replaced the problem list of Weed's format (King, 1985a, 1987). The components of the GONR are summarized in Table 4–1.

King (1981) presented an example of use of the GONR for a 60-year-old man who had had a cerebral vascular accident. She also presented an example of use of the GONR in the care of patients with end-stage renal disease (King, 1984a) and has indicated that she is developing an example of its use in oncology nursing (King, 1987). Furthermore, she explained how the GONR can be used when caring for families (King, 1983a, 1983b, 1983c). Moreover, Gonot (1983) presented a brief example of use of the GONR in a psychiatric/mental health setting. Gonot (1986) also derived a theoretical model of family therapy from King's conceptual framework, her theory of goal attainment, and her views of the family.

King (1986b) described the use of her theory of goal attainment by a graduate student who was caring for a comatose patient. Because the patient could not communicate verbally, mutual goals were set with the patient's husband. The student, however, communicated verbally with the patient and observed and recorded her nonverbal responses. The student ascertained that goals set with the husband were attained after the patient regained consciousness and returned to her home.

King (1986b) also described use of the goal attainment theory by a clinical specialist who was working with a 43-year-old man who had had coronary artery bypass surgery. Moreover, King (1984b) discussed the application of her conceptual framework and theory in community health nursing.

Barger (1985) presented several examples of care of patients in a psychiatric setting, including a suicidal patient and a patient who was hallucinating. She noted the value of King's nursing process in helping the nurse focus on the patient's perceptions as well as his or her own perceptions of the situation. In addition, Smith and Alligood (1985) discussed the use of King's conceptual framework to guide nursing care of a couple expecting their first child.

TABLE 4–1.   Components of the Goal-Oriented Nursing Record

  I. Data base
    A. Composed of all information gathered about a person on entry into the health care system
       1. Nursing history and health assessment
       2. Physician history and physical examination
       3. Results of laboratory tests and x-ray examinations
       4. Information from sources such as family and social workers
    B. Classification of client
       1. According to severity of illness
       2. According to ability to perform activities of daily living
 II. Nursing diagnosis
    A. List of nursing diagnoses
    B. Purposes
       1. Provides a consistent approach that may be used by many nurses to implement a plan of nursing care
       2. Serves as a guide for continuous assessment of signs and symptoms of a disturbance or interference in client's ability to function in usual roles
       3. Serves as a guide to plan for the client's immediate nursing care
       4. Provides an approach for coordination of nursing diagnoses with medical and allied professionals' problem lists
III. Goal list
    A. List of nursing goals
    B. Purposes
       1. Provides a consistent and systematic approach to help individuals move toward a healthy state
       2. Serves as a guide to nurses in monitoring the disturbances and interferences in clients and to be alert for any new client information
       3. Provides a means for nurses and clients to interact, to share information, to set mutual goals, to explore means and agree on means to achieve goals
       4. Provides for continuity of care
       5. Serves to focus attention on clients' participation in decisions about their care
       6. Provides for growth and learning for both nurse and client through the interaction required to set goals

TABLE 4–1. *Continued*

IV. Plan
    A. Plan is based on assessment and nursing diagnoses
    B. Means agreed upon to resolve the problem reflected in each nursing diagnosis and attain goals
    C. May include client education as an integral component
V. Progress notes
    A. Narrative notes
        1. Concise summary of client's progress
        2. Written when flow sheets indicate changes in the client
    B. Flow sheets
        1. Used to record routine information
        2. Used for continuous or repetitive recording of specific information
        3. Used to record daily routine care
        4. Used to record cumulative data
    C. Final summary or discharge notes
        1. Discussion of each nursing diagnosis
        2. Statement of each goal
        3. Statement regarding attainment of goal
        4. Identification of future goals

Adapted from King, I.M. (1981). A theory for nursing. Systems, concepts, process. New York: John Wiley & Sons, pp. 164–176; and from King, I.M. (1985a, May). Panel discussion with theorists. Nurse Theorist Conference, Pittsburgh, PA. (Cassette recording)

King's conceptual framework has documented utility for nursing education. Daubenmire (1985) presented some rules for nursing education, stating that the conceptual framework leads to a focus on the dynamic interaction of the nurse-client dyad. Given this focus, emphasis is placed on nursing student behavior as well as client behavior. She also indicated that the conceptual framework acts as the decision base for what is and is not taught and for the sequence of courses in a curriculum. King's (1986a) recent book on curriculum development presents a clear and detailed description of how her work can be used to develop baccalaureate and associate degree nursing education programs. King stated that the concepts related to the personal, interpersonal, and social systems serve as content for nursing courses. She explained that

> in my conceptual framework, the concepts are the specific content to be learned and this represents theoretical knowledge if one develops each concept. This theoretical knowledge is used by students when teachers plan learning experiences for them in concrete nursing situations. (p. 81)

King's conceptual framework has been used as a guide for curriculum design in a few schools of nursing. The Ohio State University School of Nursing in Columbus has used the conceptual framework as a guide for the baccalaureate curriculum since 1972. Components of that curriculum were described by Daubenmire and King (1973), King (1984b), Daubenmire (1985), and Daubenmire and Malone (1986). The master's program at Loyola University of Chicago School of Nursing also has used King's conceptual framework (King, personal communication, February 23, 1982). Furthermore, Olivet Nazarene College in Kankakee, Illinois (Asay & Ossler, 1984) and a hospital based school of nursing in Winnipeg, Manitoba, Canada have used the conceptual framework as a curriculum guide (Fromen & Sanderson, 1985).

Brown and Lee (1980) proposed a model for continuing nursing education based on King's conceptual framework. They presented the following rationale for using King's framework as the foundation for the continuing education model:

> The concepts—social systems, health, perception, and interpersonal relationships—are relevant in every nursing situation; the interacting levels of operation—individuals, groups, and society—depict a reciprocal relationship between human behaviour and the environment; and the triad of elements—continuing nursing education, nursing practice, and nursing research—are interrelated in the nursing profession (p. 473).

King has begun to demonstrate the utility of her conceptual framework for nursing administration, although rules for administration have not yet been formulated. King (in press) discussed use of the theory of goal attainment in nursing administration. Elberson (in press) described use of King's conceptual framework in nursing administration. Furthermore, the Goal-Oriented Nursing Record (GONR) system is being implemented in several nursing service areas (King, personal communication, July 18, 1987). King (1981) claimed that use of the GONR would facilitate nursing audits. Such a measure of quality of nursing care would operationalize Chance's (1982) proposal concerning the use of nursing models for establishing standards of professional accountability. Given the focus of the theory of goal attainment on process (action, reaction, interaction) and outcome (transaction or goal attainment regarding functional ability), quality assurance programs based on King's work certainly could be developed.

Contributions to Nursing Knowledge

King's Interacting Systems Framework and her theory of goal attainment represent substantial contributions to nursing knowledge. The concepts and propositions of the framework, together with the content related to each concept of the personal, interpersonal, and social systems, form the beginning of conceptual-theoretical systems of nursing knowledge needed for various nursing activities. Furthermore, the theory of goal attainment is a major contribution to the body of distinctive nursing theory. The fact that this theory has been tested empirically and has received initial support is especially significant. However, additional tests of the theory of goal attainment are needed. Furthermore, the credibility of the conceptual framework requires investigation by means of empirical studies designed to test theories that provide further specification of its concepts and propositions.

The emphasis on client participation in the conceptual framework and theory, including mutual goal setting and exploration of means to achieve goals, should be attractive to the many nurses who are consumer advocates. Some authors have maintained that this emphasis imposes a limitation on use of the conceptual framework and theory in situations where clients cannot participate, such as infants and patients who are comatose or irrational (Austin & Champion, 1983; Stevens, 1984). In contrast, the evidence given in the section on social utility indicates that the framework and theory can be used with individuals who cannot interact verbally. However, as noted in the section on social congruence, the conceptual framework may not be appropriate for use with clients who have external locus of control.

The many concepts comprising King's conceptual model make up an extensive vocabulary. However, the concepts and their definitions were taken from well-known works. Thus, mastery of the vocabulary should not pose a major problem for potential users of the model.

King (cited in Ackerman, et al., 1986) summarized the contributions of her work by noting that her approach to nursing is the only one that "has provided a theory that deals with choices, alternatives, participation of all individuals in decision making and specifically deals with outcomes of nursing care" (p. 241).

REFERENCES

Ackerman, M.L., Brink, S.A., Jones, C.G., Moody, S.L., Perlich, G.L., & Prusinski, B.B. (1986). Imogene King. Theory of goal attainment. In A. Marriner, Nursing theorists and their work (pp. 231–245). St. Louis: CV Mosby.

Asay, M.K., & Ossler, C.C. (Eds.) (1984). Conceptual models of nursing. Applications in community health nursing. Proceedings of the Eighth Annual Community Health Nursing Conference. Chapel Hill, NC: Department of Public Health Nursing, School of Public Health, University of North Carolina.

Austin, J.K., & Champion, V.L. (1983). King's theory for nursing: Explication and evaluation. In P.L. Chinn (Ed.), Advances in nursing theory development (pp. 47–61). Rockville, MD: Aspen.

Barger, D.F. (1985, September). King's interaction model as practiced in an inpatient psychiatric setting. Paper presented at program on Conceptual Models of Nursing and their Application, Veterans Administration Medical Center, Coatesville, PA.

Benne, R.D., & Bennis, W.G. (1959). The role of the professional nurse. American Journal of Nursing, 59, 380–383.

Bross, I. (1953). Design for decision. New York: Macmillan.

Brower, H.T. (1981). Social organization and nurses' attitudes toward older persons. Journal of Gerontological Nursing, 7, 293–298.

Brown, S.T., & Lee, B.T. (1980). Imogene King's conceptual framework: A proposed model for continuing nursing education. Journal of Advanced Nursing, 5, 467–473.

Bruner, J.S., & Krech, W. (Eds.). (1968). Perception and personality. New York: Greenwood Press.

Byers, P. (1985, August). Application of Imogene King's framework. Paper presented at conference on Nursing Theory in Action, Edmonton, Alberta, Canada. (Cassette recording)

Chance, K.S. (1982). Nursing models: A requisite for professional accountability. Advances in Nursing Science 4(2), 57–65.

Cherry, C. (1966). On human communication. Cambridge, MA: MIT Press.

Daubenmire, M.J. (1985, August). Application of Imogene King's framework. Paper presented at conference on Nursing Theory in Action, Edmonton, Alberta, Canada. (Cassette recording)

Daubenmire, M.J., & King, I.M. (1973). Nursing process models: A systems approach. Nursing Outlook, 21, 512–517.

Daubenmire, M.J., & Malone, J. (1986, April). Strategies for teaching nursing models. King's model. Paper presented at Sigma Theta Tau conference on Nursing Knowledge: Improving Education Through Theory, Cleveland, OH.

Dewey, J. (1963). Experience and education. New York: Collier Books.

DiVincenti, M. (1977). Administering nursing service (2nd ed.). Boston: Little, Brown & Co.

Elberson, K. (in press). Applying King's model to nursing administration. In B. Henry, M. DiVincenti, C. Arndt, & A. Marriner (Eds.). Dimensions of nursing administration. Theory, research, education, and practice. Boston: Blackwell Scientific Publications.

Erikson, E. (1950). Childhood and society. New York: Norton.

Etzioni, A.A. (1975). Comparative analysis of complex organizations (rev. ed.). New York: The Free Press.

Fisher, S., & Cleveland, S. (1968). Body image and personality. New York: Dover.

Fraser, J.T. (Ed.). (1972). The voices of time. New York: George Braziller.

Freud, S. (1966). Introductory lectures on psychoanalysis (J. Strachey, Ed. and trans.) New York: Norton.

Fromen, D., & Sanderson, H. (1985, August). Application of Imogene King's framework. Paper presented at conference on Nursing Theory in Action, Edmonton, Alberta, Canada. (Cassette recording.)

Gesell, A. (1952). Infant development. New York: Harper.

Gibson, J. (1966). The senses considered as perceptual systems. Boston: Houghton Mifflin.

Gonot, P.J. (1983). Imogene M. King: A theory for nursing. In J.J. Fitzpatrick & A.L. Whall, Conceptual models of nursing: Analysis and application (pp. 221–243). Bowie, MD: Brady.

Gonot, P.W. (1986). Family therapy as derived from King's conceptual model. In A.L. Whall, Family therapy theory for nursing. Four approaches (pp. 33–48). Norwalk, CT: Appleton-Century-Crofts.

Griffiths, D. (1959). Administrative theory. Englewood Cliffs, NJ: Prentice-Hall.

Haas, J.E. (1964). Role conception and group consensus: A study of disharmony in hospital work groups. Columbus, OH: Ohio State University College of Commerce and Administration, Bureau of Business Research, 1964.

Hall, E. (1959). The silent language. Greenwich, CT: Fawcett.

Havighurst, R. (1953). Human development and education. New York: McKay.

Heiss, J. (1981). The social psychology of interaction. Englewood Cliffs, NJ: Prentice-Hall.

Ittleson, W., & Cantril, H. (1954). Perception: A transactional approach. Garden City, NY: Doubleday & Co.

Janis, I. (1958). Psychological stress. New York: John Wiley & Sons.

Jersild, A.T. (1952). In search of self. New York: Columbia University Teachers College Press.

Katz, D., & Kahn, R.L. (1966). The social psychology of organizations. New York: John Wiley & Sons.

King, I.M. (1964). Nursing theory—problems and prospect. Nursing Science, 2, 394–403.

King, I.M. (1968). A conceptual frame of reference for nursing. Nursing Research, 17, 27–31.

King, I.M. (1971). Toward a theory of nursing. General concepts of human behavior. New York: John Wiley & Sons.

King, I.M. (1975). A process for developing concepts for nursing through research. In P.J. Verhonick (Ed.), Nursing research I (pp. 25–43). Boston, Little, Brown & Co.

King, I.M. (1976). The health care system: Nursing intervention subsystem. In H. Werley, A Zuzich, M. Zajkowski, & A.D. Zagornik (Eds.), Health research: The systems approach (pp. 51–60). New York: Springer.

King, I.M. (1978, December). King's conceptual model of nursing. Paper presented at Second Annual Nurse Educator Conference, New York. (Cassette recording)

King, I.M. (1981). A theory for nursing. Systems, concepts, process. New York: John Wiley & Sons.

King, I.M. (1983a). King's theory of nursing. In I.W. Clements & F.B. Roberts, Family health. A theoretical approach to nursing care (pp. 177–188). New York: John Wiley & Sons.

King, I.M. (1983b). The family coping with a medical illness. Analysis and application of King's theory of goal attainment. In I.W. Clements & F.B. Roberts, Family health. A theoretical approach to nursing care (pp. 383–385). New York: John Wiley & Sons.

King, I.M. (1983c). The family with an elderly member. Analysis and application of King's theory of goal attainment. In I.W. Clements & F.B. Roberts, Family health. A theoretical approach to nursing care (pp. 341–345). New York: John Wiley & Sons.

King, I.M. (1984a). A theory for nursing. King's conceptual model applied in community health nursing. In M.K. Asay & C.C. Ossler (Eds.), Conceptual models of nursing. Applications in community health nursing. Proceedings of the Eighth Annual Community Health Nursing Conference (pp. 13–34). Chapel Hill, NC: Department of Public Health Nursing, School of Public Health, University of North Carolina.

King, I.M. (1984b). Effectiveness of nursing care: Use of a goal oriented nursing record in end stage renal disease. American Association of Nephrology Nurses and Technicians Journal, 11(2), 11–17, 60.

King, I.M. (1985a, May). Panel discussion with theorists. Nurse Theorist Conference, Pittsburgh, PA. (Cassette recording)

King, I.M. (1985b, August). Imogene King. Paper presented at conference on Nursing Theory in Action, Edmonton, Alberta, Canada. (Cassette recording)

King, I.M. (1986a). Curriculum and instruction in nursing. Norwalk, CT: Appleton-Century-Crofts.

King, I.M. (1986b). King's theory of goal attainment. In P. Winstead-Fry (Ed.), Case studies in nursing theory (pp. 197–213). New York: National League for Nursing.

King, I.M. (1987, May). King's theory. Paper presented at Nurse Theorist Conference, Pittsburgh, PA. (Cassette recording)

King, I.M. (in press). Theories and hypotheses for nursing administration. In B. Henry, M. DiVincenti, C. Arndt, & A. Marriner (Eds.), Dimensions of nursing administration. Theory, research, education, and practice. Boston: Blackwell Scientific Publications.

Klein, G. (1970). Perception, motivation and personality. New York: Knopf.

Linton, R. (1963). The study of man. New York: Appleton-Century-Crofts.

Lyman, S., & Scott, M. (1967). Territoriality: A neglected sociological dimension. Social Problems, 15, 236–249.

Magan, S.J. (1987). A critique of King's theory. In R. R. Parse, Nursing science. Major paradigms, theories, and critiques (pp. 115–133). Philadelphia: WB Saunders.

Marriner, A. (1986). Nursing theorists and their work. St. Louis: CV Mosby.

Meleis, A.I. (1985). Theoretical nursing. Development and progress. Philadelphia: JB Lippincott.

Monet, A., & Lazarus, R.S. (Eds.). (1977). Stress and coping. New York: Columbia University Press.

Moore, M.A. (1968). Nursing: A scientific discipline? Nursing Forum, 7, 340–348.

Moore, M.A. (1969). The professional practice of nursing: The knowledge and how it is used. Nursing Forum, 8, 361–373.

Orme, J.E. (1969). Time, experience and behavior. New York: American Elsevier.

Parse, R.R. (1987). Nursing science. Major paradigms, theories, and critiques. Philadelphia: WB Saunders.

Parsons, T. (1951). The social system. Glencoe, IL: The Free Press.

Piaget, J. (1969). The mechanisms of perception. New York: Basic Books.

Rosendahl, P.B., & Ross, V. (1982). Does your behavior affect your patient's response? Journal of Gerontological Nursing, 8, 572–575.

Ruesch, J., & Kees, W. (1972). Nonverbal communication. Los Angeles: University of California Press.

Schilder, P. (1951). The image and appearance of the human body. New York: International Universities Press.

Selye, H. (1956). The stress of life. New York: McGraw-Hill.

Shontz, F. (1969). Perceptual and cognitive aspects of body experience. New York: Academic Press.

Simon, H.A. (1957). Administrative behavior (2nd ed.). New York: Macmillan.

Simon, Y.R. (1962). A general theory of authority. South Bend, IN: University of Notre Dame Press.

Smith, D.P., & Alligood, M.R. (1985, October). Matching nursing models to clinical practice: King. Paper presented at Sigma Theta Tau conference on Nursing Knowledge: Improving Practice Through Theory, Atlanta, GA.

Sommer, R. (1969). Personal space. Englewood Cliffs, NJ: Prentice-Hall.

Stevens, B.J. (1984). Nursing theory. Analysis, application, evaluation (2nd ed.). Boston: Little, Brown & Co.

Walker, L.O., & Nicholson, R. (1980). Criteria for evaluating nursing process models. Nurse Educator, 5(5), 8–9.

Wapner, S., & Werner, H. (Eds.). (1965). The body percept. New York: Random House.

Watzlawick, P. Beavin, J.H., & Jackson, D.D. (1967). Pragmatics of human communication. New York: Norton.

Weed, L.L. (1969). Medical records, medical education, and patient care. Cleveland: Case Western Reserve University Press.

Zald, M.N. (Ed.). (1970). Power in organization. Nashville, TN: Vanderbilt University Press.

ANNOTATED BIBLIOGRAPHY

Ackerman, M.L., Brink, S.A., Jones, C.G., Moody, S.L., Perlich, G.L., & Prusinski, B.B. (1986). Imogene King. Theory of goal attainment. In A. Marriner, Nursing theorists and their work (pp. 231–245). St. Louis: CV Mosby.
This book chapter presents an overview of King's theory of goal attainment.

Austin, J.K., & Champion, V.L. (1983). King's theory for nursing: Explication and evaluation. In P.L. Chinn (Ed.), Advances in nursing theory development (pp. 49–61). Rockville, MD: Aspen.
This book chapter presents an overview of King's theory of goal attainment. The evaluation includes diagrams of the propositions of the theory.

Brower, H.T. (1981). Social organization and nurses' attitudes toward older persons. Journal of Gerontological Nursing, 7, 293–298.
This article presents the report of a study that tested the hypothesis that nurses' attitudes toward older persons are dependent upon the type of institution in which they work. Study findings revealed that nurses employed in visiting nurse home health agencies and nurses employed in hospitals had more favorable attitudes toward the aged than nurses employed in private home health agencies. Interaction theory served as the theoretical framework of the study, and King's concept of social systems was incorporated into the theoretical framework.

Brown, S.T., & Lee, B.T. (1980). Imogene King's conceptual framework: A proposed model for continuing nursing education. Journal of Advanced Nursing, 5, 467–473.
King's conceptual framework is used as the basis for development of a continuing education model. Concepts addressed by King are discussed, followed by a presen-

tation of the continuing education model. The proposed model is analyzed for utility and found to be a helpful guide for development of continuing education programs.

Buchanan, B.F. (1987). Conceptual models: An assessment framework. Journal of Nursing Administration, 17(10), 22–26.
King's conceptual framework is analyzed using the framework developed by the author of this article.

Daubenmire, M.J., & King, I.M. (1973). Nursing process models: A systems approach. Nursing Outlook, 21, 512–517.
King's conceptual framework is discussed and integrated with the nursing process as a framework for undergraduate curriculum development. A methodology is presented for student learning of the nursing process. Specific skills to be mastered in each phase of the methodology are identified.

Elberson, K. (in press). Applying King's model to nursing administration. In B. Henry, M. DiVincenti, C. Arndt, & A. Marriner (Eds.), Dimensions of nursing administration. Theory, research, education, and practice. Boston: Blackwell Scientific Publications.
Discussion of the use of King's work in administration of nursing services is discussed in this book chapter.

Fitzpatrick, J.J., Whall, A.L., Johnston, R.L., & Floyd, J.A. (1982). Nursing models and their psychiatric mental health applications. Bowie, MD: Brady, 1982.
This book presents a brief analysis of King's conceptual framework, among others. Reformulated theoretical approaches, consistent with King's conceptual framework, in individual psychotherapy and family therapy are discussed.

George, J.B. (1980). Imogene M. King. In Nursing Theories Conference Group, Nursing theories. The base for professional nursing practice (pp. 184–198). Englewood Cliffs, NJ: Prentice-Hall.

George, J.B. (1985). Imogene M. King. In Nursing Theories Conference Group, Nursing theories. The base for professional nursing practice (2nd ed., pp. 235–257). Englewood Cliffs, NJ: Prentice-Hall.
An overview of King's conceptual framework is presented. Definitions of major concepts and a comparison of the conceptual framework to the nursing process are included. Criticisms of the conceptual framework are offered. The 1980 chapter is based on King's 1971 book and the 1985 chapter is based on King's 1981 book.

Gonot, P.J. (1983). Imogene M. King: A theory for nursing. In J.J. Fitzpatrick & A.L. Whall, Conceptual models of nursing: Analysis and application (pp. 221–243). Bowie, MD: Brady.
This book chapter presents an analysis and brief evaluation of King's conceptual framework.

Gonot, P.W. (1986). Family therapy as derived from King's conceptual model. In A.L. Whall, Family therapy theory for nursing. Four approaches (pp. 33–48). Norwalk, CT: Appleton-Century-Crofts.
The author presents a theoretical model for family therapy that was deduced from King's conceptual framework and theory of goal attainment.

King, I.M. (1964). Nursing theory—problems and prospect. Nursing Science, 2, 394–403.
The development of nursing theory is discussed. The need for a unifying framework for nursing knowledge is supported. Major and minor propositions regarding nursing and the nursing process are presented. These are proposed to be a guide for conceptualization of relevant concepts in nursing.

King, I.M. (1968). A conceptual frame of reference for nursing. Nursing Research, 17, 27–31.
Major concepts of King's conceptual framework are defined. The utility of the conceptual framework for nursing practice, research, and education is explored.

King, I.M. (1971). Toward a theory of nursing. General concepts of human behavior. New York: John Wiley & Sons.
This book presents King's conceptual framework in its entirety. Four main con-

cepts relevant to nursing—social systems, health, perception, and interpersonal relationships—are discussed. The importance of the framework for nursing is outlined.

King, I.M. (1975). A process for developing concepts for nursing through research. In P.J. Verhonick (Ed.), Nursing research I (pp. 25–43). Boston: Little, Brown & Co.
A general discussion of concepts and the importance of concept development in nursing is presented. The function of concepts in building knowledge is discussed. A method is proposed for the development of nursing concepts. The process is applied to research using King's conceptual framework as the example.

King, I.M. (1976). The health care system: Nursing intervention subsystem. In H. Werley, A. Zuzich, M. Zajkowski, & A.D. Zagornik (Eds.), Health research: The systems approach (pp. 51–60). New York: Springer.
General system theory and its relation to King's conceptual framework are discussed. The importance of system theory in nursing is delineated. Specific examples of nursing situations that reinforce the need for a systems approach are offered.

King, I.M. (1978). JANFORUM: U.S.A.: Loyola University of Chicago School of Nursing. Journal of Advanced Nursing, 3, 390.
This brief commentary focuses on the university as a social system. Awareness of the interrelationships among academic departments of nursing, the nursing profession, and society is emphasized.

King, I.M. (1978). The "why" of theory development. In Theory development: What, why, how? (pp. 11–16). New York: National League for Nursing.
The importance of theory development in nursing is discussed. The functions and usefulness of theory are explored and exemplified by reference to King's conceptual framework. Relationships among science, theory, and research are examined. It is concluded that nursing must develop theory through research in order to advance the profession.

King, I.M. (1981). A theory for nursing. Systems, concepts, process. New York: John Wiley & Sons.
This book presents revisions in King's conceptual framework and a theory of goal attainment derived from the conceptual framework. Concepts associated with personal, interpersonal, and social systems are discussed in detail. The development and testing of the theory of goal attainment is described. The theory is used to develop the Goal-Oriented Nursing Record.

King, I.M. (1983). King's theory of nursing. In I.W. Clements & F.B. Roberts, Family health. A theoretical approach to nursing care (pp. 177–188). New York: John Wiley & Sons.
This chapter presents a brief description of King's conceptual framework as it applies to families. The chapter emphasizes the interaction process and provides an overview of the Goal-Oriented Nursing Record.

King, I.M. (1983). The family coping with a medical illness. Analysis and application of King's theory of goal attainment. In I.W. Clements & F.B. Roberts, Family health. A theoretical approach to nursing care (pp. 383–385). New York: John Wiley & Sons.
Concepts from King's theory of goal attainment are applied to a family in which the father is suffering from leukemia. The communication process and the process of transaction are emphasized.

King, I.M. (1983). The family with an elderly member. Analysis and application of King's theory of goal attainment. In I.W. Clements & F.B. Roberts, Family health. A theoretical approach to nursing care (pp. 341–345). New York: John Wiley & Sons.
This chapter presents a discussion of concepts from King's theory of goal attainment in relation to a family with multiple problems. Suggestions derived from King's theory are given for dealing with the problems.

King, I.M. (1984). A theory for nursing. King's conceptual model applied in community health nursing. In M.K. Asay & C.C. Ossler (Eds.), Conceptual models of nursing. Applications in community health nursing. Proceedings of the Eighth Annual Community Health Nursing Conference (pp. 13–34). Chapel Hill, NC: Department of Public Health Nursing, School of Public Health, University of North Carolina.

King presents an overview of her conceptual framework and a discussion of how her work is used to guide development of curriculum content related to health and public health.

King, I.M. (1984). Effectiveness of nursing care: Use of a goal-oriented nursing record in end stage renal disease. American Association of Nephrology Nurses and Technicians Journal, 11(2), 11–17, 60.

King presents a discussion of the application of concepts of her theory of goal attainment to the care of patients with end stage renal disease. Examples are given of application of her Goal-Oriented Nursing Record.

King, I.M. (1986). Curriculum and instruction in nursing. Norwalk, CT: Appleton-Century-Crofts.

King's book focuses on the process of curriculum development in nursing. One section includes a review of King's work and how it can be used to guide course content.

King, I.M. (1986). King's theory of goal attainment. In P. Winstead-Fry (Ed.), Case studies in nursing theory (pp. 197–213). New York: National League for Nursing.

King discusses her theory of goal attainment. Research designed to test the theory of goal attainment is described and testable hypotheses are presented. A case study of an interaction between a nurse and a comatose patient guided by the theory is presented.

King, I.M. (1987). King's theory of goal attainment. In R.R. Parse, Nursing science. Major paradigms, theories, and critiques (pp. 107–113). Philadelphia: WB Saunders.

This chapter is the publication of King's presentation at the Nurse Theorist Conference held in Pittsburgh, Pennsylvania, in May 1985.

King, I.M. (in press). Theories and hypotheses for nursing administration. In B. Henry, M. DiVincenti, C. Arndt, & A. Marriner (Eds.), Dimensions of nursing administration. Theory, research, education, and practice. Boston: Blackwell Scientific Publications.

King presents a discussion of the use of her work in nursing administration situations.

Magan, S.J. (1987). A critique of King's theory. In R.R. Parse, Nursing science. Major paradigms, theories, and critiques (pp. 115–133). Philadelphia: WB Saunders.

This chapter is the publication of a critique of King's work that was presented at the Nurse Theorist Conference held in Pittsburgh, Pennsylvania, in May 1985.

Rosendahl, P.B., & Ross, V. (1982). Does your behavior affect your patient's response? Journal of Gerontological Nursing, 8, 572–575.

This article presents the report of a study that tested the effect of the investigator's attending behavior (making eye contact and making comments that reflected the topic introduced by the subject) on the subject's mental status. King's process of action, reaction, interaction, and transaction was used as a framework for the study.

Uys, L.R. (1987). Foundational studies in nursing. Journal of Advanced Nursing, 12, 275–280.

This article presents a brief discussion of King's conceptual framework within the context of a language critique, with emphasis on analysis of concepts and the way in which they were used in the framework.

CHAPTER

5

Levine's Conservation Model_____

This chapter presents an analysis and evaluation of Myra E. Levine's Conservation Model. Levine's work clearly fits the definition of a conceptual model of nursing used in this book. Indeed, Levine (1985) regards her work as "a generalization" that subsumes more specific theories.

The key terms of Levine's conceptual model are listed below. These terms were taken from various presentations of elements of the model.

KEY TERMS_____

Holism
Wholeness
Change
Adaptation
Integrity
Internal Environment
    Homeostasis
    Homeorhesis
External Environment
    Operational
    Perceptual
    Conceptual

Levels of Organismic Response
    Fight or Flight
    Inflammatory Response
    Stress
    Perceptual Awareness
Perceptual Systems
    Basic Orienting System
    Visual System
    Auditory System
    Haptic System
    Taste-Smell System
Conservation

Health as Patterns of Adaptive Change	Conservation Principles—*Cont.* Conservation of Personal Integrity
Goal of Nursing Promotion of Wholeness	Conservation of Social Integrity
Trophicognosis	Theory of Therapeutic Intention
Conservation Principles Conservation of Energy Conservation of Structural Integrity	Theory of Redundancy

ANALYSIS OF LEVINE'S CONSERVATION MODEL

This section presents an analysis of Levine's Conservation Model. The analysis draws from several of Levine's publications, including a recent book chapter, "The four conservation principles: Twenty years later" (Levine, in press).

Development of the Model

Levine presented the rudiments of her conceptual model in an article entitled "Adaptation and assessment: A rationale for nursing intervention" (Levine, 1966a). Additional elements of the model were presented in two other articles, "The four conservation principles of nursing" (Levine, 1967), and "The pursuit of wholeness" (Levine, 1969b). A comprehensive discussion of the model was presented in the book, *Introduction to clinical nursing* (1969a). The second edition of this book was published in 1973. Other features of the model were given in Levine's 1971 publication, "Holistic nursing," and her presentations at conferences (Levine, 1978a, 1984a, 1986). The most recent explication of Levine's conceptual model is the book chapter, "The four conservation principles: Twenty years later" (Levine, in press). Levine (personal communication, July 15, 1987) regarded the book chapter as "a significant restatement of the model . . . a natural evolutionary statement of how the basic concepts are related to each other."

Levine (1969a) commented that she developed her model as a starting point for the theory development needed to provide the "why's" of nursing activities. She stated, "The serious study of any discipline requires a theoretical baseline which gives it substance and meaning" (p. ix). Although Levine did not underestimate the importance of technical skills, she pointed out:

> Nursing . . . remain[s] characterized by a rigid dependence on procedures. The "why" is not entirely neglected, but it is often applied after

the fact, as if such justification invested the procedure with a special scientific holiness. Nurses cherish "applied science principles" in an era when nursing is deeply involved in scientific research, but even the lessons learned from nurse researchers are too often ignored. (p. vii)

Levine's attention to the theoretical basis for nurses' actions came at a time when nursing was beginning to recognize the need for substantive knowledge (Newman, 1972). A major feature of her work is the explication of the scientific concepts underlying nursing processes. In fact, she deliberately set out to provide "an intellectual framework for analysis and understanding of the scientific nature of nursing activity" (Levine, 1969a, p. viii).

Levine (1973) developed her model from the basic assumption that nursing intervention is a conservation activity. Drawing from Tillich (1961), she assumed that the "multidimensional unity of life" must be conserved. She also assumed that "the human being responds to the forces in his environment in a singular yet integrated fashion" (p. 6). Elaborating, Levine explained:

> The holistic nature of the human response to the environment provides the rationale for substantive principles of nursing. A principle is a fundamental concept that forms the basis for a chain of reasoning. Formulated on a broad base, it establishes the relationships between apparently otherwise unrelated facts. Nursing principles are fundamental assumptions which provide a unifying structure for understanding a wide variety of nursing activities. Nursing principles are all "conservation" principles. (p. 13)

Levine (personal communication, February 2, 1982) stated that she "did not invent the notion of Conservation—I simply live in a natural world where it is a characteristic of experience." Levine is known for her careful citations of the many scientists from various disciplines whose work has influenced her thinking. She acknowledged the contributions to her thinking made by the work of Kurt Goldstein (1963), Rene Dubos (1961, 1965), James E. Gibson (1966), Erik Erikson (1964), Sir Arthur Sherrington (1906), and Irene Beland (1971), among others. However, she disclaimed, "even with some vigor," any dependence on Maslow and other more recent authors whose work focuses on holism.

Levine's use of knowledge from a variety of disciplines indicates that she used a deductive approach to develop her conceptual model. This approach is further illustrated in the following comment:

> The essential science concepts develop the rationale [for nursing actions], using ideas from all areas of knowledge that contribute to the development of the nursing process in the specific area of the model. (Levine, 1969a, p. viii)

Content of the Model: Concepts

Person

Levine's model focuses on the individual person, described as a holistic being. Citing Erikson's (1964) definition of wholeness, Levine (1969b) stated, "From the moment of birth until the instant of death, every individual cherishes and defends his 'wholeness'" (p. 93). Levine (1973, in press) pointed out that Erikson's definition emphasizes the mutuality between diversified functions and parts within an entirety. This definition also maintains that the boundaries between parts are open and fluid, such that the parts "have a yearning for each other" (Levine, 1978a). Wholeness, according to Levine (in press), "can be used as a starting point of analysis only if it can be converted into manageable parts ... but none of the isolated aspects of 'wholeness' can have meaning outside of the context within which the individual experiences his life. ... Only then are the 'open and fluid' boundaries established."

Levine (1973) further described the person as an organism that is a system of systems. She stated:

> The total life process of the entire organism is dependent upon the inter-relatedness of its component systems. In fact, the organism is a system of systems, and in its wholeness expresses the organization of all the contributing parts. (pp. 8–9)

Levine (1973) characterized the life process as unceasing change that has direction, purpose, and meaning. She explained:

> The organism represents a pattern of orderly, sequential change. Because it is both ordered and sequential, the pattern is a message. So long as the pattern is consistent, it is also understandable. ... The change which supports the well-being of the organism can be predicted, measured, and observed, and therefore is a cogent message. (pp. 9–10)

According to Levine (1973), change occurs through adaptation. She explained, "The organism retains its integrity in both the internal and external environment through its adaptive capability" (p. 10). She went on to say:

> Adaptation is the process of change whereby the individual retains his integrity within the realities of his environments. Adaptation is basic to survival, and it is an expression of the integration of the entire organism. (pp. 10–11)

In fact, Levine (in press) maintained that "the life process is the process of adaptation."

Further discussion of the person and adaptation within the context of Levine's conceptual model requires consideration of the relationship between the person and the environment. The next section focuses on Levine's view of environment. It is followed by consideration of the person-environment relationship and additional discussion of adaptation.

Environment

Levine referred to an internal environment and an external environment. She maintained that "the integrated response of the individual aris[es] from the internal environment" (Levine, 1973, p. 12). Drawing upon the concept of the "milieu interne" that Claude Bernard discussed in the late nineteenth century, Levine (1973) explained:

> Bernard identified the primordial seas, captured within the integument of the human body and providing the organism with a tightly regulated solution of substances essential to its continuing well-being. . . . Man carried the essentials with him, safely packaged inside his skin. But it was apparent to Bernard, and to the army of investigators who followed him, that the internal environment was susceptible to constant change. (p. 7)

Levine (1973) traced the further development of the concept of internal environment to Cannon's (1939) formulation of homeostasis and finally to Waddington's (1968) idea of homeorhesis. Homeostasis, maintained Levine (in press), should not be viewed as a system of balance and quiescence but rather as "a state of energy-sparing which also provides the necessary baselines for a multitude of synchronized physiological and psychological factors." Levine (personal communication, August 13, 1987) explained that homeostasis reflects congruence of the person with the environment.

Homeorhesis, as described by Levine (1973), is

> a stabilized flow rather than a static state. Such a concept emphasizes the fluidity of change within a space-time continuum and more nearly describes the remarkable patterns of adaptation which permit the individual's body to sustain its well-being within the vast changes which encroach upon it from the environment. (p. 7)

The internal environment is subject to continuous change from the challenges of the external environment, which always are a form of energy. The maintenance of the integration of bodily functions in the face of these changes depends on multiple negative feedback loops, which are control mechanisms that result in autoregulation of the internal environment (Levine, 1973). Synchronization of multiple negative feedback loops is accomplished through homeostasis (Levine, in press).

Levine (1973) rejected the "simplistic view of the external environment" as "a kind of stage setting against which the individual plays out his life" (p. 12). Rather, she adopted Bates's (1967) formulation of external environment as perceptual, operational, and conceptual.

The perceptual environment encompasses "that portion of the environment to which the individual responds with his sense organs" (Levine, 1973, p. 12). It includes "those factors which can be recorded on the sensory system—the energies of light, sound, touch, temperature, and chemical change that is smelled or tasted, as well as position sense and balance" (Levine, in press). Levine (1971) pointed out that the person "is not a passive recipient of sensory input. [Rather], he seeks, selects, and tests information from the environment in the context of his definition of himself, and so constantly defends his safety, his identity, and in a larger sense, his purpose" (p. 262).

The operational environment is "that which interacts with living tissue even though the individual does not possess sensory organs which can record the presence of these external factors" (Levine, in press). Thus, the operational environment is not directly perceived by the individual. It encompasses "every unseen, and unheard aspect of the individual's life-space" including all forms of radiation, microorganisms, and odorless and colorless pollutants (Levine, in press). Although this aspect of the environment cannot be apprehended by the senses or anticipated symbolically, it is of vital concern because of its potential danger to the well-being of the individual (Levine, 1971).

The conceptual environment is "the environment of language, ideas, symbols, concepts and invention" (Levine, in press). It encompasses "the exchange of language, the ability to think and to experience emotion . . . value systems, religious beliefs, ethnic and cultural traditions, and the individual psychological patterns that come from life experiences" (Levine, 1973, p. 12). This aspect of the environment takes into account the fact that "human beings are sentient, thinking, future-oriented and past-aware individuals" (Levine, in press).

Levine (1973) mentioned the importance of both internal and external environments and noted that the interface between the two is involved in the person's adaptation. She explained:

> Separate consideration of either the internal or external environments can provide only a partial view of the complex interaction that is taking place between them. It is, in fact, at the interface where the exchange between internal and external environments occurs that the determinants for nursing intervention are found. In this broader sense, all adaptations represent the accommodation that is possible between the internal and external environments. (p. 12)

Person and Environment

Levine (in press) maintained that the person is not separate from the environment. She stated, "The person cannot be described apart from the specific environment in which he is found. The precise environment necessarily completes the 'wholeness' of the individual." Levine further stated:

> The interaction at the interface between individual and environment is an orderly, sometimes predictable, but always a limited process. The consequence of the interaction is invariably the product of the characteristics of the living individual *and* the external factors. . . . The *process* of the interaction is *adaptation*.

Levine (in press) explained that adaptation can be thought of as a way in which the person and the environment become congruent over time or as the "fit" of the person with his or her "predicament of time and space." The fundamental nature of adaptation, then, is "a consequence of an historical progression: the evolution of the species through time, reflecting the sequence of change in the genetic patterns which have recorded the change in the historical environments."

Adaptation is characterized by specificity. Each body system has specific tasks involving biochemical changes in response to environmental challenges. Although the tasks are specific, they are synchronized with each other and serve the individual as a whole. Specificity in biochemistry is dependent upon sequential change that occurs in cascades. The cascade "is characterized by the intermingling of the steps with each other—the precursor is not entirely exhausted when the intermediate forms develop and the final stage is congruent with the steps that precede it" (Levine, in press).

Levine (in press) explained that the cascade of adaptations is characterized by redundancy, which refers to the series of wave-like adaptive responses that are available to the individual when environmental challenges arise. Some redundant systems respond instantly to threatened shifts in physiological parameters. Others are corrective and utilize the time interval provided by the instantaneous response to correct imbalances. Still other redundant systems function by re-establishing a previously failed response.

Redundancy also is seen in four levels of organismic responses to environmental challenges. These responses are considered to be

> coexistent in a single individual, and in fact, often influence each other. They represent, however, an assembly of parts which have indeed entered into fruitful association and organization. Together they permit the person to protect and maintain his integrity as an individual. (Levine, 1969b, p. 98)

Levine (in press) pointed out that because the responses are redundant "they do not follow one another in a prescribed sequence, but are integrated in the individual by his cognitive abilities, the wealth of his previous experience, his ability to define his relationships to the events and the strengths of his adaptive capabilities." She further noted that although some responses can be considered physiological and some, behavioral, "the integration of living processes argues that they are one and the same—not merely parallel and not merely simultaneous—but essential portions of the same activity."

The most primitive level of organismic response is the fight-or-flight mechanism. This adrenocortical-sympathetic reaction is an instantaneous response to a real or imagined threat. The fight-or-flight mechanism swiftly provides a condition of physiological and behavioral readiness for sudden and unexplained environmental challenges.

The second level is the inflammatory-immune response. This response to injury is important for maintenance of structural continuity and promotion of healing. It "assures restoration of physical wholeness and the expectation of complete healing" (Levine, in press).

The third level is the stress response. Drawing from Selye's (1956) description of stress, Levine (in press) stated that this response is "recorded over time and is influenced by the accumulated experience of the individual."

The fourth level of organismic response is perceptual awareness as mediated through the sense organs. This sensory response is concerned with gathering information from the environment and converting it to meaningful experience (Levine, 1969b; in press). Perceptual awareness is described in some detail by Levine (1973). She stated, "The human being is a sentient being, and the ability to interact with the environment seems ineluctably tied to his sensory organs" (p. 446). Drawing upon Gibson's (1966) formulation of perceptual systems to explain the mediation of behavior by sensory organs, Levine (1969b) commented, "Individual identity arises out of information received through these intact and functional perceptual systems" (p. 97).

Gibson (1966) proposed five perceptual systems. The basic orienting system provides a general orientation to the environment and is essential to the function of the other perceptual systems. The anatomical organ of this system is the balancing portion of the inner ear, which responds to changes in gravity, acceleration, and movement. The visual system permits the person to look, and the auditory system permits listening to sounds as well as identifying the direction from which they are coming. The haptic system responds to touch through reception of sensations by the skin, joints, and muscles. The taste-smell system provides information about chemical stimuli and facilitates safe nourishment (Levine, 1969b, 1973). Levine (in press) pointed out that for Gibson, "the individual does not merely 'see'— he *looks*; he does not merely 'hear'—he *listens*. Thus equipped with the ability to select information from the environment, the individual is an active, seeking participant in it—not merely reacting but influencing, changing and creating the parameters of his life."

The product of adaptation, according to Levine (in press), is conservation. She explained:

Survival depends on the adaptive ability to use responses that *cost the least* to the individual in expense of effort and demand on his well-being. That is, of course, the essence of *conservation*. . . . Conservation is clearly the consequence of the multiple, interacting and synchronized negative feedback systems that, acting together provide for the stability of the living organism. . . . [Indeed,] homeostasis might be called conservation.

Health

Levine (1973, 1984a) characterized health and disease as patterns of adaptive change. She commented that adaptation is not an all-or-none process; rather, it is a matter of degree—some adaptations are successful and some are not; some work and some do not. There are, however, no maladaptations. Thus, adaptation has no value attached to it; it just is. Levine (1973) went on to explain:

The measure of effective adaptation is compatibility with life. A poor adaptation may threaten life itself, but at the same time the degree of adaptive potential available to the individual may be sufficient to maintain life at a different level of effectiveness. . . . All the processes of living are processes of adaptation. Survival itself depends upon the quality of the adaptation possible for the individual. (p. 11)

Levine (in press) further explained, "The most successful adaptations are those that best fit the organism in its environment. A 'best fit' is accomplished with the least expenditure of effort, with sufficient protective devices built in so that the goal is achieved in as economic and expeditious a manner as possible."

Levine (1984b) indicated that she does not like the term wellness and prefers the word healthy. It may be inferred from her description of health as "wholeness" (Levine, 1973, p. 11) and as "successful adaptation" (Levine, 1966a, p. 2452) that she used the term health to mean wellness.

It also may be inferred that wellness means social well-being. This inference is supported by the following statement: "One criterion of successful adaptation is the attainment of social well-being, but there is tremendous variation in the degree to which this is achieved" (Levine, 1966a, p. 2452). Indeed, Levine (1984b) has stated that health is socially defined in the sense of "Do I continue to function in a reasonably normal fashion?"

Levine used Wolf's (1961) concept of disease as adaptation to noxious environmental forces for her description of illness. She explained, "disease represents efforts of the individual to protect his integrity" (Levine, 1971, p. 257). Disease also was described as undisciplined and unregulated change, a disruption in the orderly sequential pattern of change that is characteristic of life. This anarchy of pattern may not be successful in supporting life. Levine (1973) maintained that "Such anarchy, in fact, occurs in disease processes and unless the pattern can be restored, the organism will die" (p. 9).

The anarchy of disease processes is a positive feedback mechanism. Levine (1973) noted that positive feedback "results in an increasing rate of function without the regulatory control that restores balance. Thus a 'vicious cycle' is instituted which produces more and more disruption of function" (p. 10).

Levine (1973) pointed out that individuals acknowledge illness through their perceptual systems. She stated:

> Physical well-being is dependent upon an experienced body which is communicating the "right" signals. The constancy of awareness of the internal feeling of the body is the baseline against which well-being is measured. . . . Individuals can acknowledge "illness" only in recognizing an alteration in their perception of internal feelings. (pp. 455–456)

The foregoing description of health indicates that Levine conceptualized this concept as a continuum. This interpretation is supported by the following comment:

> Adaptation . . . is susceptible to an infinite range within the limits of life compatibility. Within that range there are numerous possible degrees of adaptation. Thus, the dynamic processes establishing balance along the continuum are adaptation. (Levine, 1973, p. 11)

Nursing

Levine (1973) described nursing as a human interaction. "It is a discipline rooted in the organic dependency of the individual human being on his relationships with other human beings" (p. 1). She further described nursing as "a subculture, possessing ideas and values which are unique to nurses, even though they mirror the social template which created them" (p. 3).

The goal of nursing, according to Levine (1984a), is the promotion of wholeness for all people, well or sick. She maintained:

> The goal of all nursing care should be to promote wholeness, realizing that for every individual that requires a unique and separate cluster of activities. The individual's integrity—his one-ness, his identify as an individual, his wholeness—is his abiding concern, and it is the nurse's responsibility to assist him to defend and to seek its realization. (Levine, 1971, p. 258)

Levine repeatedly emphasized the importance of deriving nursing processes from scientific knowledge, as well as from the messages given by the patient. This is illustrated in the following quotations:

> Ultimately, decisions for nursing intervention must be based on the unique behavior of the individual patient. It is the nurse's task to bring

a body of scientific principles on which decisions depend into the precise situation which she shares with the patient. (Levine, 1966a, p. 2452)

The integrated response of the individual to any stimulus results in a realignment of his very substance, and in a sense this creates a message which others may learn to understand. Each message, in turn, is the result of observation, selection of relevant data, and assessment of the priorities demanded by such knowledge. . . . Understanding the message and responding to it accurately constitute the substance of nursing science. (Levine, 1967, pp. 46–47)

The nursing process of Levine's conceptual model is conservation. Levine (in press) defined conservation as "keeping together" and stated that conservation—the "keeping together" function—should be the major guideline for all nursing intervention. She emphasized the roles of both nurse and patient in conservation, as illustrated in the following statement:

"To keep together" means to maintain a proper balance between active nursing intervention coupled with patient participation on the one hand and the safe limits of the patient's ability to participate on the other. (Levine, 1973, p. 13)

In fact, Levine (1984b) stated that she regards patients as partners or participants in nursing care. She views the person who is a patient as being temporarily dependent on the nurse. The nurse's goal is to end the dependence, that is, the patient status of the person, as quickly as possible. As part of the patient's environment, the nurse brings to nursing care situations his or her "own cascading repertoire of skill, knowledge, and compassion. It is a shared enterprise and each participant is rewarded" (Levine, in press).

Although Levine did not identify an explicit nursing process, it is possible to extract a format from several of her publications. Levine (1966a) referred to assessment of the patient's nursing requirements, stating "Sensitive observation and the selection of relevant data form the basis for [the nurse's] assessment of [the patient's] nursing requirements" (p. 2452). The elements of assessment are delineated in Levine's discussion of identification of nursing care needs. She called this "trophicognosis," which is defined as "a nursing care judgment arrived at by the scientific method" (Levine, 1966b, p. 57).

Levine (1966b) presented trophicognosis as an alternative to nursing diagnosis. Tracing the development of nursing diagnosis and its legal interpretation, she pointed out that the term always referred to "diagnosis of disease made by a nurse" (p. 55). Then, citing the only dictionary definition of diagnosis, she maintained that it is "incorrect to use the term diagnosis as a synonym for observations, judgments, problems, needs or assessments" (pp. 56–57). In concluding her argument, Levine stated:

> Because the term, nursing diagnosis, is now susceptible of legal inter-
> pretation, and other usages of the term are semantically incorrect, it is
> proposed that a new nursing term be used to describe the scientific ap-
> proach in the determination of nursing care. Such a method of ascrib-
> ing nursing care needs may be called trophicognosis. (p. 57)

The elements of trophicognosis are presented in Table 5–1.
Levine (personal communication, August 13, 1987) stated that she and
her colleagues are developing a taxonomy of trophicognoses.

According to Levine (1973), "nursing intervention must be designed so that it fosters successful adaptation whenever possible" (p.
13). Indeed, "nursing must view the individual so that the 'best fit'
available to him can be sustained" (Levine, in press). Nursing intervention may be therapeutic or supportive. Levine (1973) explained:

> When nursing intervention influences adaptation favorably, or toward
> renewed social well-being, then the nurse is acting in a therapeutic
> sense. When nursing intervention cannot alter the course of the adap-
> tation—when her best efforts can only maintain the status quo or fail
> to halt a downward course—then the nurse is acting in a supportive
> sense. (p. 13)

Nursing intervention is structured according to four conservation
principles, including conservation of energy, conservation of structural integrity, conservation of personal integrity, and conservation of
social integrity. Levine (in press) explained that the conservation of
energy is a natural law "found to hold everywhere in the universe for
all animate and inanimate entities." Energy "is eminently identifiable,
measurable, and manageable." Energy parameters of concern to nurses
include body temperature; pulse, respiratory, and metabolic rates;
blood gases; and blood pressure, among others. Individuals conserve
their energy, but even at perfect rest, energy from life-sustaining activities, such as biochemical changes, is expended. Levine (in press)
commented,

> The conservation of energy is clearly evident in the very sick, whose
> lethargy, withdrawal and self-concern are manifested while, in its wis-
> dom, the body is spending its energy resource on the processes of
> healing.

Conservation of structural integrity focuses on healing. Levine
pointed out that we expect and have confidence in the ability of our
bodies to heal. Healing, according to Levine (in press), "is the defense
of wholeness . . . [and] a consequence of an effective immune
system."

Conservation of personal integrity focuses on the fact that the self
is "more than a physical experience of the whole body—although it is
unquestionably a part of that awareness." This principle emphasizes

TABLE 5–1.   Elements of Trophicognosis

I. Establishing an objective and scientific rationale for nursing care
  A. Basis for implementation of prescribed medical regimen
    1. Knowledge and understanding of the medical diagnosis
    2. Evaluation of the medical history with specific reference to areas influencing the nursing care plan
    3. Knowledge of laboratory and x-ray reports emphasizing factors that influence nursing care
    4. Consultation with physician to share information and clarify nursing care decisions
    5. Knowledge of aspects of prescribed medical regimen (expected and untoward effects) as contribution to the evaluation of the effectiveness of the therapy
  B. Basis for implementation of prescribed paramedical regimen
    1. Knowledge of paramedical diagnoses and prescriptions for care
    2. Clear definition of nurse's role in paramedical prescriptions
  C. Determination of nursing processes demanded by medical treatment
    1. Observation of effects of prescribed medical aspects of patient's care on individual progress
    2. Adaptation of nursing techniques to the unique cluster of needs demonstrated in the individual patient
  D. Basis for implementation of the unique nursing needs of the individual patient
    1. Knowledge and understanding of the principles of nursing science
    2. Provision for gathering a nursing history with specific reference to aspects that will influence the nursing care plan
    3. Accurate recording and transmittal of observations and evaluation of patient's response to nursing processes
    4. Utilization of knowledge gained in consultation with family members or other individuals concerned with the patient including the religious counselor
II. Implementation of nursing care within the structure of administrative policy, availability of equipment, and established standards of nursing care

Levine, M.E. (1966b). Trophicognosis: An alternative to nursing diagnosis. In American Nurses' Association Regional Clinical Conference (Vol. 2, pp. 59–60). New York: American Nurses' Association, with permission.

individuals' perseverance in retaining their identities. "Everyone seeks to defend his identify as a 'self,' in both that hidden, intensely private person that dwells within and in the public faces assumed as individuals move through their relationships with others" (Levine, in press).

Conservation of social integrity emphasizes the fact that "selfhood needs definition beyond the individual . . . [and that] the individual is created by his environment, and in turn creates within it." This principle states that each individual's identity places him or her "in a family, a community, a cultural heritage, a religious belief, a socioeconomic slot, an educational background, a vocational choice" (Levine, in press).

Levine (in press) pointed out that the conservation principles do not operate singly but rather are "joined within the individual as a cascade of life events, churning and changing as the environmental challenge is confronted and resolved in each individual's unique way." Use of the four conservation principles in the nursing process is outlined in Table 5–2.

TABLE 5–2. Levine's Conservation Principles

I. Principle of Conservation of Energy: Nursing intervention is based on the conservation of the individual patient's energy
  A. Relevant scientific considerations
    1. The ability of the human body to perform work is dependent upon its energy balance—the supply of energy-producing nutrients measured against the rate of energy-using activities
    2. The energy required by alterations in physiological function during illness represents an additional demand made on the energy production systems
    3. Fatigue, often experienced with illness, is an empirical measure of the additional energy demand
  B. Nursing intervention
    1. General considerations
      a. Nursing intervention is based on the balancing of energy input with energy output
      b. Assessment of patient's ability to perform necessary activities without producing excessive fatigue
        (1) Vital signs
        (2) Patient's general condition
        (3) Patient's behavior
        (4) Patient's tolerance of nursing activities required by his or her condition
      c. Allowable activity for patient based on his or her energy resources
      d. Interventions designed to provide an adequate deposit of energy resource and regulate expenditure of energy
    2. Examples of specific interventions
      a. Provision for rest
      b. Maintenance of adequate nutrition
II. Principle of Conservation of Structural Integrity: Nursing intervention is based on the conservation of the individual patient's structural integrity
  A. Relevant scientific considerations
    1. Structural change results in a change of function
    2. Pathophysiological processes present a threat to structural integrity
    3. Healing processes restore structural integrity
    4. Surgical procedures are designed to restore structural integrity
    5. Structural integrity is restored when the scar is organized and integrated in the continuity of the part affected
  B. Nursing intervention
    1. General considerations
      a. Limit amount of tissue involvement in infection and disease
      b. Prevent trophicogenic (nurse-induced) disease

TABLE 5–2. *Continued*

    2. Examples of specific nursing interventions
      a. Anatomical positioning of patient
      b. Physiological positioning of patient
      c. Maintenance of patient's personal hygiene
      d. Assist patient with range of motion exercises and passive exercises

III. Principle of Conservation of Personal Integrity: Nursing intervention is based on the conservation of the patient's personal integrity
  A. Relevant scientific considerations
    1. There is always a privacy to individual life
    2. Assumption of responsibility for one's own decisions develops with maturation
    3. Self-identify and self-respect are the foundations of a sense of personal integrity
    4. Illness threatens self-identity and self-respect
    5. Hospitalization may compound and exaggerate the threat to personal integrity
    6. Individuals possess a lifetime commitment to the value systems and social patterns of their subcultural affiliations
  B. Nursing intervention
    1. General considerations
      a. Respect from the nurse is essential to the patient's self-respect
      b. Accept the patient the way he is
      c. Foster patient participation in decision making within safe limits
      d. Determine and take into account patient's moral and ethical values
    2. Examples of specific nursing interventions
      a. Recognize and protect patient's space needs
      b. Assure privacy during performance of body functions and therapeutic procedures
      c. Respect importance patient places on personal possessions
      d. Use appropriate mode of address when dealing with patient
      e. Support patient's defense mechanisms as appropriate

IV. Principle of Conservation of Social Integrity: Nursing intervention is based on the conservation of the individual patient's social integrity
  A. Relevant scientific considerations
    1. The social integrity of individuals is tied to the viability of the entire social system
    2. Individual life has meaning only in the context of social life
    3. The way in which individuals relate to various social groups influences their behavior
    4. Individual recognition of wholeness is measured against relationships with others
    5. Interactions with others become more important in times of stress
    6. The patient's family may be deeply affected by the changes resulting from illness
    7. Hospitalization is characterized by isolation from family and friends
  B. Nursing intervention
    1. General considerations
      a. A failure to consider the patient's family and friends is a failure to provide excellent nursing care

TABLE 5-2.   *Continued*

---

  b. The social system of the hospital is artificial
  c. Concern for holistic well-being of individuals demands attention to community attitudes, resources, and provision of health care in the community
  d. The nurse-patient interaction is a social relationship which is disciplined and controlled by the professional role of the nurse
2. Examples of specific nursing interventions
  a. Consider patients' social needs when placing them in the nursing unit
  b. Position patient in bed to foster social interaction with other patients
  c. Avoid sensory deprivation for the patient
  d. Promote the patient's use of newspapers, magazines, radio, and television as appropriate
  e. Provide family with knowledgeable support and assistance
  f. Teach family members to perform functions for the patient as necessary

---

Adapted from Levine, M.E. (1967). The four conservation principles of nursing. Nursing Forum, 6, 47–59; and Levine, M.E. (1973). Introduction to clinical nursing (2nd ed., pp. 13–18). Philadelphia: FA Davis.

Content of the Model: Propositions

The propositions of Levine's Conservation Model link the metaparadigm concepts of person, environment, health, and nursing. The person is repeatedly placed in the context of the environment, as is illustrated in the following quotations:

> The individual is always within an environmental milieu, and the consequences of his awareness of his environment persistently influence his behavior at any given moment. (Levine, 1973, p. 444)

> [The person's] presence in the environment also influences it and thereby the kind of information available from it. (Levine, 1973, p. 446)

> The individual protects and defends himself within his environment by gaining all the information he can about it. (Levine, 1973, p. 451)

The linkages among all four metaparadigm concepts are stated in the following quotations:

> The nurse participates actively in every patient's environment, and much of what she does supports his adaptations as he struggles in the predicament of illness. (Levine, 1973, p. 13)

> But even in the presence of disease, the organism responds wholly to the environmental interaction in which it is involved, and a considerable element of nursing care is devoted to restoring the symmetry of response—symmetry that is essential to the well-being of the organism. (Levine, 1969b, p. 98)

Areas of Concern

The major area of concern addressed by Levine's Conservation Model is the maintenance of the person's wholeness. Levine focuses on adaptation as the process by which individuals maintain their wholeness or integrity. Thus, the model emphasizes the effectiveness of the person's adaptations. Furthermore, this conceptual model focuses the nurse's attention on the person and the complexity of his or her relationships with the internal and external environments. The model also emphasizes the nurse's responsibility for conservation of the patient's energy, as well as his or her structural, personal, and social integrity.

The source of threats to the person's wholeness or integrity is environmental challenge. Apparently, challenges may come from the internal or external environment. This interpretation of Levine's ideas is supported by the following comment:

> The exquisite internal balance responds constantly to the external forces. . . . There is an intimate relationship between the internal and the external environments, much of it vividly understood in recent years by research in physiological periodicity and the circadian cycles. (Levine, 1973, p. 8)

This interpretation is supported further by Levine's (1973) reference to positive feedback in the internal environment, which is manifested when pathological processes occur and can be responsible for pathology.

EVALUATION OF LEVINE'S CONSERVATION MODEL

This section presents an evaluation of Levine's Conservation Model. The evaluation is based on the results of the analysis of the model as well as publications and presentations by others who have used or commented on this conceptual model.

Explication of Assumptions

Levine explicitly identified the assumptions underlying her conceptual model. Her presentation of the model indicates that she values a holistic approach to the nursing care of all people, well or sick. She also values the unique individuality of each person, as noted in comments such as:

> Ultimately, decisions for nursing intervention must be based on the unique behavior of the individual patient. . . . A theory of nursing must recognize the importance of unique detail of care for a single pa-

tient within an empiric framework which successfully describes the requirements of all patients. (Levine, 1973, p. 6)

Patient centered nursing care means individualized nursing care. It is predicated on the reality of common experience: every man is a unique individual, and as such he requires a unique constellation of skills, techniques, and ideas designed specifically for him. (Levine, 1973, p. 23)

Furthermore, although Levine (1973) commented that human beings are dependent on their relationships with other human beings, she values the patient's participation in nursing care. This is attested to by the following comment:

"To keep together" means to maintain a proper balance between active nursing intervention coupled with patient participation on the one hand and the safe limits of the patient's ability to participate on the other. (p. 13)

Comprehensiveness of Concepts and Propositions

Levine's descriptions of the person, the environment, health, and nursing are comprehensive and essentially complete. Consequently, there is little need for inference in this conceptual model.

The nursing process extracted from Levine's writings meets Walker and Nicholson's (1980) criteria. Levine repeatedly emphasized the need for a scientific knowledge base for nursing judgments. Moreover, Levine's frequent citations of relevant research support the consistency of this model with scientific findings on human behavior. These features of the model are evident in statements such as:

It is the nurse's task to bring a body of scientific principles on which decisions depend into the precise situation which she shares with the patient. (Levine, 1966a, p. 2452)

The modern nurse has available rich knowledge of human anatomy, physiology, and adaptability. (Levine, 1966a, p. 2453)

Furthermore, Levine emphasized a concern for the individual person reflecting the ethical standards of nursing. She expressed her ethical standards in the article, "Nursing ethics and the ethical nurse." She concluded that publication by stating:

The wholeness which is part of our awareness of ourselves is shared best with others when no act diminishes another person and no moment of indifference leaves him with less of himself. Every moment of moral injustice extracts a price from both patient and nurse, just as every moment of moral responsibility gives each strength to grow in his wholeness. (Levine, 1977, p. 849)

Levine's attention to ethical standards also is reflected in the following statements:

> Nursing intervention must deal with the rights and privileges of the individual in tangible ways. . . . The emphasis on patient teaching recognizes the individual's right to be assisted in understanding the implications of his disease, his treatment, and his care. He must also be assured that his medical and social problems will remain privileged and confidential. (Levine, 1967, p. 54)

> True conservation demands that the nurse accept the patient the way he is. (Levine, 1967, p. 55)

The generality of the nursing process is partially documented in Levine's (1973) book. This text includes nursing processes appropriate for patients who have a failure of nervous system integration, hormonal disturbances, fluid and electrolyte imbalances, aberrant cellular growth, and several other pathological states. In addition, the applicability of the nursing process in various settings is documented below in the section on social utility.

The dynamic nature of the nursing process is evident in Levine's (1973) statement that nursing care plans "must allow for progress and change and project into the future the patient's response to treatment" (p. 46), as well as in Levine's (in press) presentation of nursing care as use of a "cascading repertoire of skill, knowledge, and compassion." Given Levine's explanation of cascades as nonlinear interacting and evolving processes, the nursing process clearly is dynamic.

The criterion for comprehensiveness of propositions stipulates that all four metaparadigm concepts be linked. The statements presented in the analysis section attest to the satisfaction of this criterion.

Logical Congruence

World Views

Levine's conceptual model clearly reflects the organismic view of the world. She regards the person as a holistic being who constantly strives to preserve wholeness and integrity. Furthermore, although Levine (in press) discusses physiological and behavioral responses, she regarded these as "one and the same—not merely parallel and not merely simultaneous—but essential portions of the same activity." Moreover, although she identified four principles of conservation, she viewed them as joined, not isolated or separate.

The elements of organicism are exemplified explicitly in the following quotations:

> Nursing intervention, traditionally directed by procedures or manifestations of disease symptoms, needs new directions if the holistic approach is to be utilized. The individual must be recognized in his wholeness, and the powerful influence of adaptation recognized as a dynamic and ever-present factor in evaluating his care. Instead of list-

ing "needs" or "symptoms," it should be possible to identify for each individual the patterns of his adaptive response, and to tailor intervention to enhance their effectiveness. (Levine, 1971, pp. 257–258)

All nursing care is focused on man and the complexity of his relationships with his environment, both internal and external, and common experience emphasizes that every response to every environmental stimulus results from the integrated and unified nature of the human organism. In other words, every response is an organismic one—no other kind is possible—and every adaptive change is accomplished by the entire individual. (Levine, 1967, p. 46)

Organicism also is reflected in Levine's characterization of the person as an active participant in interactions with the environment. This is seen especially in her statement that "The individual can . . . never be passive. He is an active participant in his environment, not only altering it by his presence but also actively and constantly seeking information from it" (Levine, 1969b, p. 96). The active organism viewpoint also is reflected in Levine's discussion of the perceptual systems. For example, Levine (1973) commented, "The human being is a sentient being, and the ability to interact with the environment seems ineluctably tied to his sensory organs" (p. 446). She also noted, "The perceptual systems provide information to the individual; usually this is knowledge sought by the individual" (Levine, 1973, p. 450).

There is little evidence of a mechanistic world view in the model. In fact, Levine (1971) explicitly rejected mechanism, stating "The mechanistic view of the body and mind does little to restore to the individual the wholeness he recognizes in himself" (p. 254). However, at one point Levine did present a somewhat reactive mechanistic view of the person. She stated, "The human being responds to the forces in his environment in singular yet integrated fashion" (Levine, 1966a, p. 2452). Here, Levine appears to be attempting to translate the mechanistic idea of reaction to the environment by bringing in the idea of a more holistic, integrated response. Furthermore, this comment is offset by Levine's explicit statements about the active nature of the person, as noted above.

Levine's model seems to reflect the world view of change. This viewpoint is evident in statements such as:

Change is the essence of life, and it is unceasing as long as life goes on. (Levine, 1973, p. 10)

Change is characteristic of life. (Levine, 1973, p. 10)

In contrast, the emphasis on homeostasis and conservation suggests that Levine's model reflects the persistence view of the world. Levine (in press) regarded homeostasis as "a state of energy-sparing"; it even "might be called conservation." The essence of conservation, in turn, is use of responses "that *cost the least* to the individual in expense of effort and demand on his well-being."

Given Levine's primary focus on conservation, it seems more appropriate to classify this conceptual model as within the persistence view of the world. Apparently, Levine regards the many changes that must occur as the person faces environmental challenges as necessary for survival. Conservation facilitates and maintains the patterns and routines of human behavior, and adaptive changes represent invention of new routines to avoid extinction.

Classification of the Model

Close examination of the content of Levine's Conservation Model indicates that the systems category is an appropriate classification. The characteristic of integration of parts is reflected in the following quotations:

> The total life process of the entire organism is dependent upon the inter-relatedness of its component systems. In fact, the organism is a system of systems. (Levine, 1973, pp. 8–9)

> Human life must be described in the language of "wholes." . . . perceiving the "wholes" depends upon recognizing the organization and interdependence of observable phenomena. (Levine, 1971, p. 255)

Other than her comment regarding the organism as a system of systems, Levine does not explicitly address the characteristic of system. Environment, however, is addressed repeatedly and is viewed as both internal and external. The relationship of the person to environment is expressed clearly in the following statement: "The person cannot be described apart from the specific environment in which he is found" (Levine, in press).

Levine (1973) related the idea of "wholeness" to that of the open system. Citing Erikson (1968), she stated that a whole is an open system and explained, "The unceasing interaction of the individual organism with its environments does represent an 'open and fluid' system" (p. 11).

The characteristic of boundary is explicitly addressed in this conceptual model in the discussion of individual territoriality. Levine (1973) commented, "every individual requires space and both the establishment of his personal boundaries and their defense are essential components of his behavior" (p. 459). Levine (1973) went on to cite Hall's (1966) work on human territorial behavior, with its identification of the intimate, personal distance, social distance, and public distance zones maintained between people.

The systems model characteristic of tension, stress, strain, and conflict is alluded to by Levine in her discussion of adaptation. She stated,

> Change is characteristic of life, and adaptation is the method of change. The organism retains its integrity in both the internal and ex-

ternal environment through its adaptive capability. Adaptation is the process of change whereby the individual retains his integrity within the realities of his environment. (Levine, 1973, pp. 10–11)

Levine's (in press) use of the term environment challenge suggests that this is what represents the factors or forces that are responsible for initiating change and adaptation.

Levine (1973) referred to the characteristic of steady state when she discussed homeorhesis. This term denotes "a stabilized flow rather than a static state" (p. 7). Levine (1973) commented, "The concept of stabilized flow more accurately reflects the reality of daily change as well as the alterations in physiological activity that characterize the processes of growth and development" (pp. 7–8). In her most recent work, however, Levine (in press) seemed to favor homeostasis as the best descriptor of internal environment, regarding it as a state that "provides the necessary baselines for a multitude of synchronized physiological and psychological factors," rather than a system of balance and quiescence. In fact, Levine (personal communication, August 13, 1987) indicated that homeostasis is the appropriate view of the internal environment because it captures the notion of the congruence of the person with the environment.

The characteristic of feedback is addressed in this conceptual model in terms of physiological and pathological processes. In keeping with systems models, Levine (1973, in press) associated negative feedback with autoregulation of physiological systems and positive feedback with disruption of function seen in pathological processes.

Meleis (1985) classified Levine's conceptual model within the outcome category. She noted that Levine's work focuses on nursing activities and actions designed to care for people. Marriner (1986) placed Levine's work within her energy fields category. Stevens (1984) classified Levine's model in the conservation category. Interestingly, J.P. Riehl-Sisca (personal communication, July 23, 1987) indicated that Levine apparently regards her conceptual model as an interaction model. The content of Levine's model does not, however, address any of the characteristics of that category as described in this book. Certainly, Levine's work deals with the interaction between person and environment, but that is not the same as the symbolic interactionism emphasis of the interaction category. When asked about the interaction classification, Levine (personal communication, August 13, 1987) agreed that her conceptual model does not reflect symbolic interactionism. She went on to say that hers is "an adaptation model." She also acknowledged some systems elements in her work.

Generation and Testing of Theory

Levine (1978a) stated that she was trying to develop two theories, which she called therapeutic intention and redundancy. Work on the theory of therapeutic intention began in the early 1970s. Levine (personal communication to L. Criddle, July 22, 1987) indicated that she "was seeking a way of organizing nursing intervention growing out of the reality of the *biological* realities which nurses had to confront." Her thinking about therapeutic intention is summarized in the following statements that describe broad areas of therapeutic intervention and create parameters of nursing intervention.

1. Therapeutic regimes which support the integrated healing processes of the body and permit optimal restoration of structure and function through natural response to disease.
2. Therapeutic regimes which substitute an external servomechanism for a failure of autoregulation of an essential integrating system.
3. Therapeutic regimes which focus on specific causes, and by surgical restructuring or drug therapy, restore individual integrity and well-being.
4. Therapeutic regimes which cannot alter or substitute for the pathology so that only supportive measures are possible to promote comfort and humane concern.
5. Therapeutic regimes which balance a significant toxic risk against the threat of the disease process.
6. Therapeutic regimes which simulate physiological processes and reinforce or antagonize usual responses in order to create a therapeutic change in function.
7. Therapeutic regimes which provide manipulation of diet and activity to correct metabolic imbalances related to nutrition and/or exercise. (Levine, personal communication to L. Criddle, July 22, 1987)

Levine (personal communication, August 13, 1987) regarded the seven areas of therapeutic intention as an "imperfect list that is not yet complete."

Although the theory of therapeutic intention seems to extend the nursing process component of the Conservation Model, Levine (personal communication to L. Criddle, July 22, 1987) stated that she never associated the idea of therapeutic intention with the principles of conservation. She explained, "I suppose it would be a claim to some greater wisdom to suggest that every idea I ever had was in some way associated with the Conservation Principles—but that is simply not true. My thought habits are fairly consistent but I have devoted them to many areas which are not organically related."

Levine (1978a) noted that she and a colleague had been working on the theory of redundancy for some time. This "completely untested, completely speculative" theory has "redefined aging and almost everything else that has to do with human life." She proposed that "aging is the diminished availability of redundant systems necessary for effective maintenance of physical and social well-being" (Levine, 1978b). This theory seems to extend the discussion of redundancy related to specificity of adaptation and organismic responses.

Social Considerations

Social Congruence

Although Levine's conceptual model was initially formulated many years ago, it is congruent with the present-day emphasis on holistic approaches to health care and consideration of the person as a unique individual. Levine developed her model at a time when nursing activities in acute care settings were becoming more mechanical, owing to the rapid increase in medical technology. She spoke out against the growing functionalism of nursing and reoriented nurses to the patient as a whole being, as is evident in the following comment:

> Discovering ways to perceive and cherish the essential wholeness of man becomes imperative with the rapid growth of automation in modern disciplines which possess a technology. Nursing is one of them, and nurses will not escape the sweeping changes that automation promises. But nurses do know that the integrated human being is not merely "programmed' to respond to life in automatic ways. . . . It is the task of nursing to recognize and value the wondrous variety of all mankind while offering ministrations that conserve the unique and special integrity of every man. (Levine, 1966a, p. 2453)

Levine (1973) noted that "the whole man is the focus of nursing intervention—in health and sickness, in tragedy and joy, in hospitals and clinics and in the community" (p. vii). Although little discussion of the use of this conceptual model in health promotion and illness prevention situations is available, its broad focus is congruent with society's increasing interest in promotion of health and prevention of illness.

Social Significance

Hirschfeld (1976) provided some evidence of the social significance of Levine's Conservation Model. She noted, "Myra Levine's four principles of conservation are useful in deciding what will help the cognitively impaired aged person and determining what the priorities should be in his or her care" (p. 1981). She went on to describe application of the principles of conservation to the care of several patients who had cognitive impairments. In concluding her article, Hirschfeld stated,

> Surely, nursing care that incorporates Levine's four conservation principles can make a difference to the individual and family equilibrium that are disturbed by events as devastating as mental impairment. (p. 1984)

Additional evidence of social significance was provided by V.G. Lathrop (personal communication, May 5, 1982), who used Levine's model to guide the nursing care of patients in the Intensive Treatment Unit for Mentally Ill Offenders at Saint Elizabeth's Hospital in Washington, D.C. According to Lathrop, nursing audits based on the American Nurses' Association Psychiatric/Mental Health Standards of Nursing Practice revealed that "treatment provided was more holistic in nature."

Social Utility

The utility of Levine's Conservation Model for nursing research is documented by several studies. The rules for research regarding phenomena to be studied and how they are to be studied have been proposed by Levine (personal communication to L. Criddle, July 22, 1987), who stated, "I do not believe that the Conservation Principles can be used as a research model *one at a time.* They intersect with each other and must be viewed in context." Levine (personal communication, August 13, 1987) did, however, indicate that it would be appropriate to develop instruments that deal with just one conservation principle. Levine (1978a) provided further specification of phenomena to be studied when she noted that a needed area of nursing research is the investigation of the interface between the internal and external environments of the person. Other rules must be developed.

Four doctoral dissertations based on Levine's conservation principles were recently completed at the University of Illinois at Chicago. Cox (1987) studied pregnancy, anxiety, and time perception. Fleming (1987) compared women with different perineal conditions after childbirth. Foreman (1987) described the development of confusion in elderly patients. MacLean (1987) described cues used by nurses for identification of activity intolerance. In addition, Blasage's (1987) dissertation research, at Loyola University of Chicago, examined and identified trends in Levine's writings.

Other research based on Levine's conceptual model includes studies by Newport (1984), Yeates and Roberts (1984), and Winslow and her associates (1984, 1985). Newport compared the body temperatures of infants who had been placed on their mothers' chests immediately after birth with those of infants who were placed in a warmer. Yeates and Roberts compared the effects of two bearing-down techniques during the second stage of labor on labor progress.

Winslow (personal communication to M.E. Levine, October 6, 1982) indicated that her research on energy utilization during toileting and bathing is based on Levine's principle of conservation of energy. However, the published reports of this research do not cite Levine (Winslow, 1983; Winslow, Lane, & Gaffney, 1984, 1985).

Geden's (1982) report of her study of energy expenditure during lifting cited notions of energy mentioned in some nursing models, including Levine's. There is no evidence, however, that this research was an explicit test of Levine's principle of conservation of energy. In fact, Geden (1985) interpreted her work within the context of Orem's general theory of nursing.

Tompkins (1980) cited a few conceptual models of nursing, including Levine's, in the discussion of findings from her study of the effect of restricted mobility and leg dominance on perceived duration of time. This research was not, however, derived from Levine's model.

The utility of Levine's conceptual model for nursing practice has been documented and rules for practice are becoming evident. First, it is clear that the focus of all nursing care is conservation of the patient's wholeness. Second, it is clear that legitimate recipients of nursing care encompass individuals who are sick and those who are well. And third, it is clear that the nursing process is guided by the principles of conservation.

Levine's conceptual model has been used in various clinical settings and situations. Hirschfeld (1975) linked the principles of conservation with theories of pathophysiology, aging, and cognitive impairment to develop nursing interventions for several patients who were cognitively impaired as a result of illness. Herbst (1981) linked the principles of conservation with knowledge of the pathophysiology of cancer and presented a comprehensive description of nursing that takes into account the wholeness of the patient, the nurse, and the disease process. Brunner (1985) used the conservation principles and knowledge of cardiac pathology to formulate a nursing care plan for cardiac patients. Crawford-Gamble (1986) described the use of the four conservation principles, linked with knowledge of the effects of surgery, in the care of a woman undergoing reimplantation of digits of her hand. Fawcett and her associates (1987) used knowledge of end-stage heart disease and critical care unit environments to formulate trophicognoses for a 57-year-old man.

Furthermore, Cox (1985) described the use of Levine's Conservation Model to guide nursing care of elderly residents of The Alverno Health Care Facility in Clinton, Iowa. Her discussion underscored the utility of Levine's model for health promotion and illness prevention. In addition, Pond (1985) reported her use of the conceptual model in the Emergency Department of the Hospital of the University of Pennsylvania in Philadelphia. And M. Mercer (personal communication, December 10, 1983) outlined an assessment format based on Levine's model that she used in the critical care unit at Chester County Hospital in West Chester, Pennsylvania.

Use of the conceptual model as a guide for nursing practice also was reported by V.G. Lathrop and M.J. Stafford. As noted in the section on social significance, Lathrop (personal communication, May 5, 1982) used Levine's Conservation Model in a psychiatric-mental health setting. Furthermore, Stafford (personal communication, June 2, 1982), a clinical specialist in cardiac nursing, used Levine's Conservation Model for nursing care of patients at the Hines Veterans Administration Hospital in Hines, Illinois.

The utility of Levine's conceptual model for nursing education also is documented. The rule for education regarding curriculum content is partially specified in Levine's (1969a, 1973) book. Although her book was written and revised many years ago, the content areas identified as appropriate for an introductory nursing course are just as relevant today. The areas are vital signs, body movement and positioning, personal hygiene, fluids, nutrition, pressure gradient systems, application of heat and cold, medications, and asepsis. Other rules for education have not yet been formulated.

No publications describing the use of the model in specific nursing education programs could be located, although Stevens (1984) offered a hypothetical curriculum design based on Levine's model. However, findings from surveys of baccalaureate nursing programs conducted by Hall (1979) and Riehl (1980) revealed that Levine's conceptual model is used as a guideline for curriculum development. In particular, Riehl found that Levine's model is "popular with faculty, especially in the Chicago area" (p. 396). The names of the schools of nursing using Levine's model were not given in the survey reports. In another survey, Allentown College of St. Francis de Sales in Center Valley, Pennsylvania, was identified as having a nursing curriculum based on Levine's model (Asay & Ossler, 1984).

In addition, L. Zwanger (personal communication, June 4, 1982) reported that Levine's Conservation Model is used in nursing education programs sponsored by Kapat-Holim, the Health Insurance Institution of the General Federation of Labour in Israel, based in Tel-Aviv. Moreover, M.J. Stafford (personal communication, June 2, 1982) stated that she used the model "in teaching formal and informal classes such as the Critical Care Nursing course, Pacemaker Therapy, and The Nurse's Role in Electrocardiography" at the Hines Veterans Administration Hospital in Hines, Illinois.

Levine's Conservation Model has documented utility for nursing service administration. One rule for administration was suggested by Levine (1969b) when she indicated that the person's perceptual system could serve as the basis for organization of hospital units. Levine explained that the patient's ability to receive information and interpret it must be taken into account, as well as territorial needs. Other rules have not yet been developed.

The utility of Levine's conceptual model for various administrative endeavors is evident. Taylor (1974) developed a form for evaluation of the quality of nursing care of neurological patients. The conservation principles served as the goals of nursing care and were used as the frame of reference for "defining commonly recurring nursing problems on the neurological service" (p. 342). In addition, M.J. Stafford (personal communication, June 2, 1982) commented that she used Levine's Conservation Model to identify process and outcome criteria in the nursing care of patients with cardiovascular problems. Furthermore, the utility of Levine's conceptual model for nursing administration is documented by its use at The Alverno Health Care Facility in Clinton, Iowa. Here, the conservation principles structure the format of the nursing care plan and provide guidelines for staff development. The nursing care plan contains an extensive summary of the patient's trophicognosis and care is organized according to the four conservation principles (Cox, 1985).

Contributions to Nursing Knowledge

Levine's Conservation Model makes a substantial contribution to nursing knowledge by focusing attention on the whole person. Levine moved beyond the idea of the total person to the concept of the person as a holistic being. Pointing to the limitations of the so-called total person approach, she noted:

> Nurses have long known that patients are complete persons, not groups of parts. It is out of this realization that the attempts toward "comprehensive care" and "total care" have come, and it is because we have been frustrated by failing to achieve the ideal of completion that the search for a more definitive approach to bedside care has continued. (Levine, 1969b, p. 94)

This conceptual model is consistent in its approach to the person as a holistic being. Physiological and behavioral responses are regarded as one and the same and conservation principles are joined. Moreover, Levine's principles of conservation provide a framework for holistic nursing care. These principles focus attention on the patient as a unique individual.

The Conservation Model has a distinctive and extensive vocabulary that requires some study for mastery. However, Levine was careful to provide adequate definitions of most terms, so that there should be minimal confusion about the meaning of her ideas.

Although documentation of the utility of Levine's conceptual model for nursing activities is increasing, its credibility must be established. More systematic evaluations of the use of the model in various clinical situations are needed, as are empirical studies that test theories directly derived from or linked with the conservation principles.

In conclusion, Levine's Conservation Model provides nursing with a logically congruent, holistic view of the person. Two theories related to the model have been formulated but they require further development and empirical testing. The lack of major limitations suggests that this conceptual model may be an effective guide for nursing actions.

REFERENCES

Asay, M.K., & Ossler, C.C. (Eds.). (1984). Conceptual models of nursing. Applications in community health nursing. Proceedings of the Eighth Annual Community Health Nursing Conference. Chapel Hill: Department of Public Health Nursing, School of Public Health, University of North Carolina.

Bates, M. (1967). A naturalist at large. Natural History, 76(6), 8–16.

Beland, I. (1971). Clinical nursing: Pathophysiological and psychosocial implications (2nd ed.). New York: Macmillan.

Blasage, M.C. (1987). Toward a general understanding of nursing education: A critical analysis of the work of Myra Estrin Levine. Dissertation Abstracts International, 47, 4467B.

Brunner, M. (1985). A conceptual approach to critical care. Focus on Critical Care, 12(2), 39–44.

Cannon, W.B. (1939). The wisdom of the body. New York: Norton.

Cox, B. (1987). Pregnancy, anxiety, and time perception. Doctoral dissertation, University of Illinois at Chicago.

Cox, R. (1985). Application of Levine's Conservation Model. Paper presented at conference on Nursing Theory in Action, Edmonton, Alberta, Canada. (Cassette recording)

Crawford-Gamble, P.E. (1986). An application of Levine's conceptual model. Perioperative Nursing Quarterly, 2(1), 64–70.

Dubos, R. (1961). Mirage of health. New York: Doubleday.

Dubos, R. (1965). Man adapting. New Haven: Yale University Press.

Erikson, E.H. (1964). Insight and responsibility. New York: Norton.

Erikson, E.H. (1968). Identity: Youth and crisis. New York: Norton.

Fawcett, J., Cariello, F.P., Davis, D.A., Farley, J., Zimmaro, D.M., & Watts, R.J. (198). Conceptual models of nursing: Application to critical care nursing practice. Dimensions of Critical Care Nursing, 6, 202–213.

Fleming, N. (1987). Comparison of women with different perineal conditions after childbirth. Doctoral dissertation, University of Illinois at Chicago.

Foreman, M. (1987). The development of confusion in the hospitalized elderly. Doctoral dissertation, University of Illinois at Chicago.

Geden, E. (1982). Effects of lifting techniques on energy expenditure: A preliminary investigation. Nursing Research, 31, 214–218.

Geden, E. (1985). The relationship between self-care theory and empirical research. In J. Riehl-Sisca, The science and art of self-care (pp. 265–270). Norwalk, CT: Appleton-Century-Crofts.

Gibson, J.E. (1966). The senses considered as perceptual systems. Boston: Houghton-Mifflin.

Goldstein, K. (1963). The organism. Boston: Beacon Press.

Hall, E.T. (1966). The hidden dimension. Garden City, NY: Doubleday & Co.

Hall, K.V. (1979). Current trends in the use of conceptual frameworks in nursing education. Journal of Nursing Education, 18(4), 26–29.

Herbst, S. (1981). Impairments as a result of cancer. In N. Martin, N. Holt, & D. Hicks, (Eds.), Comprehensive rehabilitation nursing (pp. 553–578). New York: McGraw-Hill.

Hirschfeld, M.J. (1976). The cognitively impaired older adult. American Journal of Nursing, 76, 1981–1984.

Levine, M.E. (1966a). Adaptation and assessment: A rationale for nursing intervention. American Journal of Nursing, 66, 2450–2453.

Levine, M.E. (1966b). Trophicognosis: An alternative to nursing diagnosis. In American Nurses' Association Regional Clinical Conference (Vol. 2, pp. 55–70). New York: American Nurses' Association.

Levine, M.E. (1967). The four conservation principles of nursing. Nursing Forum, 6, 45–59.

Levine, M.E. (1969a). Introduction to clinical nursing. Philadelphia: FA Davis.

Levine, M.E. (1969b). The pursuit of wholeness. American Journal of Nursing, 69, 93–98.

Levine, M.E. (1971). Holistic nursing. Nursing Clinics of North America, 6, 253–264.

Levine, M.E. (1973). Introduction to clinical nursing (2nd ed.). Philadelphia: FA Davis.

Levine, M.E. (1977). Nursing ethics and the ethical nurse. American Journal of Nursing, 77, 845–849.

Levine, M.E. (1978a, December). The four conservation principles of nursing. Paper presented at Second Annual Nurse Educator Conference, New York. (Cassette recording)

Levine, M.E. (1978b, December). Application to education and service. Paper presented at the Second Annual Nurse Educator Conference, New York. (Cassette recording)

Levine, M.E. (1984a, August). Myra Levine. Paper presented at the Nurse Theorist Conference, Edmonton, Alberta, Canada. (Cassette recording)

Levine, M.E. (1984b, August). Concurrent sessions. M. Levine. Discussion at the Nurse Theorist Conference, Edmonton, Alberta, Canada. (Cassette recording)

Levine, M.E. (1985, August). Myra Levine. Paper presented at conference on Nursing Theory in Action, Edmonton, Alberta, Canada. (Cassette recording)

Levine, M.E. (1986, August). Myra Levine. Paper presented at Nursing Theory Congress: Theoretical pluralism: Direction for a practice discipline, Toronto, Ontario, Canada. (Cassette recording)

Levine, M.E. (in press). The four conservation principles: Twenty years later. In J.P. Riehl, Conceptual models for nursing practice (3rd ed.). Norwalk, CT: Appleton and Lange.

MacLean, S. (1987). Description of cues nurses use for diagnosing activity intolerance. Doctoral dissertation, University of Illinois at Chicago.

Marriner, A (1986). Nursing theorists and their work. St. Louis: CV Mosby.

Meleis, A.I. (1985). Theoretical nursing: Development and progress. Philadelphia: JB Lippincott.

Newman, M.A. (1972). Nursing's theoretical evolution. Nursing Outlook, 20, 449–453.

Newport, M.A. (1984). Conserving thermal energy and social integrity in the newborn. Western Journal of Nursing Research, 6, 176–197.

Pond, J. (1985, August). Application of Levine's Conservation Model. Paper presented at conference on Nursing Theory in Action, Edmonton, Alberta, Canada. (Cassette recording)

Riehl, J.P. (1980). Nursing models in current use. In J.P. Riehl & C. Roy, Conceptual models for nursing practice (2nd ed., pp. 393–398). New York: Appleton-Century-Crofts.

Selye, H. (1956). The stress of life. New York: McGraw-Hill.

Sherrington, A. (1906). Integrative function of the nervous system. New York: Scribner's.

Stevens, B.J. (1984). Nursing theory. Analysis, application, evaluation (2nd ed.). Boston: Little, Brown & Co.

Taylor, J.W. (1974). Measuring the outcomes of nursing care. Nursing Clinics of North America, 9, 337–348.

Tillich, P. (1961). The meaning of health. Perspectives in Biology and Medicine, 5, 92–100.

Tompkins, E.S. (1980). Effect of restricted mobility and dominance on perceived duration. Nursing Research, 29, 333–338.

Waddington, C.H. (Ed.). (1968). Towards a theoretical biology. I. Prolegomena. Chicago: Aldine.

Walker, L.O., & Nicholson, R. (1980). Criteria for evaluating nursing process models. Nurse Educator, 5(5), 8–9.

Winslow, E.H. (1983). Oxygen consumption and cardiovascular response in normal subjects and in acute myocardial infarction patients during basin bath, tub bath, and shower. Dissertation Abstracts International, 43, 2856B.

Winslow, E.H., Lane, L.D., & Gaffney, F.A. (1984). Oxygen consumption and cardiovascular response in patients and normal adults during in-bed and out-of-bed toileting. Journal of Cardiac Rehabilitation, 4, 348–354.

Winslow, E.H., Lane, L.D., & Gaffney, F.A. (1985). Oxygen consumption and cardiovascular response in control adults and acute myocardial infarction patients during bathing. Nursing Research, 34, 164–169.

Wolf, S. (1961). Disease as a way of life: Neural integration in systemic pathology. Perspectives in Biology and Medicine, 4, 288–305.

Yeates, D.A., & Roberts, J.E. (1984). A comparison of two bearing-down techniques during the second stage of labor. Journal of Nurse-Midwifery, 29, 3–11.

ANNOTATED BIBLIOGRAPHY

Brunner, M. (1985). A conceptual approach to critical care nursing using Levine's model. Focus on Critical Care, 12(2), 39–44.
This article presents an example of Levine's conceptual model for the care of a cardiac patient. One modification of the conceptual model is the use of nursing diagnoses, rather than trophicognoses. A nursing care plan is given.

Crawford-Gamble, P.E. (1986). An application of Levine's conceptual model. Perioperative Nursing Quarterly, 2(1), 64–70.
Levine's conservation model is used as a framework to guide care of a patient undergoing reimplantation of digits of her right hand. The four conservation principles are used as a basis for nursing care throughout the surgical experience.

Esposito, C.H., & Leonard, M.K. (1980). Myra Estrin Levine. In Nursing Theories Conference Group, Nursing theories. The base for professional nursing practice (pp. 150–163). Englewood Cliffs, NJ: Prentice-Hall.
An overview of Levine's model is presented. Nursing is defined and a description of the four conservation principles is included. The nursing process is described in detail and an application of the model to a clinical situation is offered. Limitations of the model are identified. This review suggests that the authors misinterpreted much of Levine's work.

Fawcett, J., Cariello, F.P., Davis, D.A., Farley, J., Zimmaro, D.M., & Watts, R.J. (1987). Conceptual models of nursing: Application to critical care nursing practice. Dimensions of Critical Care Nursing, 6, 202–213.
This article includes a brief analysis of Levine's conceptual model and identification of trophicognoses for a 57-year-old man who was dying from cardiac disease.

Foli, K.J., Johnson, T., Marriner, A., Poat, M.C., Poppa, L., & Zoretich, S.T. (1986). Myra Estrin Levine. Four conservation principles. In A. Marriner, Nursing theorists and their work (pp. 335–344). St. Louis: CV Mosby.
This chapter presents an overview of Levine's conservation model.

Herbst, S. (1981). Impairments as a result of cancer. In N. Martin, N. Holt & D. Hicks (Eds.), Comprehensive rehabilitation nursing (pp. 553–578). New York: McGraw-Hill.
This book chapter presents an overview of Levine's conservation principles. The conservation principles are then applied to the problems the cancer patient experiences.

Hirschfeld, M.J. (1976). The cognitively impaired older adult. American Journal of Nursing, 76, 1981–1984.
Care of the cognitively impaired older adult is discussed in the context of Levine's conservation principles. Theories of aging and cognitive impairment are incorporated into the discussion.

Leonard, M.K. (1985). Myra Estrin Levine. In Nursing Theories Conference Group, Nursing theories. The base for professional nursing practice (2nd ed., pp. 180–194). Englewood Cliffs, NJ: Prentice-Hall.
This book chapter presents a review of Levine's conservation model. The review does not present an accurate account of the model inasmuch as several aspects of Levine's work were misinterpreted.

Levine, M.E. (1966). Adaptation and assessment: A rationale for nursing intervention. American Journal of Nursing, 66, 2450–2453.
Historical developments that influenced nursing are reviewed. The role of the

nurse in promoting adaptation to disease is addressed. Emphasis is placed on scientific knowledge as well as awareness of individual responses as the basis for assessment.

Levine, M.E. (1966). Trophicognosis: An alternative to nursing diagnosis. In American Nurses' Association Regional Clinical Conference (Vol. 2, pp. 55–70). New York: American Nurses' Association.
Trophicognosis is offered as a more accurate term to describe nursing judgments than diagnosis. The term is defined and described in detail and is contrasted with nursing diagnosis. A comprehensive clinical example is included.

Levine, M.E. (1967). The four conservation principles of nursing. Nursing Forum, 6, 45–59.
The conservation principles central to Levine's conceptual model are presented in detail. General clinical examples are included to augment understanding of the principles.

Levine, M.E. (1969). The pursuit of wholeness. American Journal of Nursing, 69, 93–98.
The concepts of wholeness and interaction of person and environment are discussed. Four levels of organismic response are described and examples of each are offered. Five perceptual systems are discussed and possible dysfunctions are considered. The holistic approach to nursing is presented.

Levine, M.E. (1969). Introduction to clinical nursing. Philadelphia: FA Davis.
This book contains the first comprehensive presentation of Levine's Conservation Model. The first and last chapters present the major concepts of the model. Designed as a beginning level medical-surgical nursing text, the book includes several other chapters considering nursing care of patients with failure of nervous system integration; failure of integration resulting from hormonal disturbance; disturbances of homeostasis in terms of fluid and electrolyte imbalance, nutritional needs, systemic oxygen needs, and cellular oxygen needs; aberrant cellular growth; and an inflammatory process. Each of these chapters includes a list of objectives, essential science concepts, and the relevant nursing process.

Levine, M.E. (1971). Holistic nursing. Nursing Clinics of North America, 6, 253–264.
The concept of holism is discussed and contrasted with dualistic, mechanistic approaches. The four conservation principles are delineated. The importance of organismic generalizations in nursing is presented.

Levine, M.E. (1971). ReNewal for nursing. Philadelphia: FA Davis.
This book was written for the nurse returning to nursing practice. Levine maintains that the returning nurse has retained her identity as a nurse, has matured, and has considerably more knowledge and skill than she may credit herself. In the first chapter, Levine describes the patient in terms of current concepts, such as "the patient is a person." She uses her conceptual model definition of health as wholeness throughout the book. The content follows the format of Levine's text, Introduction to clinical nursing. Each chapter identifies relevant pragmatics, including related diagnostic entities, related nursing procedures, and appropriate drug therapy. The concluding chapter focuses on the implications of recent research for improved nursing care.

Levine, M.E. (1973). Introduction to clinical nursing (2nd ed.). Philadelphia: F.A. Davis.
The second edition of Levine's textbook. Format is similar to the first edition. Content is updated and greater emphasis is placed on the changing role of the nurse.

Levine, M.E. (in press). The four conservation principles: Twenty years later. In J.P. Riehl, Conceptual models for nursing practice (3rd ed.). Norwalk, CT: Appleton and Lange.
This book chapter presents a revision and expansion of several concepts and propositions of Levine's conceptual model. Emphasis is placed on the concepts of conservation and adaptation and the four conservation principles.

Newport, M.A. (1984). Conserving thermal energy and social integrity in the newborn. Western Journal of Nursing Research, 6, 176–197.
Levine's principles of conservation of energy and social integrity provided the conceptual base for the study reported in this article. The investigator compared tem-

peratures of infants placed in a warmer immediately after birth with those of infants placed on their mothers' chests immediately after birth. No temperature differences were found between the two groups of infants.

Pieper, B.A. (1983). Levine's nursing model. In J.J. Fitzpatrick & A.L. Whall, Conceptual models of nursing: Analysis and application (pp. 101–115). Bowie, MD: Brady.
This book chapter presents an overview of Levine's conservation model.

Taylor, J.W. (1974). Measuring the outcomes of nursing care. Nursing Clinics of North America, 9, 337–348.
A pilot project to develop criterion measures of patient outcomes of nursing care is described in a step-by-step manner. Levine's four conservation principles are used as the frame of reference for defining common nursing problems in the care of neurological patients.

Winslow, E.H., Lane, L.D., & Gaffney, F.A. (1984). Oxygen consumption and cardiovascular response in patients and normal adults during in-bed and out-of-bed toileting. Journal of Cardiac Rehabilitation, 4, 348–354.

Winslow, E.H., Lane, L.D., & Gaffney, F.A. (1985). Oxygen consumption and cardiovascular response in control adults and acute myocardial infarction patients during bathing. Nursing Research, 34, 164–169.
These two reports focus on the results of studies based on Levine's principle of the conservation of energy.

Yeates, D.A., & Roberts, J.E. (1984). A comparison of two bearing-down techniques during the second stage of labor. Journal of Nurse-Midwifery, 29, 3–11.
This article presents the report of a pilot study designed to determine the differences in progression of second stage labor for women who followed their involuntary urge to bear down and women who used sustained breath-holding techniques. The study, which was derived from Levine's conceptual model, revealed no differences between the two groups of women in terms of second stage labor progression.

CHAPTER

6

Neuman's Systems Model_____

This chapter presents an analysis and evaluation of Betty Neuman's Systems Model. Neuman's work clearly fits the definition of a conceptual model of nursing. In fact, Neuman (in press) explicitly referred to her work as a model or conceptual framework.

The key terms of Neuman's conceptual model are listed below. These terms were taken from the second edition of Neuman's (in press) book, *The Neuman Systems Model. Application to nursing education and practice.*

KEY TERMS_____

Client/Client System	Lines of Resistance
Individual	Environment
Family	Internal
Community	External
Variables	Created
Physiological	Stressors
Psychological	Intrapersonal
Sociocultural	Interpersonal
Developmental	Extrapersonal
Spiritual	Client System Stability
Central Core	Variances from Wellness
Flexible Line of Defense	Reconstitution
Normal Line of Defense	Goal of Nursing

Goal of Nursing—*Cont.*	Prevention as Intervention
Retain, Attain, and Maintain	Format
Optimal Client Wellness	Primary Prevention
Nursing Process Format	Secondary Prevention
Nursing Diagnosis	Tertiary Prevention
Nursing Goals	Theory of Optimal Client System
Nursing Outcomes	Stability

ANALYSIS OF NEUMAN'S SYSTEMS MODEL

This section presents an analysis of Neuman's Systems Model. The analysis draws heavily from the recent refinements and revisions of the model (Neuman, in press).

Development of the Model

Neuman's conceptual model was first presented in 1972, in an article entitled, "A model for teaching total person approach to patient problems" (Neuman & Young, 1972). A refinement of the model was published in the 1974 edition of Riehl and Roy's book, *Conceptual models for nursing practice* and reprinted in their 1980 edition (Neuman, 1974, 1980). Further refinements were presented in a chapter of the first edition of Neuman's (1982) book, *The Neuman Systems Model. Application to nursing education and practice.* The most recent version of the model is presented in a chapter of the second edition of Neuman's (in press) book. Another chapter in this book includes Neuman's autobiography and the history of the evolution of the Neuman Systems Model.

The Neuman Systems Model was developed in response to expressed needs of graduate students at the School of Nursing, University of California, Los Angeles, for course content that would present the breadth of nursing problems prior to content emphasizing specific nursing problem areas (Neuman & Young, 1972). Neuman (1985) claimed she had no intention of creating a specific conceptual model for the nursing community when she developed her model. It is, however, interesting to note that her model was formulated at the time when several other conceptual models of nursing had just been published (e.g., King, 1971; Orem, 1971; Rogers, 1970). Moreover, as Peterson (1977) pointed out, this was the time when the criteria for National League for Nursing accreditation first stipulated that nursing education programs should be based on conceptual models.

Neuman (in press) maintained that her model is a comprehensive, holistic view of the client system, including individuals, groups, communities, and society. Although Neuman (1974) asserted that nursing is a unique profession, she considered her model "appropriate for providers of health care in disciplines other than nursing" (p. 99).

The Neuman Systems Model is based on open systems thinking. Neuman (in press) asserted that "The systems concept adequately provides the most tangible structure within which the plethora of phenomena in nursing can be dealt with to meet its desired goal of client/client system stability." Neuman (in press) noted that the following statements are the assumptions of her conceptual model:

1. Though each individual client or group as a client system is unique, each system is a composite of common known factors or innate characteristics within a normal, given range of response, contained within a basic structure.

2. Many known, unknown, and universal stressors exist. Each differs in its potential for disturbing a client's stability or normal line of defense. The particular interrelationship of client variables—physiological, psychological, sociocultural, developmental, and spiritual—at any point in time can affect the degree to which a client is protected by the flexible line of defense against possible reaction to a single stressor or combination of stressors.

3. Each individual client/client system, over time, has evolved a normal range of response to the environment which is referred to as a normal line of defense or usual wellness/stability state.

4. When the cushioning, accordion-like effect of the flexible line of defense is no longer capable of protecting the client/client system against an environmental stressor, the stressor breaks through the normal line of defense. The interrelationship of variables . . . determines the nature and degree of the system reaction or possible reaction to the stressor.

5. The client in a state of wellness or illness is a dynamic composite of the interrelationship of variables. . . . Wellness is on a continuum of available energy to support the system in its optimal state.

6. Implicit within each client system is a set of internal resistance factors known as lines of resistance, which function to stabilize and return the client to the usual wellness state (normal line of defense) or stability following an environmental stressor reaction.

7. Primary prevention relates to general knowledge that is applied in client assessment/intervention in identification and reduction or mitigation of risk factors associated with environmental stressors.

8. Secondary prevention relates to symptomatology following a reaction to stressors, appropriate ranking of intervention priorities, and treatment to reduce symptoms.

9. Tertiary prevention relates to the adjustive processes taking place as reconstitution begins and the maintenance factors that move the client back in a circular manner toward primary prevention.

Neuman (1974, 1985) stated that her conceptual model arose from observations made during her clinical experiences in mental health nursing, as well as from a synthesis of knowledge from several other disciplines. The model is derived from Chardin's (1955) philosophical beliefs about the wholeness of life, Marxist philosophical views of the oneness of man and nature (Cornu, 1957), Gestalt and field theories of the interaction between person and environment (Edelson, 1970), general system theory of the nature of living open systems (Bertalanffy, 1968), Putt's (1972) ideas of entropy and evolution in systems, Selye's (1950) conceptualization of stress, and Caplan's (1964) formulation of levels of prevention. Thus, both inductive and deductive strategies were used to develop this conceptual model.

Content of the Model: Concepts

Person

The person in Neuman's conceptual model is defined as a client/ client system that is a composite of physiological, psychological, sociocultural, developmental, and spiritual variables. The term client is used "because it honors respect for the client, caregiver collaborative relationships, and wellness perspectives of the model" (Neuman, in press). The client system is viewed as an open system in interaction with the environment. Physiological variables refer to bodily structure and function; psychological variables refer to mental processes and relationships; sociocultural variables refer to social and cultural functions; developmental variables refer to the developmental processes of life; and spiritual variables refer to aspects of spirituality. Neuman (in press) noted that the client may never recognize or develop the spiritual variables, although they permeate all other client system variables. Spiritual variables are viewed as a continuum from complete unawareness or denial to a consciously developed high level of spiritual understanding. The five variable areas are interrelated in each client system. Ideally, the variables function harmoniously in relation to environmental stressor influences. Furthermore, Neuman (in press) noted that although all five variable areas are encompassed by each client system, they exhibit "varying degrees of development and a wide range of interactive styles and potential."

As illustrated in Figure 6–1, the client/client system is depicted as a central core surrounded by concentric rings. The central core is a basic structure of survival factors "common to the species, such as variables contained within, innate or genetic factors, and strength and weakness of the system parts" (Neuman, in press). When the client is the individual, the basic survival factors are exemplified by temperature range, genetic response patterns, ego structure, and strengths and weaknesses of body organs. Certain unique features or baseline char-

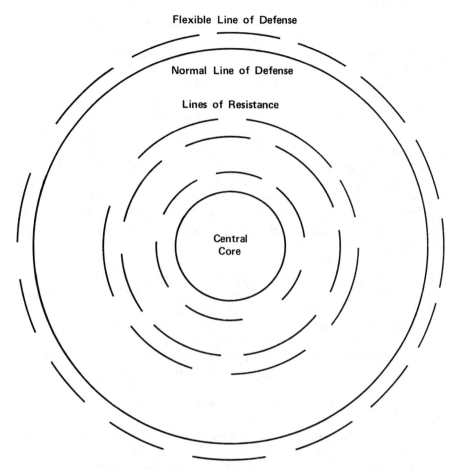

Figure 6–1.   Graphic representation of the client system. (Adapted from Neuman, B & Young, RJ (1972). A model for teaching total person approach to patient problems. Nursing Research, 21, 265.)

acteristics, such as cognitive ability, also are contained within the central core (Neuman, in press). Thus, the five variable areas—physiological, psychological, sociocultural, developmental, and spiritual—are part of the basic structure (Neuman, 1985).

The concentric rings shown in Figure 6–1 represent three mechanisms that protect the basic structure. The outermost ring is the flexible line of defense. This mechanism is a protective buffer for the client's normal or stable state. Ideally, it prevents invasion of stressors and keeps the client system free from stressor reactions or symptomatology. The flexible line of defense is thought of as a dynamic accordion-like mechanism, rapidly expanding away from or drawing closer to the normal line of defense. When the flexible line has expanded away from the normal line of defense, greater protection against stressor invasion is provided; when it draws closer to the normal line, less protection is provided (Neuman, in press).

The normal line of defense lies between the flexible line of defense and the lines of resistance. This second protective mechanism is the client/client system's normal or usual wellness state. It reflects "what the client has become or evolved to over time [and] is the result of adjustment between client system variables and environmental stressors" (Neuman, in press). In effect, the normal line of defense is a standard against which variances from wellness can be judged. The normal line of defense, like the flexible line, can expand or contract, but apparently does so more slowly. Expansion of the normal line of defense reflects an enhanced wellness state; contraction, a diminished state of wellness (Neuman, in press).

The innermost concentric rings are the line of resistance. This third protective mechanism is involuntarily activated when a stressor invades the normal line of defense. The lines of resistance attempt to stabilize the client system and foster a return to the normal line of defense. These lines contain internal factors that support the basic structure and the normal line of defense, such as mobilization of white blood cells. If the lines of resistance are effective, the system can reconstitute; if they are ineffective, death may ensue (Neuman, 1985, in press).

Neuman (1985) explained that the flexible line of defense protects the normal line of defense, and the lines of resistance protect the basic structure. The flexible line of defense is immediately called into action when the client system encounters a stressor and attempts to maintain stability. If the flexible line of defense is not effective, the normal line of defense breaks down and a stressor reaction, or symptoms, occurs. The lines of resistance then are activated and, if effective, pull the client back toward wellness. The condition of the flexible line of defense, then, determines whether a reaction is likely when a stressor is encountered.

More specifically, the client/client system's reaction to a stressor is determined in part by natural and learned resistance, which is manifested by the strength of the flexible and normal lines of defense and the lines of resistance. The amount of resistance, in turn, is determined by the interrelationship of the five variable areas of the client system. Reaction also is determined by the time of encounter with a stressor, as well as by its nature and intensity. Other factors influencing reaction to a stressor include idiosyncrasies in the basic structure, past and present conditions of the client system, available energy resources, the amount of energy required for adaptation, and the client system's perception of the stressor (Neuman, 1974, 1985, in press).

Environment

Neuman (1974) identified man and environment as the basic phenomena of her conceptual model. Indeed, "consideration of environment is critical since health and wellness vary as to needs, predisposition, perception and goals of all identifiable systems; environment is that viable arena which has relevance to the life space of the system" (Neuman, in press). Environment is defined as "all internal and external factors or influences surrounding the identified client/client system" (Neuman, in press). The relationship between the client/client system and the environment is reciprocal. "Input, output and feedback between the client and environment is of a circular nature [such that] the client may influence or be influenced by environmental forces" (Neuman, in press). Three relevant environments have been identified by Neuman (in press). The internal environment "consists of all forces or interactive influences internal to or contained solely within the boundaries of the defined client/client system." It is intrapersonal in nature. The external environment "consists of all forces or interaction influences external to or existing outside the defined client/client system" and is interpersonal and extrapersonal in nature. The created-environment is subconsciously developed by the client as "a symbolic expression of system wholeness." It is intrapersonal, interpersonal, and extrapersonal in nature. The created-environment supersedes and encompasses both internal and external environments. Neuman (in press) went on to explain that the created-environment

> acts as an immediate or long range "safe" reservoir for existence or maintenance of system integrity expressed either consciously, unconsciously, or both simultaneously. The created-environment is dynamic and represents the client's subconscious mobilization of all system variables including the basic structure energy factors, toward system integration, stability and integrity. It is inherently purposeful, though subconsciously developed, since its function is to offer a protective shield or safe arena for system function. It pervades all systems, large and small, to at least some degree; it is either spontaneously created, increased or decreased as warranted for the need condition of an especially created-environment. . . . All basic structure factors and system variables influence or are influenced by the created-environment, which is developed and maintained, in varying degrees of protectiveness, at any given point in time. . . . The created-environment is based on the unseen unconscious knowledge, self esteem and belief influences, energy exchanges, system variables and predisposition; it is a process based concept of perpetual adjustment within which a client may either increase or decrease the wellness state.

Neuman (in press) drew from Selye's (1950) work to define stressors as "tension producing stimuli or forces occurring both within the internal and external environmental boundaries of the client/client system." She classified stressors as intrapersonal, interpersonal, and extrapersonal. Intrapersonal stressors are within the internal environment of the client/client system and include forces such as conditioned and autoimmune responses. Interpersonal stressors are in the external environment. They occur at the boundary between the client/client system and the proximal external environment and include forces such as role expectations and communication patterns. Extrapersonal stressors also are in the external environment. They occur at the boundary of the client/client system and the distal external environment and include forces such as financial concerns or social policies. Neuman (1985) maintained that stressors are neutral, but the outcome of an encounter with a stressor may be beneficial or noxious, positive or negative.

Health

Neuman (in press) equated health with wellness and defined it as the condition of optimal stability of the client/client system. Optimal system stability, she explained, "is the best possible health state at any given point in time." Neuman described optimal system stability as "the condition in which all . . . system variables are in balance or harmony with the whole of the client/client system." She went on to say that health "is reflected in the level of wellness. When system needs are met, a state of optimal wellness exists, conversely, unmet needs reduce the wellness state."

The emphasis in Neuman's conceptual model is on wellness. Although she used the term illness, she more frequently spoke of variance from wellness, which she described as "the difference from the normal or usual wellness condition" (Neuman, in press). A variance from wellness is determined by comparing the normal health state with what is taking place at a given time (Neuman, 1985).

Reconstitution occurs after the person's reaction to stressors. More specifically, reconstitution involves the "return and maintenance of system stability following treatment of stressor reaction" (Neuman, in press). If reconstitution does not occur, death ensues. Reconstitution can lead to client system stability and a level of wellness that is the same as it was prior to the stressor reaction, progress to a higher than usual wellness level, or result in a lower than usual wellness level. Health of the client/client system, therefore, "is envisioned as being at various and changing levels, within normal range, higher or lower, throughout the life span, due to basic structure factors and satisfactory adjustment or lack of it to environmental stressors" (Neuman, in press).

Neuman (in press) placed health or wellness on a continuum "dichotomous with illness." Drawing from Putt's (1972) view of systems thinking, Neuman noted that the wellness-illness continuum

> implies that energy flow is continuous between the client system and environment. To conceptualize wellness, then, is to determine actual or possible effects of stressor invasion in terms of existing client system energy levels as follows: client movement is toward negentropy when more energy is being generated than used; when more energy is required than is being generated, movement is toward entropy or illness, or possible death.

Drawing further from systems thinking, Neuman (in press) also described health as "a continuum from wellness to illness." She went on to say that wellness and illness "are dichotomous in that Wellness is considered to be a state of saturation or inertness—one free of disrupting needs—while Illness is a state of insufficiency—disrupting needs are yet to be satisfied." Moreover, Neuman equated wellness with negentropy and illness with entropy.

Nursing

Neuman (1974) viewed nursing as a "unique profession" that "is concerned with all the variables affecting an individual's response to stressors" (p. 102). The major concern for nursing is "keeping the client system stable through accuracy in both assessment of effects and possible effects of environmental stressors and assisting client adjustments required for an optimal wellness level" (Neuman, in press).

The goal of nursing, according to Neuman (in press), is "to facilitate for the client, optimal wellness through either retention, attainment or maintenance of client system stability." More specifically, the goal of nursing actions is "to assist the client in creating and shaping reality in a desired direction, related to retention, attainment and/or maintenance of optimal system wellness through purposeful interventions . . . directed at mitigation or reduction of stress factors and adverse conditions which affect or could affect optimal client functioning, at any given point in time."

Neuman (in press) presented a nursing process format that encompasses three steps or categories: nursing diagnosis, nursing goals, and nursing outcomes. The first step, nursing diagnosis, includes acquisition of an appropriate data base that identifies, assesses, classifies, and evaluates the dynamic interactions among the physiological, psychological, sociocultural, developmental, and spiritual variables comprising the client system. This step of the nursing process takes into account the perceptions of both the client and the caregiver. Neuman (in press) underscored this point by identifying the following considerations to be taken into account when collecting data: (1)

proper assessment includes knowledge of all factors influencing a client's perceptual field, and (2) the meaning of a stressor should be validated by both client and caregiver. Neuman added that when these considerations are taken into account, "factors within the caregiver's perceptual field influencing assessment of the client situation should become apparent."

The first step of the nursing process is concluded when a nursing diagnostic statement is formulated. This statement includes identification of actual or potential variances from wellness and available resources, as well as identification of hypothetical interventions postulated to assist the client reach the desired system stability or wellness level. The diagnostic statement is based on a synthesis of client data and relevant theory. Neuman (in press) recommended that the diagnostic statement use "available and relevant diagnostic nomenclature, adding to it as required."

The second step of the nursing process is the formulation of nursing goals, which are negotiated with the client for desired prescriptive changes to correct variances from wellness. Intervention strategies postulated to retain, attain, and/or maintain client system stability also are formulated at this time. The second step, then, encompasses specification of outcome goals and intervention strategies designed to achieve the goals.

The third nursing process step is nursing outcomes. Intervention strategies, using one or more prevention as intervention modalities, are implemented at this step. Neuman's (in press) prevention as intervention format specifies three modalities. Primary prevention is described as the action required to retain client system stability. Secondary prevention is the action required to attain system stability. And tertiary prevention is the action required to maintain system stability.

Neuman (in press) stated that "intervention can begin at any point at which a stressor is either suspected or identified." Intervention involving primary prevention is selected when the risk of or hazard from a stressor is known but a reaction has not yet occurred. Interventions attempt to reduce the possibility of the client's encounter with the stressor or strengthen the flexible line of defense to decrease the possibility of a reaction when the stressor is encountered. Health promotion, according to Neuman (in press), is a component of primary prevention, "with the basic purpose of preventing illness by increasing the wellness potential."

Intervention involving secondary prevention is selected when a reaction to a stressor has already occurred. Interventions deal with existing symptoms and attempt to strengthen the lines of resistance through use of the client's internal and external resources. Neuman (1974) introduced the idea of priorities in this prevention modality by stating, "ranking of need priority can occur . . . only by proper assessment of internal as well as external resources, that is, getting at the total meaning of the experience for the individual" (p. 105). If secondary prevention interventions are effective, reconstitution occurs. If they are not effective, "death occurs as a result of failure of the basic structure" (Neuman, in press).

Intervention involving tertiary prevention is selected when some degree of client system stability and reconstitution has occurred following secondary prevention interventions. Tertiary prevention interventions maintain reconstitution when client resources are mobilized to prevent additional reactions to stressors or regression from the current wellness level. Neuman (in press) pointed out that "tertiary prevention tends to lead back, in circular fashion, toward primary prevention."

Neuman (in press) pointed out that the prevention as intervention modalities represents a typology of nursing care that identifies the client's entry point into the health care system as well as the type of intervention needed. She also pointed out that more than one prevention modality may be used simultaneously if the client's condition warrants multi-level intervention.

The final step of the nursing process concludes when the results of intervention, termed outcome goals, are evaluated to confirm their attainment or to guide reformulation of nursing goals. The entire nursing process format for Neuman's model is presented in Table 6–1. This table incorporates Neuman's nursing process format and prevention as intervention format.

Neuman's (in press) approach to nursing process reflects systems thinking. She stated, "Using a systems holistic approach to protect and promote client welfare, nursing action must be skillfully related to the meaningful and dynamic organization of . . . the whole." She went on to say, "Both system processes and nursing actions are purposeful and goal directed. That is, nursing vigorously attempts to control variables affecting client care."

TABLE 6–1.   The Neuman Systems Model: Nursing Process Format

I. Nursing diagnosis determined by
   A. Data base that includes the simultaneous consideration of the dynamic interactions of physiological, psychological, sociocultural, developmental, and spiritual variables in the areas of
      1. Identification and evaluation of potential or actual stressors that pose a threat to the stability of the client system
      2. Assessment of condition and strength of basic structure factors and energy resources
         a. Collect biographic data
         b. Identify referral source

TABLE 6–1. *Continued*

3. Assessment of characteristics of the flexible and normal lines of defense, lines of resistance, degree of potential reaction, reaction, and/or potential for reconstitution following a reaction
4. Identification, classification, and evaluation of potential and/or actual intrapersonal, interpersonal, and extrapersonal interactions between the client and the environment, considering all five variable areas
5. Evaluation of past, present, and possible future life process and coping patterns influence on client system stability
6. Identification and evaluation of actual and potential internal and external resources for optimal state of wellness
7. Identification and resolution of perceptual differences between care-givers and client system
   a. Assess client's perception of stressors
      (1) Identify client's major problem, stress area, or areas of concern
      (2) Identify client's perceptions of how present circumstances differ from usual pattern of living
      (3) Identify ways in which client handled similar problems in the past
      (4) Identify what client anticipates for self in the future as a consequence of the present situation
      (5) Determine what client is doing and what he or she can do to help himself or herself
      (6) Determine what client expects care-givers, family, friends, or others to do for him or her
   b. Assess care-giver's perception of stressor (repeat 7.a.(1)–(6) from care-giver's perspective)
B. Variances from wellness determined by considering that
   1. Synthesis of theory with the data base allows for client problem definition and prioritization, determination of client system level of wellness, system stability needs, and total available resources to accomplish desired outcomes
   2. Hypothetical interventions are postulated to reach the desired client stability or wellness level, i.e., to maintain the flexible and normal lines of defense
II. Nursing goals determined by
   A. Negotiation with the client for desired prescriptive change to correct variances from wellness, based on classified needs and resources identified in the nursing diagnosis
   B. Appropriate intervention strategies that are postulated for retention, attainment and/or maintenance of client system stability as desired outcome goals
III. Nursing outcomes determined by
   A. Nursing intervention that is accomplished through use of one or more of three prevention modes—primary prevention (action to retain system stability), secondary prevention (action to attain system stability), tertiary prevention (action to maintain system stability, usually following secondary prevention)
      1. Nursing actions in primary prevention
         a. Classify stressors as to client system threat to stability and prevent stressor invasion

TABLE 6–1. *Continued*

b. Provide information to maintain or strengthen existing client system strengths
c. Support positive coping and functioning
d. Desensitize existing or possible noxious stressors
e. Motivate toward wellness
f. Coordinate/integrate interdisciplinary theories and epidemiological input
g. Educate/reeducate
h. Use stress as a positive intervention strategy
2. Nursing actions in secondary prevention
a. Following stressor invasion, protect basic structure
b. Mobilize and maximize internal/external resources toward stability and energy conservation
c. Facilitate purposeful manipulation of stressors and reactions to stressors
d. Motivate, educate, and involve client system in health care goals
e. Facilitate appropriate treatment/intervention measures
f. Promote advocacy by coordination/integration
g. Provide primary prevention/intervention as required
3. Nursing actions in tertiary prevention
a. During reconstitution, attain/maintain maximum level of wellness and stability
b. Educate, reeducate, and/or reorient as needed
c. Support client system in appropriate goal directedness and change efforts
d. Coordinate and integrate health service resources
e. Provide primary and/or secondary prevention/intervention as needed
B. Evaluation of outcome goals following intervention, which either confirms outcome goals or serves as a basis for reformulation of subsequent nursing goals
C. Intermediate and long-range goals for subsequent nursing action that are structured in relation to short-term goal outcomes
D. Client outcome that validates the nursing process

Adapted from Neuman, B. (1982). The Neuman Systems Model: Application to nursing education and practice (pp. 18–28). Norwalk, CT: Appleton-Century-Crofts.

Content of the Model: Propositions

The relationship between the person and the environment is mentioned repeatedly in the Neuman Systems Model. The reciprocal nature of this relationship is seen in the following quotations:

> The client is an interacting open system in total interface with both internal and external environmental forces or stressors. The client is viewed as in constant change, with reciprocal environmental interaction and at all times moving toward either a dynamic state of wellness or illness in varying degrees. (Neuman, in press)

> The client is a system capable of both input and output related to the intra-, inter-, and extrapersonal environmental influences; interacting with the environment by adjusting to it or adjusting the environment to itself, as a system. The process of interaction and adjustment results in varying degrees of harmony, stability or balance between the client and environment. Ideally, it is one of optimal client system stability. (Neuman, in press)

The relationship between person, environment, and nursing is exemplified by the comment that nursing is concerned with "keeping the client system stable through accuracy in both assessment of effects and possible effects of environmental stressors" (Neuman, in press).

All four metaparadigm concepts—person, environment, health, and nursing—are linked in Neuman's statements about primary, secondary, and tertiary prevention. Although environment is more implicit than explicit in these statements, it is taken into account. Indeed, as Neuman (in press) pointed out, "In keeping the systems stable, the nurse creates a linkage between the client, environment, health and nursing." The linkages are reflected in the following quotations:

> The *Primary Prevention as Intervention* modality is used for *Primary Prevention as wellness retention,* that is, to protect the client system normal line of defense or usual wellness state by strengthening the flexible line of defense. The *goal* is to promote client wellness by stress prevention and reduction of risk factors. (Neuman, in press)

> The *Secondary Prevention as Intervention* modality is used for *Secondary Prevention as wellness attainment,* that is, to protect the basic structure by strengthening the internal lines of resistance. The *goal* is to provide appropriate treatment of symptoms to attain optimal client system stability or wellness and energy conservation. (Neuman, in press)

> The *Tertiary Prevention as Intervention* modality is used for *Tertiary Prevention as wellness maintenance,* that is, to protect client system reconstitution or wellness level following treatment. Reconstitution may be viewed as feedback from the input/output of secondary intervention. The *goal* is maintenance of an optimal wellness level by supporting existing strengths and conservation of client system energy. (Neuman, in press)

Areas of Concern

The areas of concern or problems that Neuman's conceptual model addresses are reactions to stressors, variances from wellness, and retention, attainment, and maintenance of client system stability. The sources of these problems are the intrapersonal, interpersonal, and extrapersonal stressors arising in the internal and external environments. Indeed, Neuman (1985) commented that problems originate in internal and external environmental stressors and the client's response to those stressors.

EVALUATION OF NEUMAN'S SYSTEMS MODEL

This section presents an evaluation of Neuman's conceptual model. The evaluation is based on the results of the analysis, as well as publications and presentations by others who have used or commented on this conceptual model.

Explication of Assumptions

Neuman (in press) explicitly identified assumptions underlying her conceptual model. These assumptions indicate that Neuman values a holistic, systems based approach to the care of clients. Neuman's choice of a systems approach to health care reflects her assumption that systems thinking is a comprehensive way of viewing clients and their environments.

Neuman also values intervention prior to manifestations of variances from wellness, as well as after these occur. She emphasized the need to consider both the client's and the caregiver's perceptions of stressors. Furthermore, she assumes that nursing goals are established effectively when negotiated with the client. These aspects of the conceptual model indicate her respect for the perceptions and rights of each client. In fact, she deliberately labeled the person as a client to denote her respect for those for whom nurses care and her concern for collaborative goal setting. Furthermore, Neuman values wellness. In fact, Neuman (in press) regards her work as "a wellness model."

Neuman assumes that the environment is the source of stressors. But she regards stressors as neutral. The outcome of encounters with stressors is what has a negative or positive valence.

It should be noted that the nine statements Neuman (in press) identified as the assumptions of her conceptual model are propositions that define, describe, and link the concepts of the model. Strictly speaking, then, these statements are not assumptions upon which the model was based.

Comprehensiveness of Concepts and Propositions

The revisions and refinements evident in Neuman's (in press) most recent version of her conceptual model have clarified several areas of confusion found in earlier versions of the model and have improved the adequacy of concept definitions and descriptions. The revisions and refinements certainly suggest that Neuman has been responsive to critiques of her work, such as the chapter on analysis and evaluation of the model by Fawcett and colleagues (1982) published in the first edition of Neuman's book. Indeed, Stevens (1982) commended Neuman for the scholarly attitude and scientific detachment demonstrated by inclusion of the critique in the book.

Given the abstract and general nature of conceptual models, Neuman's descriptions of the person, the environment, health, and nursing are generally adequate. The concept of health, however, could be clarified with regard to Neuman's (in press) view of wellness and illness as a continuum and a dichotomy. Given Neuman's apparent emphasis on a continuum, it would be more appropriate to identify wellness and illness as the polar ends of the continuum, rather than dichotomous conditions. Another aspect of health that could be clarified is Neuman's view of wellness as negentropy and illness as entropy. This is because general system theory, upon which Neuman based a substantial portion of her model, views the living open system as negentropic. Entropy, according to Bertalanffy (1968), is a characteristic only of closed systems.

Neuman's description of the nursing process generally meets the criteria proposed by Walker and Nicholson (1980). Nursing diagnoses are based on knowledge derived from a synthesis of theory with the data base of client factors. The nursing process is dynamic in that evaluation of outcomes either confirms goals or serves as a basis for reformulation of new goals. Neuman does not, however, provide for continual movement from collection of data base factors to tentative diagnoses and back to collection of data. As is seen in the section on social utility, the nursing process is useful in a variety of situations. Moreover, the emphasis on the client's view of the situation and the negotiation needed for identification of appropriate interventions reflects a concern for ethical standards. Finally, the entire conceptual model is based on reputable scientific findings from several disciplines.

The statements linking person, environment, health, and nursing leave no gaps among these concepts. As seen in the analysis section, Neuman's statements about primary, secondary, and tertiary prevention provide the required general linkages among the concepts of the model.

Logical Congruence

World Views

The Neuman Systems Model reflects a primarily organismic world view. This view of the world is represented by Neuman's use of Gestalt and field theories, as well as philosophies that emphasize the unity of the person. Neuman's holistic approach also reflects this view of the world. Holism, according to Neuman (in press), is implicit in the conceptual model. She considered holism as "both a philosophical and biological concept, implying relationships, processes, interactions, wholeness, dynamic freedom and creativity in adjusting to stress in both the internal and external environment." Moreover, Neuman viewed the client system as active, in that it has the ability to adjust the environment to itself.

Furthermore, although Neuman identified five different variables comprising the client (physiological, psychological, sociocultural, developmental, and spiritual), she emphasized the need to consider all of them at any given time. To underscore this, Neuman (1974) stated, "the wholeness concept . . . is based upon the appropriate interrelationship of variables" (p. 103).

Though the primary focus of the Neuman Systems Model is the organismic view, mechanism is introduced in Neuman's description of the created-environment as a conscious and unconscious structure, which implies a psychoanalytic orientation. Mechanism also is introduced with Neuman's use of Selye's (1950) mechanistic theory of stress and adaptation and her view of illness as entropy. Logical translation of the contrasting and incompatible mechanistic ideas in the model is required. This could be accomplished by rethinking the created-environment, by incorporating a more dynamic view of stress than Selye's such as Lazarus's (1981) notions of stress and coping, and by redefining illness within an open systems perspective.

Neuman's emphasis on client system stability seems to reflect the persistence view of the world. This view also is reflected in the focus on protection of the central core of the client system by the various lines of defense and resistance. These lines serve to minimize changes and maximize stability.

However, Neuman's conceptual model also reflects the change view of the world. This is noted in Neuman's (in press) contention that "the client is viewed as in constant change." This statement suggests that Neuman does not regard change as necessary only for survival, but as a continual part of life. Logical translation of the incompatible views of stability and change are required.

Classification of the Model

Neuman's conceptual model clearly fits within the systems category of conceptual models (Marriner, 1986; Riehl & Roy, 1980; Stevens, 1984). Neuman (personal communication, November 6 and 13, 1980) commented that she did not take classification into account when formulating her model, but that she now agrees this is the appropriate category. In fact, she recently stated, "The Neuman Systems

Model is an open systems model that views nursing as primarily concerned with appropriate nursing action in relation to reactions or possible reactions of the client and client system" (Neuman, in press).

The Neuman Systems Model addresses system in the discussion of the person. The definition of person as an interacting open client system that is a dynamic composite of the interrelationship of physiological, psychological, sociocultural, developmental, and spiritual variables fits the requirement that a systems view treats phenomena as organized, integrated entities. The model addresses environment in detail, with descriptions of the internal, external, and created environments. Moreover, the internal and external environments are the source of stressors that influence the client system.

Neuman (in press) maintained that boundary must be described for each client system. She explained, "The Neuman Systems Model considers the 'client' as a system whether it is defined as one or many, proximal or distal. This implies that each system boundary must be identified or defined as well as the parts contained within it." In general, the flexible line of defense is the boundary between the client system and environmental stressors. Boundary permeability is considered in Neuman's discussion of factors that influence stressor invasion and reactions to stressors.

Neuman's discussion of environmental stressors encompasses the systems models characteristic of tension, stress, strain, and conflict. Neuman (in press) explicitly identified stressors as the forces that operate within or upon the system.

Neuman (in press) views client system stability as a steady state. More specifically, the normal line of defense is regarded as analogous to the steady state of systems thinking.

The systems characteristic of feedback is addressed in Neuman's (in press) discussion of client system processes. She stated, "Feedback of output into input makes the system self-regulated in relation to either maintenance of a desired health state or goal outcome."

Although Neuman's model includes developmental variables, they are viewed as changes in the client system over time. Thus, there is no evidence of logical incompatibility with regard to different categories of models.

Meleis (1985) did not classify Neuman's model. Stevens (1984) considered the model within the systems category; she did not place it within her classification scheme of intervention, substitution, conservation, sustenance, and enhancement categories.

Generation and Testing of Theory

No empirically testable theories have yet been derived directly from the Neuman Systems Model. Neuman (in press) recently stated that she and her colleague, Audrey Koertvelyessy, "jointly identified the major theory for the model . . . as the *Theory of Optimal Client System Stability*." She went on to say, "Several other theories are inherent within the model which could be clarified with the goal of optimizing health for the client." Neuman did not identify any concepts or propositions for the theory of optimal client system stability, nor did she provide any direction for generation of other theories.

Although Neuman did not identify it as such, her proposition of prevention as intervention could be considered the beginning of a theory. She postulated that modes of intervention are structured within primary, secondary, and tertiary prevention, and that these prevention modes facilitate the integrative processes necessary to attain and maintain client system stability. The concepts of this theory must be operationally defined and linked by specific propositions before it can be empirically tested.

Hoffman (1982) has begun the task of operationally defining the concepts of the Neuman Systems Model. For example, she proposed that one possible definition of internal environment could be strength or weakness of various body parts or organs. Hoffman's attempt is a noteworthy first step, but it fails to identify the methods needed to empirically measure the concepts. Measurement of strength or weakness of body parts, for example, must be described in observable terms if the concept of internal environment is to be empirically tested.

Ziemer's (1983) study of the effects of preoperative information on postoperative recovery of abdominal surgery patients was based on Neuman's conceptual model. Ziemer used surgery to represent a stressor; the reported frequency of coping behaviors to represent lines of defense; provision of information to represent primary prevention; and pain intensity, distress, and the presence of symptoms indicating complications of surgery to represent impact of stressors. The theoretical structure for the study was developed from theories of stress and coping borrowed from other disciplines. Study findings did not support the conceptual model level proposition that primary prevention, in the form of preoperative information, would decrease the impact of stressors. Although the validity of Ziemer's measures of stressor impact must be questioned, the results of this study suggest that a basic proposition of Neuman's model may not be credible.

Social Considerations

Social Congruence

The Neuman Systems Model is generally congruent with current societal expectations of nursing care. The present emphasis on primary prevention seen in the news media and in numerous self-help books and articles is increasing consumers' awareness of the contributions of all health care workers, including nurses, to promotion of wellness and prevention of illness. As more nurses move into ambulatory care settings, their roles in primary prevention should become a typical expectation of consumers. Indeed, Neuman (in press) commented, "Primary Prevention as Intervention is an expanding futuristic concept with which the nursing field must become increasingly concerned. It has unlimited potential for major role development which could shape the future image of nursing."

The fact that Neuman's conceptual model emphasizes consideration of the client's perspective and negotiation of nursing goals between client and caregiver enhances its congruence with those members of society who desire input into their care. However, this emphasis may limit congruence with expectations of those who do not expect or desire to play a part in their care, such as people of some middle-eastern cultures (Meleis, 1985).

Social Significance

The social significance of the Neuman Systems Model is beginning to be established. Hoch (1987) studied the effects of a treatment protocol derived from Neuman's conceptual model on depression and life satisfaction in a sample of retired individuals. She found that the Neuman protocol group had lower depression scores and higher life satisfaction scores than a control group who received nursing intervention not based on an explicit conceptual model.

Social Utility

The social utility of the Neuman Systems Model is thoroughly documented. Two books contain numerous examples of the use of this conceptual model in nursing education, practice, administration, and research (Neuman, 1982, in press). This conceptual model is being used by nurses in the United States, Canada, England, Wales, Denmark, Sweden, Portugal, Australia, Puerto Rico, Costa Rica, Taiwan, and South Korea. The first International Nursing Symposium on the Neuman Systems Model, sponsored by Neumann College, was held in November 1986 in Aston, Pennsylvania. The Second International Symposium, sponsored by the Neuman Systems Model Trustee Group, was held in Kansas City, Missouri, in October 1988. Lists of schools of nursing that use Neuman's conceptual model were compiled by Asay and Ossler (1984), Hermiz and Meininger (1986), and Neuman (in press). Lists of clinical agencies using the model are available in Hermiz and Meininger and in Neuman. Research based on the model was identified by Neuman.

The concepts and propositions of the Neuman Systems Model are beginning to provide guidelines for nursing research, and rules for research are beginning to be formulated. Neuman (1985) indicated that the model lends itself to both inductive and deductive research and that theories can be directly derived from the model or existing theories can be linked to it. These research rules require further specification, and other rules have to be developed.

Some reports of research based on Neuman's conceptual model are available. Ziegler (1982) discussed a descriptive-formative/summative evaluation study dealing with utilization of a nursing diagnosis taxonomy deduced from the Neuman Systems Model. Ziemer (1983) used concepts of the conceptual model to guide her study of the effects of preoperative information on postoperative recovery. Capers (1987) used Neuman's model to guide her study of the relationship between cultural variables and perceptions of problematical behavior held by lay black adults and black and white registered nurses. Burritt (1988) used Neuman's model to guide her investigation of the effects of social support on the relationships between job stress and job satisfaction and job performance. Wilson (1987) used Neuman's model as a guide for her study of the relationship between patients' psychological responses to the surgical intensive care unit and their identification of stressors.

The utility of Neuman's conceptual model for nursing practice is well documented. Some rules for practice may be extracted from the model. Clearly, the purpose of nursing practice is to assist clients to retain, attain, or maintain optimal system stability. Clinical problems of interest are those related to actual or potential reactions to stressors. The nursing process is described as the three step format of nursing diagnosis, nursing goals, and nursing outcomes. Interventions take the form of primary, secondary, and tertiary prevention. An assessment/intervention tool was presented by Neuman (in press), along with directions for its use.

A major focus of Neuman's (1982, in press) books is use of the model as a guide for clinical nursing practice. The first edition of the book included several descriptions of the model in various clinical situations. Goldblum-Graff and Graff (1982) adapted the model to family therapy by linking its concepts and propositions to those of a theory of contextual family therapy. Benedict and Sproles (1982) applied the model to general nursing health care delivery in community settings. In doing so, they added the following basic premise to Neuman's assumptions:

> A population possesses characteristics reflective of the community as an entity in itself. These characteristics usually are represented as group-specific tendencies. They define a population-at-risk or determine a priority high-risk group. Just as there are common "knowns"

for all individuals and their response ranges, so too there are separate sets of commonalities for health risk populations and/or subgroups such as the aged, the worker, or the handicapped. (p. 224)

Baker (1982b) used the model to plan secondary and tertiary nursing care related to the psychological needs of patients with chronic obstructive pulmonary disease. She based the care on concepts of the model as well as knowledge of the physiological and psychological aspects of COPD. Echlin (1982) described use of Neuman's model to guide the palliative care provided for patients at the Hospice of Windsor, in Ontario, Canada.

Another use of the model in nursing practice was described by Ziegler (1982). Along with other faculty members at Texas Woman's University, she developed a computerized taxonomy of nursing diagnoses deduced from Neuman's conceptual model. The following category sets were used for the taxonomy:

1. The responding subsystem: psychological, physiological, sociocultural
2. The system being diagnosed: individual, family, group or community.
3. The level of response: primary, secondary, and tertiary.
4. The source of the stressor etiology: intrasystem, intersystem, and extrasystem.
5. The type of stressor etiology: physiological, psychological, and sociocultural. (Ziegler, 1982, p. 57)

Other publications dealing with the use of Neuman's conceptual model describe the care of clients with hypertension (Johnson, 1983; Utz, 1980); acute spinal cord injuries (Sullivan, 1986); myocardial infarction (Fawcett, et al., 1987; Ross & Bourbonnais, 1985); cerebral aneurysm (Fawcett, et al., 1987); as well as applications in mental health, community health, and medical-surgical settings (Beitler, Tkachuck, & Aamodt, 1980); in rehabilitation settings (Cunningham, 1983); and in emergency nursing practice (Redheffer, 1985).

Neuman's conceptual model also has been extended for use with families and communities. Neuman (1983a, 1983b) explained how the conceptual model is used with families and described its use to guide care of a Mexican-American family following discharge of two daughters from a state mental institution. Anderson, McFarlane, and Helton (1986) adapted Neuman's model for use in community health nursing, with the community regarded as the client. And Buchanan (1987) modified Neuman's model for use with aggregates, families, and the community.

Other applications of the model are described in several chapters in Neuman's (1982) book written by nursing students who used the model as a guide for their activities in a variety of educational and clinical practice settings. Still other applications of the model to various nursing situations are described in the second edition of Neuman's (in press) book.

The utility of the Neuman Systems Model for nursing education also is well documented. Rules for education are being formulated. Mirenda's (1986) description of use of Neuman's model to guide curriculum development indicates that the curriculum content may be based on categories of stressors; the physiological, psychological, sociocultural, developmental, and spiritual variables; and primary, secondary, and tertiary prevention modalities. Mirenda's discussion also indicates that the prevention modalities may guide sequence of content. Furthermore, Neuman (1985) indicated that her conceptual model was appropriate at all levels of nursing education, including hospital-based diploma programs, associate degree programs, baccalaureate programs, and graduate programs. Further development of these rules is needed and other rules must be formulated.

The use of Neuman's conceptual model as a curriculum guide has been described in several publications and presentations. Bower (1982) presented a blueprint for curriculum development based on the model. This blueprint "is consistent with the model and . . . gives direction for the generation of terminal and level outcomes of the curriculum, the content and its organization, and the course configuration of the program" (p. 99).

Lebold and Davis (1980) described use of Neuman's model in the curriculum at St. Xavier College in Chicago. They noted that the model

> supported the development of a holistic curriculum that focuses on primary, secondary, and tertiary prevention of individuals, families, and communities in multiple and diverse systems. The resultant curriculum design facilitates learning and role induction into the profession by providing students with a structure for integrating new knowledge and skills during the program and upon its completion. (p. 157)

Mirenda (1986) described use of Neuman's model for the baccalaureate nursing program at Neumann College in Aston, Pennsylvania. She commented, "The nursing faculty at Neumann College have reported their satisfaction with this systems approach to the curriculum and to client care, and nursing students have demonstrated both professional growth and personal maturity" (p. 148).

The Neuman Systems Model also has guided development of curricula in several other nursing programs. Beitler, Tkachuck, and Aamodt (1980) described lesson plans for care of clients with personality disorders and for working with low-income families that are part of the baccalaureate program at Union College in Lincoln, Nebraska. Knox, Kilchenstein, and Yakulis (1982) and Kilchenstein and Yakulis (1984) discussed the use of the model in the baccalaureate nursing program at the University of Pittsburgh in Pennsylvania. Story and

Ross (1986) described the use of Neuman's conceptual model as a guide to content for the junior year family-centered community health nursing course at the University of Ottawa in Ontario, Canada. And Bourbonnais and Ross (1985) and Ross, Bourbonnais, and Carroll (1987) described how Neuman's model guides content for the final senior year nursing course at the University of Ottawa.

Johnson, Vaughn-Wrobel, Ziegler, Hough, Bush, and Kurtz (1982) described the development of the master's program curriculum from the Neuman Systems Model at Texas Woman's University College of Nursing. Other Texas Woman's University faculty members further described course development using the model (Conners, Harmon, & Langford, 1982). Moxley and Allen (1982) outlined the use of Neuman's model in the master's degree program at Northwestern State University in Shreveport, Louisiana. Neuman and Wyatt (1980) described the master's program in nursing service administration at Ohio University School of Nursing in Athens, Ohio. The curriculum for this program was developed from the Neuman Nursing Administration Stress/Adaptation Systems Model, a modification of Neuman's original model.

Neuman's conceptual model also has been used as the framework for the undergraduate and graduate programs at the University of Missouri–Kansas City School of Nursing. Conners (personal communication, April 22, 1982) reported that at this school, "the clinical courses and their content reflect Neuman's three levels of prevention." She also noted "The role courses use Neuman's model as a framework for assessing and understanding the systems in which role enactment takes place." Lowry (1985) described use of the model for the associate degree nursing program at Cecil Community College in North East, Maryland, and Green and Hunsicker (1895) described its use for the associate degree program at Santa Fe Community College in Gainesville, Florida.

Other nursing programs that use Neuman's model include those at Indiana University/Purdue University at Fort Wayne; Simmons College in Boston, Massachusetts; Fitchburg State College in Fitchburg, Massachusetts; Anna Maria College in Paxton, Massachusetts, the University of Nevada, Las Vegas; the University of Texas at Tyler; the University of Wyoming, Laramie (Asay & Ossler, 1984); Delta State College in Cleveland, Mississippi; the Medical University of South Carolina in Charleston; Methodist Central Hospitals of Memphis in Tennessee; the University of Puerto Rico; and Aarhus University in Aarhus, Denmark (Hermiz & Meininger, 1986). Neuman's conceptual model also is used as a curriculum guide at Lander College in Greenwood, South Carolina; Seattle Pacific University in Washington; National Yang Ming Medical College School of Nursing in Taiwan; in the baccalaureate nursing programs of the consortium of North Dakota

State University in Fargo and Concordia College in Moorhead, Minnesota, and the Minnesota Intercollegiate Nursing Consortium in St. Paul, Minnesota (College of St. Catherine, Gustavus Adolphus College, and St. Olaf College).

The Neuman Systems Model also has documented utility for continuing education in nursing. Harty (1982) demonstrated the use of the model as "a facilitating framework for accomplishing continuing education in nursing's primary goal: maintenance and reinforcement of the theoretical knowledge and clinical competence of the professional nurse" (p. 101). In addition, Baker (1982a) outlined a continuing education program for nurses in a psychiatric mental health hospital.

Documentation of the utility of Neuman's model in nursing service administration also is available. The following rules for administration were formulated by Fawcett, Botter, Burritt, Crossley, and Frink (in press):

> The distinctive focus of and purpose to be fulfilled by nursing in the clinical agency is the provision of nursing services designed to help client systems retain, attain, or maintain stability by means of primary, secondary, and tertiary prevention. The collective nursing staff is thought of as a client system that is a composite of physiological, psychological, sociocultural, developmental, and spiritual variables. The department of nursing or the larger health care institution could also be viewed as the client system. The settings for nursing services are those where primary, secondary, and tertiary prevention are appropriate. Thus, this conceptual model could be used in virtually all types of clinical agencies, including ambulatory clinics, acute care medical centers, and rehabilitation units. Management strategies focus on the staff, the department of nursing, or the total institution as the client system of the administrator, who uses management practices that promote system stability.

Pinkerton (1974) described the organization of services provided by the Allied Home Health Association of San Diego, California, according to Neuman's model. Capers, O'Brien, Quinn, Kelly, and Fenerty (1985) presented a detailed description of the planning required for implementation of Neuman's model at Mercy Catholic Medical Center, Fitzgerald Mercy Division in Darby, Pennsylvania. A symposium devoted to use of Neuman's conceptual model as a guide for nursing practice was sponsored by this agency in December 1983.

This conceptual model also is used to organize community health nursing at the Boston Department of Health and Hospitals Community Health Nursing Division in Massachusetts; to guide community health nursing in Aarhus, Denmark; and to guide care at the Rehabilitation Institute of the South in Shreveport, Louisiana (Hermiz & Meininger, 1986), and at Mount Sinai Hospital in Hartford, Connecticut (Caramanica & Thibodeau, 1987). Furthermore, the model is used as a basis for criteria for community health nursing practice throughout the provinces of Ontario and Manitoba in Canada, as well as serving as an organizational guide for the Regional Perinatal Education Program of Eastern Ontario in Ottawa, Ontario, Canada (Neuman, 1985, in press). Neuman's model also has been used to structure nursing care processes in the Obstetrical/Neonatal Nursing Department at the Hospital of the University of Pennsylvania in Philadelphia.

Arndth (1982) combined the concepts of Neuman's model with organizational theory to outline areas to consider in the analysis of nursing service organizations. Moreover, the Neuman Systems Model has proved useful for development of nursing care plans. Mayers and Watson (1982) described the adaptation of their basic nursing care planning format to accommodate Neuman's conceptual model. Neal (1982) and Capers and Kelly (1987) also described nursing care plans derived from the Neuman Systems Model.

Contributions to Nursing Knowledge

The Neuman Systems Model reflects nursing's interest in people as holistic systems, whether well or ill, and in environmental influences on health. Moreover, the use of terms such as variances from wellness and primary prevention emphasizes the wellness feature of the model. Furthermore, the focus on clients' perceptions of stressors and on negotiation of nursing care goals with the client underscores the importance of the person who is client in the nursing situation.

The multidimensional nature of the Neuman Systems Model is attractive to the many health care workers who recognize the complex nature of humans and their interactions with the environment. Although the model contains many terms, most are familiar, and, therefore, use of the model does not require mastery of an extensive new vocabulary.

The primary contribution of this conceptual model has been pragmatic, in that it has proved to be a useful guide for nursing education and nursing practice in various settings in several countries. Indeed, the model "is proving to be readily translatable to other cultures facilitating important global sharing and resolution of universal nursing concerns" (Neuman, in press). Research to generate and test theories related to this conceptual model is needed to determine its credibility beyond pragmatic considerations.

A potential contribution is the adoption of the model by other health care disciplines. This is, however, a two-edged sword, because the applicability of the model to all health care disiciplines can foster a common perspective, but in doing so may fail to point out the distinctive contribution of nursing to health care.

Neuman's (in press) own words best summarize the overall contributions of this conceptual model. She stated,

> The Neuman Systems Model fits well with the holistic client systemic concept of optimizing a dynamic yet stable interrelationship of mind, body and spirit in a constantly changing environment and society. It joins the recent World Health mandate for the year 2000 of desired unity in wellness states—wellness of body, mind, spirit and environment. It is also in unison with the American Nursing Association concern for potential stressors and primary prevention.

Neuman (personal communication, October 15, 1987) has ensured the continued evolution of her conceptual model through establishment of the Neuman Systems Model Trustee Group. Members of the Trustee Group, which is made up of nurses from the United States and other countries, have agreed "to preserve, protect, and perpetuate the integrity of the Model for the future of nursing."

REFERENCES

Anderson, E., McFarlane, J., & Helton, A. (1986). Community-as-Client: A model for practice. Nursing Outlook, 34, 220–224.

Arndth C. (1982). Systems concepts for management of stress in complex health-care organizations. In B. Neuman, The Neuman Systems Model. Application to nursing education and practice (pp. 97–114). Norwalk, CT: Appleton-Century-Crofts.

Asay, M.K., & Ossler, C.C. (Eds.). (1984). Conceptual models of nursing. Applications in community health nursing. Proceedings of the Eighth Annual Community Health Nursing Conference. Chapel Hill: Department of Public Health Nursing, School of Public Health, University of North Carolina.

Baker, N.A. (1982a). The Neuman Systems Model as a conceptual framework for continuing education in the work place. In B. Neuman, The Neuman Systems Model. Application to nursing education and practice (pp. 260–264). Norwalk, CT: Appleton-Century-Crofts.

Baker, N.A. (1982b). Use of the Neuman model in planning for the psychological needs of the respiratory disease patient. In B. Neuman, The Neuman Systems Model. Application to nursing education and practice (pp. 241–251). Norwalk, CT: Appleton-Century-Crofts.

Beitler, B., Tkachuck, B., & Aamodt, D. (1980). The Neuman Model applied to mental health, community health, and medical-surgical nursing. In J.P. Riehl & C. Roy, Conceptual models for nursing practice (2nd ed., pp. 170–178). New York: Appleton-Century-Crofts.

Benedict, M.B., & Sproles, J.B. (1982). Application of the Neuman model to public health nursing practice. In B. Neuman. The Neuman Systems Model. Application to nursing education and practice (pp. 223–240). Norwalk, CT: Appleton-Century-Crofts.

Bertalanffy, L. (1968). General system theory. New York: George Braziller.

Bourbonnais, F.F., & Ross, M.R. (1985). The Neuman Systems Model in nursing education: Course development and implementation. Journal of Advanced Nursing, 10, 117–123.

Bower, F.L. (1982). Curriculum development and the Neuman Model. In B. Neuman, The Neuman Systems Model. Application to nursing education and practice (pp. 94–99). Norwalk, CT: Appleton-Century-Crofts.

Buchanan, B.F. (1987). Human-environment interaction: A modification of the Neuman Systems Model for aggregates, families, and the community. Public Health Nursing, 4, 52–64.

Burritt, J.E. (1988). The effects of perceived social support on the relationship between job stress and job satisfaction and job performance among registered nurses employed in acute care facilities. Unpublished doctoral dissertation. University of Pennsylvania.

Capers, C.F. (1987). Perceptions of problematic behavior as held by lay black adults and registered nurses. Dissertation Abstracts International, 47, 4467B.

Capers, C.F., & Kelly, R. (1987). Neuman nursing process: A model of holistic care. Holistic Nursing Practice, 1(3), 19–26.

Capers, C.F., O'Brien, C., Quinn, R., Kelly R., & Fenerty, A. (1985). The Neuman Systems Model in practice. Planning phase. Journal of Nursing Administration, 15(5), 29–39.

Caplan, G. (1964). Principles of preventive psychiatry. New York: Basic Books.

Caramanica, L., & Thibodeau, J. (1987). Staff involvement in developing a nursing philosophy and the selection of a model for practice. Nursing Management, 18(10), 71.

Chardin, P.T. (1955). The phenomenon of man. London: Collins.

Conners, V., Harmon, V.M., & Langford, R.W. (1982). Course development and implementation using the Neuman Systems Model as a framework: Texas Woman's University (Houston Campus). In B. Neuman, The Neuman Systems Model. Application to nursing education and practice (pp. 153–158). Norwalk, CT: Appleton-Century Crofts.

Cornu, A. (1957). The origins of Marxian thought. Springfield, IL: Charles C Thomas.

Craddock, R.B., & Stanhope, M.K. (1980). The Neuman health-care systems model: Recommended adaptation. In J.P. Riehl & C. Roy, Conceptual models for nursing practice (2nd ed., pp. 159–169). New York: Appleton-Century-Crofts.

Cunningham, S.C. (1983). The Neuman Systems Model applied to a rehabilitation setting. Rehabilitation Nursing, 8(4), 20–22.

Echlin, D.J. (1982). Palliative care and the Neuman model. In B. Neuman, The Neuman Systems Model. Application to nursing education and practice (pp 257–259). Norwalk, CT: Appleton-Century-Crofts.

Edelson, M. (1970). Sociotherapy and psychotherapy. Chicago: University of Chicago Press.

Fawcett, J., Botter, M.L., Burritt, J., Crossley, J.D., & Frink, B.B. (in press). Conceptual models of nursing and organization theories. In B. Henry, M. DiVincenti, C. Arndt, & A. Marriner (Eds.), Dimensions of nursing administration. Theory, research, education, and practice. Boston: Blackwell Scientific Publications.

Fawcett, J., Cariello, F.P., Davis, D.A., Farley, J., Zimmaro, D.M., & Watts, R.J. (1987). Conceptual models of nursing: Application to critical care nursing practice. Dimensions of Critical Care Nursing, 6, 202–213.

Fawcett, J., Carpenito, J.J., Efinger, J., Goldblum-Graff, D., Groesbeck, M.J.V., Lowry, L.W., McCreary, C.S., & Wolf, Z.R. (1982). A framework for analysis and evaluation of conceptual models of nursing with an analysis and evaluation of the Neuman Systems Model. In B. Neuman, The Neuman Systems Model. Application to nursing education and practice (pp. 30–43). Norwalk, CT: Appleton-Century-Crofts.

Goldblum-Graff, D., & Graff, H. (1982). The Neuman model adapted to family therapy. In B. Neuman. The Neuman Systems Model. Application to nursing education and practice (pp. 217–222). Norwalk, CT: Appleton-Century Crofts.

Green, J., & Hunsicker, D. (1985, August). Application of Betty Neuman's framework. Paper presented at conference on Nursing Theory in Action. Edmonton, Alberta, Canada. (Cassette recording)

Harty, M.B. (1982). Continuing education in nursing and the Neuman model. In B. Neuman. The Neuman Systems Model. Application to nursing education and practice (pp. 100–106). Norwalk, CT: Appleton-Century Crofts.

Hermiz, M.E., & Meininger, M. (1986). Betty Neuman Systems Model. In A. Marriner, Nursing theorists and their work (pp. 313–331). St. Louis: CV Mosby.

Hoch, C.C. (1987). Assessing delivery of nursing care. Journal of Gerontological Nursing, 13, 10–17.

Hoffman, M.K. (1982). From model to theory construction: An analysis of the Neuman

Health-Care Systems Model. In B. Neuman, The Neuman Systems Model. Application to nursing education and practice (pp. 44–54). Norwalk, CT: Appleton-Century-Crofts.

Johnson, P. (1983). Black hypertension: A transcultural case study using the Betty Neuman model of nursing care. Issues in Health Care of Women, 4, 191–210.

Johnson, M.N., Vaughn-Wrobel, B., Ziegler, S., Hough, L., Bush, H.A., & Kurtz, P. (1982). Use of the Neuman Health-Care Systems Model in the master's curriculum: Texas Woman's University. In B. Neuman, The Neuman Systems Model. Application to nursing education and practice (pp. 130–152). Norwalk, CT: Appleton-Century-Crofts.

Kilchenstein, L., & Yakulis, I. (1984). The birth of a curriculum: Utilization of the Betty Neuman Health Care Systems Model in an integrated baccalaureate program. Journal of Nursing Education, 23, 126–127.

King, I.M. (1971). Toward a theory for nursing. New York: John Wiley & Sons.

Knox, J.E., Kilchenstein, L., & Yakulis, I.M. (1982). Utilization of the Neuman model in an integrated baccalaureate program: University of Pittsburgh. In B. Neuman, The Neuman Systems Model. Application to nursing education and practice (pp. 117–123). Norwalk, CT: Appleton-Century-Crofts.

Lazarus, R. (1981). The stress and coping paradigm. In C. Eisdorfer, D. Cohen, A. Kleinman, & P. Maxim (Eds.), Models for clinical psychopathology (pp. 177–214). New York: SP Medical and Scientific Books.

Lebold, M., & Davis, L. (1980). A baccalaureate nursing curriculum based on the Neuman Health Systems Model. In J.P. Riehl & C. Roy, Conceptual models for nursing practice (2nd ed., pp. 151–158). New York: Appleton-Century-Crofts.

Lowry, L.W. (1985, August). Application of Betty Neuman's framework. Paper presented at conference on Nursing Theory in Action, Edmonton, Alberta, Canada. (Cassette recording)

Marriner, A. (1986). Nursing theorists and their work. St. Louis: CV Mosby.

Mayers, M.A., & Watson, A.B. (1982). Nursing care plans and the Neuman Systems Model. In B. Neuman, The Neuman Systems Model. Application to nursing education and practice (pp. 69–84). Norwalk, CT: Appleton-Century-Crofts.

Meleis, A.I. (1985). Theoretical nursing. Development and progress. Philadelphia: JB Lippincott.

Mirenda, R.M. (1986). The Neuman Systems Model: Description and application. In P. Winstead-Fry (Ed.), Case studies in nursing theory (pp. 127–166). New York: National League for Nursing.

Moxley, P.A., & Allen, L.M.H. (1982). The Neuman Systems Model approach in a master's degree program: Northwestern State University. In B. Neuman, The Neuman Systems Model. Application to nursing education and practice (pp. 168–175). Norwalk, CT: Appleton-Century-Crofts.

Neal, M.C. (1982). Nursing care plans and the Neuman Systems Model: II. In B. Neuman, The Neuman Systems Model. Application to nursing education and practice (pp. 85–93). Norwalk, CT: Appleton-Century-Crofts.

Neuman, B. (1974). The Betty Neuman Health-Care Systems Model: A total person approach to patient problems. In J.P. Riehl & C. Roy. Conceptual models for nursing practice (pp. 99–114). New York: Appleton-Century-Crofts.

Neuman, B. (1980). The Betty Neuman Health-Care Systems Model: A total person approach to patient problems. In J.P. Riehl & C. Roy, Conceptual models for nursing practice (2nd ed., pp. 119–134). New York: Appleton-Century-Crofts.

Neuman, B. (1982). The Neuman Systems Model. Application to nursing education and practice. Norwalk, CT: Appleton-Century-Crofts.

Neuman, B. (1983a). Family intervention using the Betty Neuman Health Care Systems Model. In I.W. Clements & F.B. Roberts, Family health. A theoretical approach to nursing care (pp. 239–254). New York: John Wiley & Sons.

Neuman, B. (1983b). The family experiencing emotional crisis. Analysis and application of Neuman's Health Care Systems Model. In I.W. Clements & F.B. Roberts. Family health. A theoretical approach to nursing care (pp. 353–367). New York: John Wiley & Sons.

Neuman, B. (1985, August). Betty Neuman. Paper presented at conference on Nursing Theory in Action, Edmonton, Alberta, Canada. (Cassette recording)

Neuman, B. (in press). The Neuman Systems Model. Application to nursing education and practice (2nd ed.). Norwalk, CT: Appleton and Lange.

Neuman, B., & Wyatt, M. (1980). The Neuman Stress/Adaptation systems approach to education for nurse administrators. In J.P. Riehl & C. Roy, Conceptual models for nursing practice (2nd ed., pp. 142–150). New York: Appleton-Century-Crofts.

Neuman, B., & Young, R.J. (1972). A model for teaching total person approach to patient problems. Nursing Research, 21, 264–269.

Orem, D. (1971). Nursing: Concepts of practice. New York: McGraw-Hill.

Peterson, C.J. (1977). Questions frequently asked about the development of a conceptual framework. Journal of Nursing Education, 16(4), 22–32.

Pinkerton, A. (1974). Use of the Neuman model in a home health-care agency. In J.P. Riehl & C. Roy, Conceptual models for nursing practice (pp. 122–129). New York: Appleton-Century-Crofts.

Putt, A. (1972). Entropy, evolution and equifinality in nursing. In J. Smith (Ed.), Five years of cooperation to improve curricula in western schools of nursing. Boulder, CO: Western Interstate Commission for Higher Education.

Redheffer G. (1985). Application of Betty Neuman's Health Care Systems Model to emergency nursing practice: Case review. Point of View, 22(2), 4–6.

Riehl, J.P., & Roy, C. (1974). Conceptual models for nursing practice. New York: Appleton-Century-Crofts.

Riehl, J.P., & Roy, C. (1980). Conceptual models for nursing practice (2nd ed.). New York: Appleton-Century-Crofts.

Rogers, M.E. (1970). An introduction to the theoretical basis of nursing. Philadelphia: FA Davis.

Ross, M.M. & Bourbonnais, F.F. (1985). The Betty Neuman Systems Model in nursing practice: A case study approach. Journal of Advanced Nursing, 10, 199–207.

Ross, M.M., Bourbonnais, F.F., & Carroll, G. (1987). Curricular design and the Betty Neuman Systems Model: A new approach to learning. International Nursing Review, 34, 75–79.

Selye, H. (1950). The physiology and pathology of exposure to stress. Montreal: ACTA.

Stevens, B.J. (1982). Forward. In B. Neuman, The Neuman Systems Model. Application to nursing education and practice (pp. xiii–xiv). Norwalk, CT: Appleton-Century-Crofts.

Stevens, B.J. (1984). Nursing theory. Analysis, application, evaluation (2nd ed.). Boston: Little, Brown & Co.

Story, E.L., & Ross, M.M. (1986). Family centered community health nursing and the Betty Neuman Systems Model. Nursing Papers, 18(2), 77–88.

Sullivan, J. (1986). Using Neuman's model in the acute phase of spinal cord injury. Focus on Critical Care, 13(5), 34–41.

Utz, S.W. (1980). Applying the Neuman model to nursing practice with hypertensive clients. Cardio-Vascular Nursing, 16, 29–34.

Walker, L.O., & Nicholson, R. (1980). Criteria for evaluating nursing process models. Nurse Educator, 5(5), 8–9.

Wilson, V.S. (1987). Identification of stressors related to parents' psychologic responses to the surgical intensive care unit. Heart and Lung, 16, 267–273.

Ziegler, S.M. (1982). Taxonomy for nursing diagnosis derived from the Neuman Systems Model. In B. Neuman, The Neuman Systems Model. Application to nursing education and practice (pp. 55–68). Norwalk, CT: Appleton-Century-Crofts.

Ziemer, M.M. (1983). Effects of information on postsurgical coping. Nursing Research, 32, 282–287.

ANNOTATED BIBLIOGRAPHY

Anderson, E., McFarlane, J., & Helton, A. (1986). Community-as-Client: A model for practice. Nursing Outlook, 34, 220–224.

The Community-as-Client model, an adaptation of Neuman's conceptual model, was developed in an effort to put into practice a synthesis of public health and nursing. Definitions of person, environment, health, and nursing provide a foundation for the more specific description of this model. Components of the model are clearly described and an application of the model in a specific community is presented. The application indicates that the model can be applied to a variety of problems that affect the well-being of a specific population.

Balch, C. (1974). Breaking the lines of resistance. In J.P. Riehl & C. Roy, Conceptual models for nursing practice (pp. 130–134). New York: Appleton-Century-Crofts.
The author describes her previous interviewing techniques and contrasts them with her developing skill in using the Neuman model assessment method. Personal feelings are discussed and the attempt to validate the assessment tool is presented. Improvements in patient care are noted when the model was used as guide.

Beitler, B., Tkachuck, B., & Aamodt, D. (1980). The Neuman model applied to mental health, community health, and medical-surgical nursing. In J.P. Riehl & C. Roy, Conceptual models for nursing practice (2nd ed., pp. 170–178). New York: Appleton-Century-Crofts.
The Neuman model is applied to mental health and community health nursing through development of lesson plans based on the model. The model is applied to medical-surgical nursing settings through use of Neuman's assessment/intervention tool.

Bigbee, J. (1984). The changing role of rural women: Nursing and health implications. Health Care of Women International, 5, 307–322.
A review of the literature regarding contemporary rural women is presented in this article. Health implications are drawn using the Neuman Systems Model and are followed by a discussion of implications for nursing practice, education, and research.

Bourbonnais, F.F., & Ross, M.M. (1985). The Neuman Systems Model in nursing education: Course development and implementation. Journal of Advanced Nursing, 10, 117–123.

Ross, M.M., Bourbonnais, F.F., & Carroll, G. (1987). Curricular design and the Betty Neuman Systems Model: A new approach to learning. International Nursing Review, 34, 75–79.
These articles describe the introduction of Neuman's conceptual model to fourth-year baccalaureate students at the University of Ottawa School of Nursing in Ottawa, Ontario, Canada. Development and implementation of course content, teaching strategies, and outcomes are discussed. The authors noted that Neuman's model was an appropriate framework for organization of final-year baccalaureate nursing program content.

Buchanan, B.F. (1987). Human-environment interaction: A modification of the Neuman Systems Model for aggregates, families, and the community. Public Health Nursing, 4, 52–64.
This article presents a description of a modification of Neuman's conceptual model for use with individuals and groups. The model is a macro systems approach that provides an organizing framework that facilitates understanding of the client's relationship with the environment and intervention through preventive, corrective, and rehabilitative approaches. The client is defined as an individual, the family, aggregates, or the community.

Capers, C.F. (1986). Some basic facts about models, nursing conceptualizations, and nursing theories. Journal of Continuing Education, 16, 149–154.
The article presents an overview of conceptual models of nursing and nursing theories. Methods for teaching content about conceptual models to clinicians are given. Neuman's model is used to illustrate application of the teaching methods.

Capers, C.F., & Kelly, R. (1987). Neuman nursing process: A model of holistic care. Holistic Nursing Practice, 1(3), 19–26.
This article describes the nursing process of Neuman's conceptual model and explains the use of the process at Mercy Catholic Medical Center, Fitzgerald Mercy Division in Darby, Pennsylvania.

Capers, C.F., O'Brien, C., Quinn, R., Kelly, R., & Fenerty, A. (1985). The Neuman Systems Model in practice. Planning phase. Journal of Nursing Administration, 15(5), 29–39.

This article outlines the processes and methods used to plan implementation of Neuman's conceptual model as a guide for nursing practice at Mercy Catholic Medical Center, Fitzgerald Mercy Division in Darby, Pennsylvania.

Caramanica, L., & Thibodeau, J. (1987). Nursing philosophy and the selection of a model for practice. Nursing Management, 18(10), 71.
The formal plan used by the Department of Nursing at Mount Sinai Hospital in Hartford, Connecticut, to develop a philosophy of nursing and select a conceptual model of nursing congruent with that philosophy is described in this article. Neuman's conceptual model was selected as the basis for nursing practice.

Clark, J. (1982). Development of models and theories on the concept of nursing. Journal of Advanced Nursing, 7, 129–134.
This article illustrates the use of conceptual models of nursing as guides for nursing practice. The author, a health visitor in the United Kingdom, describes her use of Neuman's conceptual model to care for family members.

Craddock, R.B., & Stanhope, M.K. (1980). The Neuman Health-Care Systems Model: Recommended adaptation. In J.P. Riehl & C. Roy, Conceptual models for nursing practice (2nd ed., pp. 159–169). New York: Appleton-Century-Crofts.
A study of the application of Neuman's model to a home health-care agency is described. The model proved useful in collecting and analyzing data. However, a discrepancy was noted between client perception of stressors and health care provider perceptions of client stressors. Suggestions for modification of the model are offered.

Cross, J.R. (1985). Betty Neuman. In Nursing Theories Conference Group, Nursing theories. The base for professional nursing practice (pp. 258–286). Englewood Cliffs, NJ: Prentice-Hall.
This book chapter presents an overview of Neuman's conceptual model.

Cunningham, S.G. (1983). The Neuman Systems Model applied to a rehabilitation setting. Rehabilitation Nursing, 8(4), 20–22.
This article describes the use of Neuman's conceptual model for the nursing care of clients who require rehabilitation nursing.

Fawcett, J., Botter, M.L., Burritt, J., Crossley, J.D., & Fink, B.B. (in press). Conceptual models of nursing and organization theories. In B. Henry, M. DiVincenti, C. Arndt, & A. Marriner (Eds.), Dimensions of nursing administration. Theory, research, education, and practice. Boston: Blackwell Scientific Publications.
Neuman's model is reviewed and modified for nursing service administration. Conceptual-theoretical systems of knowledge for nursing administration are created by linking the model with contingency theory, role theory, and marketing theory.

Fawcett, J., Cariello, F.P., Davis, D.A., Farley, J., Zimmaro, D.M., & Watts, R.J. (1987). Conceptual models of nursing: Application to critical care nursing practice. Dimensions of Critical Care Nursing, 6, 202–213
This article includes a brief analysis of Neuman's conceptual model and applications of the model for a 36-year-old man who had had a myocardial infarction and a 19-year-old man who had a cerebral aneurysm.

Hermiz, M.E., & Meininger, M. (1986). Betty Neuman. Systems model. In A. Marriner, Nursing theorists and their work (pp. 313–331). St. Louis: CV Mosby.
This book chapter presents an overview of Neuman's conceptual model. A list of some clinical agencies that use Neuman's model is included.

Hoch, C.C. (1987). Assessing delivery of nursing care. Journal of Gerontological Nursing, 13, 10–17.
This article presents a report of a study designed to compare outcomes of nursing intervention directed by Neuman's conceptual model, Roy's model, and a control treatment directed by no explicit model. Study subjects were retired persons attending a senior citizen center. Sixteen subjects were in each of the three study groups. Findings indicated that the Neuman and Roy groups had higher life satisfaction and lower depression scores than the control group. There were no differences, however, between the Neuman and Roy groups.

Johnson, P. (1983). Black hypertension: A transcultural case study using the Betty Neuman model of nursing care. Issues in Health Care of Women, 4, 191–210.

The case study presented in this article described establishment of trust and understanding between the culturally different black client and white nurse. A 36-year-old southern black female was studied for several weeks following a hypertensive crisis episode. An ethnocare plan for the woman was developed using Neuman's model. The plan addressed six identified cultural stressors and was designed to fit the woman's perception of nursing care and its value to her.

Kilchenstein, L., & Yakulis, I (1984). The birth of a curriculum: Utilization of the Betty Neuman Health Care Systems Model in an integrated baccalaureate program. Journal of Nursing Education, 23, 126–127.
The development of an integrated baccalaureate curriculum at the University of Pittsburgh School of Nursing is described in this article. Components of Neuman's conceptual model are included in the conceptual framework for the curriculum. A diagram of the curriculum strands is provided and specific courses are discussed.

Lebold, M., & Davis, L. (1980). A baccalaureate nursing curriculum based on the Neuman Health Systems Model. In. J.P. Riehl & C. Roy, Conceptual models for nursing practice (2nd ed., pp 151–158). New York: Appleton-Century-Crofts.
Neuman's model is utilized as the foundation for baccalaureate nursing education. The model is operationalized in all aspects of curriculum development including general philosophy, content planning, and clinical experiences. Primary, secondary, and tertiary levels of prevention are emphasized as a holistic approach to nursing education.

Lowry, L. (1986). Adapted by degrees. Senior Nurse, 5(3), 25–26.
This article describes the use of Neuman's conceptual model to guide curriculum development in the associate degree nursing program at Cecil Community College in North East, Maryland.

Mirenda, R.M. (1986). The Neuman model in practice. Senior Nurse, 5(3), 26–27.
This article describes an assessment/intervention tool based on Neuman's conceptual model that is used by students at Neumann College in Aston, Pennsylvania.

Mirenda, R.M. (1986). The Neuman Systems Model: Description and application. In P. Winstead-Fry (Ed.), Case studies in nursing theory (pp. 127–166). New York: National League for Nursing.
This book chapter presents a detailed discussion of Neuman's conceptual model organized according to statements about the person, environment, health, and nursing. Use of the conceptual model to guide research, education, and practice is described. A case study dealing with application of the model as a curriculum guide at Neumann College is given. Another case study deals with model-based care of a pregnant woman with diabetes.

Mirenda, R.M., & Wright, C. (1987). Using nursing model to affirm Catholic identity. Health Progress, 68(2), 63–67, 94.
The authors compare the ideas presented in Neuman's Systems Model with the beliefs and values of the Catholic tradition of Franciscanism. They conclude that because of Neuman's emphasis on a holistic, systems approach, person as client, and flexibility, the model is compatible with the Franciscan tradition.

Neuman, B. (1974). The Betty Neuman Health-Care Systems Model: A total person approach to patient problems. In J.P. Riehl & C. Roy, Conceptual models for nursing practice (pp. 99–114). New York: Appleton-Century-Crofts. Reprinted in J.P. Riehl & C. Roy. (1980). Conceptual models for nursing practice (2nd ed., pp. 119–134). New York: Appleton-Century-Crofts.
Neuman presents her conceptual model, as well as an assessment/intervention tool.

Neuman, B. (1982). The Neuman Systems Model. Application to nursing education and practice. Norwalk, CT: Appleton-Century-Crofts.
This book presents refinements in the Neuman Systems Model, an analysis and evaluation of the model, and many applications of the model in nursing practice, education, administration, and research.

Neuman B. (1983). Family intervention using the Betty Neuman Health Care Systems Model. In I.W. Clements & F.B. Roberts, Family health. A theoretical approach to nursing care (pp. 239–254). New York: John Wiley & Sons.
The purpose of this chapter was to assist the nurse in using the Neuman Systems Model with families. The family as a system in society is described and a format

for determining family stability is presented. A classification of stressors affecting family stability is outlined. The nursing process for family intervention based on Neuman's conceptual model is included, as are an outline of the nursing process format and a schematic design of the format.

Neuman, B. (1983). The family experiencing emotional crisis. Analysis and application of Neuman's Health Care Systems Model. In I.W. Clements & F.B. Roberts, Family health. A theoretical approach to nursing care (pp. 353–367). New York: John Wiley & Sons.
A case study describing a three-generation Mexican-American family whose care had been delegated to a mental health nurse following recent discharge of both daughters from a state mental institution is presented and then analyzed using Neuman's conceptual model. The nursing process of the Neuman's Systems Model is utilized in the analysis of the family situation.

Neuman B. (1985). The Neuman Systems Model. Senior Nurse, 3(3), 20–23.
This article presents a brief description of Neuman's conceptual model.

Neuman, B. (in press). The Neuman Systems Model. Application to education and practice (2nd ed.). Norwalk, CT: Appleton and Lange.
This book presents the most recent refinements in Neuman's conceptual model, an analysis and evaluation of the model, and several applications of the conceptual model in nursing practice, education, administration, and research.

Neuman, B., & Wyatt, M. (1980). The Neuman Stress/Adaptation systems approach to education for nurse administrators. In J.P. Riehl & C. Roy, Conceptual models for nursing practice (2nd ed., pp. 142–150). New York: Appleton-Century-Crofts.
An adaptation of Neuman's model is presented as a framework for curriculum development in nursing service administration at the master's level. Incorporation of management content is described.

Neuman, B., & Young, R.J. (1972). A model for teaching total person approach to patient problems. Nursing Research, 21, 264–269.
The basic structure of Neuman's conceptual model of nursing is presented. The use of the model as a unifying framework for concepts presented in a graduate-level nursing course is described. Student evaluations revealed that the model was helpful to their understanding of course content.

Pinkerton, A. (1974). Use of the Neuman model in a home health-care agency. In J.P. Riehl & C. Roy, Conceptual models for nursing practice. New York: Appleton-Century-Crofts.
Neuman's model is applied in a home health-care setting. Specific areas of application are discussed. Significant improvements in patient care were noted after the model was adopted. A diagram indicating a conceptual approach to assessment based on the model and a theory of stress are included.

Redheffer G. (1985). Application of Betty Neuman's Health Care Systems Model to emergency nursing practice: Case review. Point of View, 22(2), 4–6.
This article presents a brief overview of Neuman's conceptual model and a discussion of the use of the model as a guide for emergency nursing practice. A case study illustrates the application of the conceptual model in the emergency room setting.

Ross, M., & Bourbonnais, F. (1985). The Betty Neuman Systems Model in nursing practice: A case study approach. Journal of Advanced Nursing, 10, 199–207.
A case study approach is used to illustrate use of Neuman's conceptual model in nursing practice. The article begins by emphasizing the importance of determining congruence between personal values and assumptions and those of a conceptual model prior to selection of the model for practice. A discussion of the conceptual basis, values, and assumptions of Neuman's model then is presented. The second part of the article provides an example of one public health nurse's use of the model in practice.

Story, E.L., & Ross, M.M. (1986). Family centered community health nursing and the Betty Neuman Systems Model. Nursing Papers, 18(2), 77–88.
This article presents an outline of the nursing curriculum at the University of Ottawa School of Nursing in Ottawa, Ontario, Canada. Various conceptual models are

used to guide curriculum construction in each year of the program. Roy's model is used in Years 1, 2, and 3; Orem's work is used in Year 3; and Neuman's model is used in Years 3 and 4. A description of Year 3 community health nursing course objectives and content based on Neuman's model is given.

Sullivan, J. (1986). Using Neuman's model in the acute phase of spinal cord injury. Focus on Critical Care, 13(5), 34–41.

This article describes the application of Neuman's conceptual model to the nursing care of a patient with acute spinal cord injury. The propositions of the model are discussed and Neuman's nursing process is described. An assessment-intervention tool based on Neuman's model and modified for critical care is presented. Tables outline stressors, nursing diagnoses, nursing goals, nursing interventions, and nursing outcomes in the secondary and tertiary prevention modes.

Thibodeau, J.A. (1983). Nursing models: Anaysis and evaluation. Monterey, CA: Wadsworth.

This book includes a chapter that presents an analysis and evaluation of Neuman's Systems Model, using an early version of the framework for analysis and evaluation of conceptual models of nursing presented in Chapter 2 of the present book.

Utz, S.W. (1980). Applying the Neuman model to nursing practice with hypertensive clients. Cardio-Vascular Nursing, 16, 29–34.

The model is applied to the care of hypertensive clients because of the emphasis it places on client perceptions of illness. The author reports successful application of the model and notes the importance of primary, secondary, and tertiary interventions in shifting the focus from illness to restoration of maximum functioning.

Venable, J.F. (1974). The Neuman Health-Care Systems Model: An analysis. In J.P. Riehl & C. Roy, Conceptual models for nursing practice (pp. 115–122). New York: Appleton-Century-Crofts. Reprinted in J.P. Riehl & C. Roy (1980). Conceptual models for nursing practice (2nd ed., pp. 135–141). New York: Appleton-Century-Crofts.

The utility of Neuman's model is analyzed according to structure, substance, and acceptability. The model is found to be clearly stated, functional in directing a broad range of nursing activities, and socially congruent, significant, and useful. The only identified deficit in the model is the apparent lack of a unique role for nursing; however, the author does not regard that as detrimental.

Walker, L.O., & Avant, K.C. (1983). Strategies for theory construction in nursing. Norwalk, CT: Appleton-Century-Crofts.

This book includes an analysis of Neuman's conceptual model from the perspective of and criteria for middle-range theory, using the theory analysis technique presented in the book. The authors maintained that "although Neuman does not claim that her model is a theory as yet, it is sufficiently developed to conduct a theory analysis" (p. 132).

Whall, A.L. (1983). The Betty Neuman Health Care System Model. In J.J. Fitzpatrick & A.L. Whall, Conceptual models of nursing. Anaysis and application (pp. 203–219). Bowie, MD: Brady.

This book chapter presents an overview of Neuman's conceptual model.

Wilson, V.S. (1987). Identification of stressors related to patients' psychologic responses to the surgical intensive care unit. Heart and Lung, 16, 267–273.

A report of a study designed to identify stressors experienced by clients manifesting transient delirium or impaired psychological response while in the surgical intensive care unit is presented in this article. The study was based on Neuman's conceptual model.

Ziemer, M.M. (1983). Effects of information on postsurgical coping. Nursing Research, 32, 282–287.

This study examined the effects of preoperative information on postoperative behavior of clients having abdominal surgery. The theoretical structure of the study was derived from Neuman Systems Model concepts, including stressor, lines of defense, primary prevention, and impact of stressors. Findings did not support the proposition that primary prevention decreases the impact of stressors.

CHAPTER

7

Orem's Self-Care Framework_____

This chapter presents an analysis and evaluation of Dorothea Orem's conceptual framework of nursing, which also has been called the self-care deficit theory of nursing and the self-care nursing theory. Orem's work now can be separated into a conceptual framework of nursing and three theories. One of these theories, the theory of nursing systems, is considered the general theory of nursing. Orem and Taylor (1986) explained that "the conceptual framework of the general theory . . . is constituted from six central or core concepts and one peripheral concept" (p. 45). The concepts and propositions of the conceptual framework are at the level of abstraction and generality usually seen in a conceptual model and are regarded as such in this chapter. In fact, Orem (personal communication, November 20, 1987) referred to her work as "the conceptual model and three theories." Inasmuch as the purpose of this book is to analyze and evaluate conceptual models of nursing, emphasis will be placed on Orem's conceptual framework. The three theories are, however, described in the evaluation section of the chapter.

The key terms of Orem's conceptual framework are listed below. These terms were taken from the third edition of Orem's (1985) book, *Nursing: Concepts of practice,* and from a book chapter entitled "Orem's general theory of nursing" (Orem & Taylor, 1986).

KEY TERMS_____

Self-Care	Self-Care Requisites
Dependent Care	Universal Self-Care Requisites

Self-Care Requisites—*Cont.*	Nursing Process—*Cont.*
Developmental Self-Care Requisites	Producing Care To Regulate Therapeutic Self-Care Demand and Self-Care Agency
Health Deviation Self-Care Requisites	
Therapeutic Self-Care Demand	Nursing Systems
Self-Care Agency	Wholly Compensatory System
Dependent-Care Agency	Partly Compensatory System
Basic Conditioning Factors	Supportive-Educating System
Power Components	Methods of Assisting
Self-Care Deficit	Acting for or Doing for Another
Dependent-Care Deficit	
Nursing Agency	Guiding Another
Goal of Nursing	Supporting Another Physically or Psychologically
To Help People Meet Their Own Therapeutic Self-Care Demands	
	Providing a Developmental Environment
Nursing Process	Teaching Another
Diagnosis and Prescription	Theory of Self-Care
Designing and Planning	Theory of Self-Care Deficits
	Theory of Nursing Systems

ANALYSIS OF OREM'S SELF-CARE FRAMEWORK

This section presents an analysis of Orem's conceptual framework. The analysis draws primarily from Orem's (1985) book, *Nursing: Concepts of practice,* and a book chapter by Orem and Taylor (1986), "Orem's general theory of nursing."

Development of the Model

The development of Orem's conceptual framework has been described in considerable detail (Nursing Development Conference Group, 1979; Orem & Taylor, 1986). Ideas that helped to shape the conceptual framework were formulated as Orem experienced a period of intensive exposure to nurses and their endeavors from 1949 to 1957, during her tenure as a nursing consultant in the Division of Hospital and Institutional Services of the Indiana State Board of Health. Her observations led to the idea that "nursing involved both a mode of thinking and a mode of communication" (Orem & Taylor, 1986, p. 41). In 1956, Orem prepared a report that contained the following definition of nursing:

1. Nurses as practitioners of nursing give specialized assistance to individuals.

2. Persons to whom nurses give specialized assistance have limitations for action of such a character that more than ordinary assistance from family or friends is necessary to meet daily needs for self-care and to intelligently participate in their medical care.
3. Nurses practice their art through their use of distinct modes of helping: by doing for persons under care, helping them do for themselves, or by helping a family member learn how to help persons with care limitations. (p. 85)

Orem's "search to know nursing in a way that would enlarge and deepen its meaning" (Orem & Taylor, 1986, p. 39) formally began in 1958 and continues to this day. Her search for the meaning of nursing has focused on the following three questions:

1. What do nurses do and what should nurses do as practitioners of nursing?
2. Why do nurses do what they do?
3. What results from what nurses do as practitioners of nursing? (Orem & Taylor, 1986, p. 39)

The answers to these questions began to emerge when Orem introduced elements of her conceptual framework in the 1959 publication, *Guides for developing curricula for the education of practical nurses*. In this report, Orem maintained that human limitations for self-care associated with health situations give rise to a requirement for nursing. She then identified areas of daily self-care, conditions that limit individuals' self-care capabilities, and methods of assisting those whose self-care abilities are limited.

The questions were answered more fully as Orem and other members of the Nursing Model Committee of The Catholic University Nursing Faculty began their work in 1965. The final report of this committee was submitted to the School of Nursing in May 1968. Orem continued her work on the conceptual framework with a group of associates who formed the Nursing Development Conference Group in September 1968. In 1971, Orem published the first edition of her book, *Nursing: Concepts of practice*. The next publication dealing with Orem's conceptual framework was authored by the Nursing Development Conference Group and appeared in 1973 under the title, *Concept formalization in nursing. Process and product*. Revisions in the conceptual framework, with more comprehensive answers to the questions, were presented by Orem in her 1978 speech at the Second Annual Nurse Educator Conference, as well as in the second editions of the books by the Nursing Development Conference Group (1979) and Orem (1980). Three theories connected to the conceptual framework were presented by Orem in her 1980 book. Refinements in the conceptual framework and the three theories are evident in the third edition of Orem's (1985) book and in the Orem and Taylor (1986) book chapter.

The initial impetus for public articulation of the conceptual framework apparently was the need to develop a curriculum for a practical nursing program (Orem, 1959). Orem (1978) commented that this task required identification of the domain and boundaries of nursing as a science and an art. Continued work on the conceptual framework was motivated by "dissatisfaction and concern due to the absence of an organizing framework for nursing knowledge and . . . the belief that a concept of nursing would aid in formalizing such a framework" (Nursing Development Conference Group, 1973, p. ix). In particular, the conceptual framework was formulated as a solution to the problem of

> the lack of specification of, and agreement about, the general elements of nursing that give direction to (1) the isolation of problems that are specifically nursing problems and (2) the organization of knowledge accruing from research in problem areas. (Nursing Development Conference Group, 1973, p. 6)

Orem's early search for the meaning of nursing led to formulation of the following assumptions that guided her subsequent work:

1. Nursing is a form of help or assistance given by nurses to persons with a legitimate need for it.
2. Nurses are characterized by their knowledge of nursing and their capabilities to use their knowledge and specialized skills to produce nursing for others in a variety of types of situations.
3. Persons with a legitimate need for nursing are characterized (a) by a demand for discernible kinds and amounts of self-care or dependent-care and (b) by health-derived or health-related limitations for the continuing production of the amount and kind of care required. In dependent-care situations the limitations of dependent-care givers are associated with the health state and the care requirements of the dependent person.
4. Results of nursing are associated with the characterizing conditions of persons in need of nursing and include (a) the meeting of existent and emerging demands for self-care and dependent care and (b) the regulation of the exercise or development of capabilities for providing care. (Orem, 1985, p. 31)

Orem (1985) noted that as she continued to develop her ideas, she accepted "the generalization that nursing is deliberate human action involving reflection [which in turn] requires the acceptance of human beings as having intrinsic activity rather than passsivity or strict reactivity to stimuli" (p. 12). Drawing from Arnold's (1960) work, she presented the following assumptions about human beings:

1. Human beings know and appraise objects, conditions, and situations in terms of their efforts on ends being sought.
2. Human beings know directly by sensing, but they also reflect, reason, and understand.

3. Human beings are capable of self-determined actions even when they feel an emotional pull in the opposite direction.
4. Human beings can prolong reflection indefinitely in deliberations about what action to take by raising questions about and directing attention to different aspects of a situation and different possibilities for action.
5. Human beings in order to act must concentrate on a suitable course of action and exclude other courses of action.
6. Purposive action requires not only that human beings be aware of objects, conditions, and situations but also that they have the ability to contend with them and treat them in some way.
7. Persons, human beings as unities, are the agents who act deliberately to attain ends or goals. (Orem, 1985, pp. 12–13)

Orem (1985) stated that her conceptual framework is based on the following proposition: "Not all people under health care, for example, from physicians, are under nursing care nor does it follow that they should be" (p. 19). She commented that the question following from this proposition was: "What condition exists in a person when that person or a family member or the attending physician or a nurse makes the judgment that the person should be under nursing care?" (p. 19). She went on to say, "The answer to the question came spontaneously with images of situations where such judgments were made and the idea that a nurse is 'another self' in a figurative sense, for the person under nursing care" (p. 19). Orem (1978) also noted that she looked to her personal and professional experiences for examples of judgments regarding the need for nursing care and the conditions of the persons when these judgments were made. The answer, she stated, finally came as a "flash of insight, an understanding that the reason why individuals could benefit from nursing was the existence of . . . self-care limitations."

More specifically, Orem (1980) stated that the unifying idea of her conceptual framework is that human beings can benefit from nursing when they have health-derived or health-related limitations for engaging in continuing care of self or care of dependent others. She identified the following five assumptions as the base upon which she developed the conceptual framework:

1. Human beings require continuous deliberate inputs to themselves and their environments in order to remain alive and function in accord with natural human endowments.
2. Human agency, the power to act deliberately, is exercised in the form of care of self and others in identifying needs for and in making needed inputs.
3. Mature human beings experience privations in the form of limitations for action in care of self and others involving the making of life-sustaining and function-regulating inputs.
4. Human agency is exercised in discovering, developing, and trans-

mitting to others ways and means to identify needs for and make
inputs to self and others.
5. Groups of human beings with structured relationships cluster tasks
and allocate responsibilities for providing care to group members
who experience privations for making required deliberate input to
self and others. (Orem, 1985, p. 33)

Orem began the development of her conceptual framework at a
time when most nursing education programs were based on conceptual models more representative of other disciplines, such as medicine, psychology, and sociology, than of nursing (Phillips, 1977).
Thus, Orem may be considered a pioneer in the development of distinctive nursing knowledge. This viewpoint is supported by the fact
that all of the aforementioned publications dealing with Orem's conceptual framework have emphasized the need for an organized body
of knowledge upon which to base programs of nursing education.

The foregoing description of the development of Orem's conceptual framework indicates that inductive reasoning was used extensively. Indeed, "it is a successful theory because it is constituted from
conceptualizations of the constant elements and relationships of nursing practice situations" (Orem & Taylor, 1986, p. 38). Deductive reasoning also is evident in Orem's description of the development of the
conceptual framework. She always has cited the works of scholars in
several disciplines and has acknowledged the contributions to her
thinking from her educational experiences. In fact, she read in a

wide range of fields, from organization and administration to social
philosophy, including the philosophic notions of points of order in
wholes composed of parts and different kinds of wholes; from hygiene
and sanitation to cultural anthropology; from the philosophic notion of
human acts to action theory as developed in sociology, psychology,
and philosophy; and from action theory to a concept of systems and
the constructs of cybernetics. (Orem & Taylor, 1986, p. 43)

Furthermore, Orem's ability to express her ideas "required self-knowledge toward clarification of my own reality of knowing nursing in a
dynamic way. B. J. F. Lonergan's work, Insight (1958), was a helpful
though difficult guide to self-knowledge" (Orem & Taylor, 1986, p. 43)

There is, however, no evidence to support contentions that the
conceptual framework is based on earlier works by Frederick and Northam (1938) or Henderson (1955). Indeed, although the idea of patient
as care agent was put forth by Frederick and Northam, the idea of self-
care originated with and was formalized by Orem (Nursing Development Conference Group, 1979). Moreover, Orem explicitly denied that
her conceptual framework was derived from Henderson's 1955 definition of nursing, though she recognized the similarities between it
and her 1956 definition of nursing (Orem & Taylor, 1986).

Contents of the Model: Concepts

Orem and Taylor (1986) stated that the six central concepts of Orem's conceptual framework are self-care, self-care agency, therapeutic self-care demand, self-care deficit, nursing agency, and nursing system. The peripheral concept is basic conditioning factors. These concepts will be discussed within the nursing metaparadigm concepts of person, environment, health, and nursing.

Person

The person of interest in Orem's conceptual framework is the nurse's patient, that is, the person who receives help and care from a nurse. Patient is used in the sense of "a receiver of care, someone who is under the care of a health care professional at this time, in some place or places" (Orem, 1985, p. 49). Orem (1985) described the person as "a human being . . . a unity that can be viewed as functioning biologically, symbolically, and socially" (p. 175). Furthermore, the human being

> is a substantial or real unity whose parts are formed and attain perfection through the differentiation of the whole during processes of development. . . . Since human beings have discernible parts (for example, arms, legs, stomach, lungs, . . . urinary systems . . . neuroendocrine systems), it is essential that parts be recognized. Each developmentally differentiated structure or functional system is an existent entity with its own operations, with relations to other differentiated parts and to their operations, and to the unitary functioning of individuals who coexist in a world with human beings. If there is acceptance of the real unity of individual human beings, there should be no difficulty in recognizing structural and functional differentiations within the unity. (pp. 179–180)

Orem focused on the person's ability to perform self-care, which is defined as

> action directed by individuals to themselves or their environments to regulate their own functioning and development in the interest of sustaining life, maintaining or restoring integrated functioning under stable or changing environmental conditions, and maintaining or bringing about a condition of well-being. (Orem & Taylor, 1986, p. 52)

Self-care is described as a goal-oriented activity that is learned. Adults care for themselves but infants, children, and socially dependent adults require varying degrees of assistance with self-care activities. When assistance that encompasses the range of actions constituting self-care is given to infants, children, and socially dependent adults by responsible adults, such as family members or significant others, it is called dependent-care (Orem & Taylor, 1986).

According to Orem (1985), self-care or dependent-care is performed in relation to three types of self-care requisites: universal, developmental, and health-deviation. Universal self-care requisites are associated with life processes and maintenance of the integrity of human structure and function. These requisites include the maintenance of a sufficient intake of air, water, and food; care associated with elimination and excrements; maintenance of a balance between activity and rest and between solitude and social interaction; prevention of hazards to human life, functioning, and well-being; and promotion of human functioning and development within social groups in accord with human potential, known limitations, and the desire to be normal. Universal self-care requisites are "common to all human beings during all stages of the life cycle, adjusted to age, developmental state, and environmental and other factors" (p. 90).

Developmental self-care requisites are associated with human developmental processes and conditions and events that occur during various stages of the life cycle, as well as with events that may adversely affect development. These requisites include universal self-care requisites particularized for developmental processes and new requisites derived from a condition, such as pregnancy or premature birth, or from an event, such as loss of a family member.

Health-deviation self-care requisites are associated with genetic and constitutional defects and human structural and functional deviations and their effects, as well as with medical diagnostic and treatment measures prescribed or performed by physicians. Health-deviation self-care requisites "exist for persons who are ill, are injured, have specific forms of pathology including defects and disabilities, and who are under medical diagnosis and treatment" (Orem, 1985, p. 97).

A more specific list of the categories of all three types of self-care requisites is presented in Table 7–1.

Orem (1985) used the term therapeutic self-care demand to refer

TABLE 7–1. Self-Care Requisites

Universal Self-Care Requisites
1. The maintenance of a sufficient intake of air
2. The maintenance of a sufficient intake of water
3. The maintenance of a sufficient intake of food
4. The provision of care associated with elimination processes and excrements
5. The maintenance of a balance between activity and rest
6. The maintenance of a balance between solitude and social interaction
7. The prevention of hazards to human life, human functioning, and human well-being
8. The promotion of human functioning and development within social groups in accord with human potential, known human limitations, and the

Orem's Self-Care Framework   **213**

TABLE 7–1. *Continued*

human desire to be normal. Normalcy is used in the sense of that which is essentially human and that which is in accord with the genetic and constitutional characteristics and the talents of individuals

Developmental Self-Care Requisites

1. The bringing about and maintenance of living conditions that support life processes and promote the processes of development, that is, human progress toward higher levels of the organization of human structures and toward maturation during:
   a. the intrauterine stages of life and the process of birth
   b. the neonatal stage of life when (1) born at term or prematurely and (2) born with normal birth weight or low birth weight
   c. infancy
   d. the developmental stages of childhood, including adolescence and entry into adulthood
   e. the developmental stages of adulthood
   f. pregnancy in either childhood or adulthood
2. Provision of care either to prevent the occurrence of deleterious effects of conditions that can affect human development or to mitigate or overcome these effects from conditions, such as:
   a. educational deprivation
   b. problems of social adaptation
   c. failures of healthy individuation
   d. loss of relatives, friends, associates
   e. loss of possessions, loss of occupational security
   f. abrupt change of residence to an unfamiliar environment
   g. status-associated problems
   h. poor health or disability
   i. oppressive living conditions
   j. terminal illness and impending death

Health-Deviation Self-Care Requisites

1. Seeking and securing appropriate medical assistance in the event of exposure to specific physical or biological agents or environmental conditions associated with human pathological events and states, or when there is evidence of genetic, physiological, or psychological conditions known to produce or be associated with human pathology
2. Being aware of and attending to the effects and results of pathological conditions and states, including effects on development
3. Effectively carrying out medically prescribed diagnostic, therapeutic, and rehabilitative measures directed to the prevention of specific types of pathology, to the pathology itself, to the regulation of human integrated functioning, to the correction of deformities or abnormalities, or to compensation for disabilities
4. Being aware of and attending to or regulating the discomforting or deleterious effects of medical care measures performed or prescribed by the physician, including effects on development
5. Modifying the self-concept (and self-image) in accepting oneself as being in a particular state of health and in need of specific forms of health care
6. Learning to live with the effects of pathological conditions and states and the effects of medical diagnostic and treatment measures in a life-style that promotes continued personal development

From Orem, D.E. (1985). Nursing: Concepts of practice (3rd ed., pp. 90–91, 96, 99). New York: McGraw-Hill, with permission.

to all self-care actions that are needed to meet the self-care requisites. More specifically, the therapeutic self-care demand is "the action demand on individuals to meet some complex of universal, developmental, and health-deviation type self-care requisites using valid and appropriate means" (Orem & Taylor, 1986, p. 52). Each person's therapeutic self-care demand varies throughout life. Calculation of this demand is explained in the section dealing with nursing.

Orem (1985) termed the capability to take action directed toward care of self as self-care agency, and the capability to take action directed toward care of others as dependent-care agency. Agency, then, is used in the sense of taking action. The person who takes action is the self-care or dependent-care agent. More specifically, self-care agency is

> a complex capability of maturing and mature individuals to (1) determine the presence and characteristics of specific requirements for regulating their own functioning and development, including prevention and amelioration of disease processes and injuries (identification and particularization of self-care requisites); (2) make judgments and decisions about what to do; and (3) perform care measures to meet specific self-care requisites in time and over time. (Orem & Taylor, p. 52)

Dependent-care agency encompasses the capabilities of self-care agency directed toward care of infants, children, and socially dependent adults.

Therapeutic self-care and self-care agency are influenced by basic conditioning factors that reflect features of individuals or their living situations. There are eight basic conditioning factors: "age, character of being male or female, health state, development state, sociocultural orientation, health care system variables, family system elements, and patterns of living" (Orem & Taylor, 1986, pp. 46–47).

Furthermore, the actions required for exercise of self-care agency are influenced by 10 enabling power components. These include ability to maintain attention to self as a self-care agent and factors significant for self-care; controlled use of available physical energy; ability to control body position; ability to reason within a self-care frame of reference; motivation; ability to make and operationalize self-care decisions; ability to acquire, retain, and operationalize technical knowledge; a repertoire of cognitive, perceptual, manipulative, communication, and interpersonal skills for performance of self-care; ability to order discrete self-care actions; and ability to consistently perform self-care actions (Nursing Development Conference Group, 1979).

When self-care agency is not sufficient to meet the therapeutic self-care demand, a self-care deficit exists. A self-care deficit, then, "expresses a relationship of inadequacy between self-care agency, an action capability, and therapeutic self-care demand, a set of action requirements for engaging in self-care" (Orem & Taylor, 1986, p. 50). A dependent-care deficit expresses the relationship between dependent-care agency and the therapeutic self-care demand of the dependent person.

Environment

Orem (1985) stated, "Requisites for self-care have their origins in human beings and their environments" (p. 36). She referred to environment through the terms environmental factor, environmental elements, environmental conditions, and developmental environment. Environmental factor was not defined, although it was depicted as outside the person. Environmental element was not defined. The term environmental conditions also was not defined, although Orem commented, "The number and nature of the inquiries the self-care provider makes about environmental conditions vary with the provider's familiarity with the surroundings" (pp. 119–120). Apparently, then, environmental conditions refer to the person's external surroundings. Furthermore, environmental conditions were described as physical and psychosocial.

Developmental environment was not explicitly defined, but was described in detail. As explained in the section on nursing, providing a developmental environment is one method a person can use to help or assist others. Such an environment "promotes personal development in relation to becoming able to meet present or future demands for action" (Orem, 1985, p. 138). A developmental environment consists of "environmental conditions that motivate the person being helped to establish appropriate goals and adjust behavior to achieve results specified by the goals. . . . It is the total environment, not any single part of it, that makes it developmental" (pp. 140–141).

Health

Orem (1985) defined health as a "state of the person that is characterized by soundness or wholeness of developed human structures and of bodily and mental functioning" (p. 179). Well-being, which is differentiated from health, focuses on the person's perception of experience. It is defined as "a state characterized by experiences of contentment, pleasure, and kinds of happiness; by spiritual experiences; by movement toward fulfillment of one's self-ideal; and by continuing personalization" (p. 179). Orem went on to explain that although well-being is associated with health, the experience of well-being may occur for an individual under adverse conditions, including disorders in human structure and functioning.

Orem (1985) also differentiated health from disease. This is clearly seen in her classification of nursing situations. The classification is based on

> (1) the presence or absence of disease, injury, disability, or disfigurement; (2) the quality of general health state described in the general sense as excellent, good, fair, poor, or in terms of the values of sets of selected characteristics that together define the person's health state; and (3) the life-cycle-oriented events and circumstances that indicate current changes and existing needs for health care. (p. 195)

Although Orem mentioned illness in her classifications system, the term was not defined. However, illness was linked to self-care in the following statement: "When self-care is not maintained, illness, disease, or death will occur" (Orem, 1985, p. 55). It may be inferred, then, that self-care is necessary for maintenance of a state of health, as that term is defined by Orem. Furthermore, wellness was not explicitly defined, although well-being was defined and described. Orem's discussion of health and well-being, and especially her classification system, suggest that she views health as a continuum from excellent to poor and disease as a separate dichotomy of presence or absence.

Nursing

Orem (1985) considered nursing to be a helping service, "a creative effort of one human being to help another human being" (p. 132). The special concern of nursing is "the individual's need for self-care action and the provision and management of it on a continuous basis in order to sustain life and health, recover from disease or injury, and cope with their effects" (p. 54). Orem (1985) noted that nursing focuses on individuals and multiperson units. She indicated that people receive nursing as individuals or as members of a multiperson unit, but "it should be recognized that only individuals have human needs that can be met through nursing" (p. 251).

Orem (1985) distinguished nursing from medicine by noting that the physician's special interests are in the patient's life processes as they have been disrupted by illness, and the nurse's special interest is the patient's continuing therapeutic care. More specifically, the nurse's perspective encompasses the patient's perspective of his or her own health situation and the physician's perspective of the patient's health situation. All three perspectives take into account four central patient components, including (1) the patient's state of health; (2) the health results sought for the patient, which may be life, normal, or near normal functioning, or effective living despite disability; (3) the therapeutic self-care demand emanating from universal, developmental, and health-deviation self-care requisites; and (4) the patient's present abilities to engage in self-care and his or her health-related disabilities in giving self-care.

Nursing is appropriate when the person is not able to engage in self-care or dependent-care. More specifically, legitimate patients of nurses "are persons whose self-care agency, because of their health situations, is not adequate for purposes of knowing or meeting their own therapeutic self-care demands" (Orem & Taylor, 1986, p. 52). Nurse-patient relationships are established, then, when an actual or potential self-care deficit is evident.

The ability to nurse is termed nursing agency, which is described as a "complex property or attribute of nurses developed through specialized education and training in the theoretical and practical nursing sciences and through their development of the art of nursing in reality situations" (Orem & Taylor, 1986, p. 53). Nursing agency is developed and activated by individual nurses. Legitimate nurses "are persons who have the sets of qualities or characteristics symbolized by the term nursing agency" (Orem & Taylor, 1986, p. 53). Nursing agency and its performance are influenced by the basic conditioning factors identified in the section describing the person, as well as the nurse's educational preparation and experience.

The goal of nursing agency is to help people meet their own therapeutic self-care demands. This goal has three components: helping the patient accomplish therapeutic self-care; helping the patient move toward responsible self-care action, which may take the form of steadily increasing independence in self-care actions or adjustment to interruptions in self-care capabilities or to steadily declining self-care capacities; and helping members of the patient's family or other person who attends the patient become competent in providing and managing the patient's care using appropriate nursing supervision and consultation (Orem, 1985).

Orem (1985) identified social, interpersonal, and technological components of nursing practice. The social components focus on the role of the nurse and of the patient. A contractual relationship is established for the purpose of obtaining nursing care. The interpersonal components of nursing practice focus on establishing an interpersonal relationship that "contributes to alleviation of the patient's stress and that of the family, enabling the patient and the family to act responsibly in matters of health and health care" (Orem, 1985, p. 215). The interpersonal relationship between nursing and patient is necessary for establishment of the social contract and for provision of care. The technological components of nursing practice encompass the nurse's actions throughout all steps of the nursing process. Attainment of the technological components "occurs within the frame of a social-contractual relationship and an interpersonal relationship" (Orem, 1985, pp. 219–220).

Orem (1985) presented the nursing process in three steps: (1) diagnosis and prescription, (2) designing and planning, and (3) producing care to regulate therapeutic self-care demand and self-care agency. The first step focuses on determining why the person needs nursing care. This requires assessment of basic conditioning factors, calculation of the person's therapeutic self-care demand, assessment of self-care agency, and identification of the self-care deficit. The nursing diagnosis in Orem's conceptual framework is stated with regard to the "existent level of self-care agency for meeting current and emergent demands and potential for continuing development or redevelopment of self-care agency" (Taylor, 1985a). The components of this step are more fully specified in Table 7–2.

The second step of the nursing process starts with the design of a system of nursing assistance. A nursing system "is a dynamic action

---

TABLE 7–2. Elements of Diagnosis and Prescription*

I. Therapeutic self-care demand
   A. Calculate the patient's present and future therapeutic self-care demand through the following operations:
      1. particularization of each universal self-care requisite and identification of and particularization of existing, emerging, or projected developmental and health-deviation self-care requisites
      2. identification of internal and external factors that will affect the way in which each self-care requisite can be met and therefore condition the selection of methods for meeting it
      3. identification of interrelationships among the universal self-care requisites, between the universal self-care requisites and the developmental and health-deviation self-care requisites, and between the developmental and health-deviation self-care requisites
      4. determination of if and how methods selected to meet specific self-care requisites will affect meeting other self-care requisites
      5. design of the courses of action through which the particular universal self-care requisites will be met in relation to courses of action for meeting developmental and health-deviation requisites
      6. formulation of a total design for self-care action that is valid for a specified duration, including points of articulation with elements of the broader system of daily living
II. Self-care agency†
   A. Determine the patient's self-care abilities by ascertaining the degree of development, the operability, and the adequacy of his or her ability to:
      1. attend to specific things and exclude other things
      2. understand the characteristics and meaning of the characteristics of specific things
      3. apprehend the need to change or regulate the things observed
      4. acquire knowledge of appropriate courses of action for regulation
      5. decide what to do
      6. act to achieve change or regulation
   B. Determine if the patient should be helped to refrain from self-care actions for therapeutic purposes
   C. Determine if the patient should be helped to protect already developed self-care capabilities for therapeutic purposes

TABLE 7–2.   *Continued*

D. Determine the patient's potential for self-care agency in the future by identifying his or her:
   1. ability to increase or deepen self-care knowledge
   2. ability to learn techniques of care
   3. willingness to engage in self-care
   4. ability to effectively and consistently incorporate essential self-care measures into daily living

III.   Self-care deficit
   A. Calculate the patient's self-care deficit by determining the qualitative or quantitative inadequacy of self-care agency in relation to the calculated therapeutic self-care demand
   B. Determine the nature and reasons for the existence of the self-care deficit

*Diagnosis and prescription pertains to self-care and dependent-care.
†Scales to assess degree of development, operability, and adequacy of self-care are presented in Nursing Development Conference Group. (1979). Concept formalization in nursing. Process and product (2nd ed., p. 205). Boston: Little, Brown & Co.
Adapted from Orem, D.E. (1985). Nursing: Concepts of practice (3rd ed., pp. 100, 105–106, 225–226). New York: McGraw-Hill.

system constituted from series and sequences of actions, produced by nurses as they engage in the diagnostic, prescriptive, and regulatory operations of nursing practice" (Orem & Taylor, 1986, p. 53). Orem (1985) identified three types of regulatory nursing systems: (1) wholly compensatory, (2) partly compensatory, and (3) supportive-educative. These three nursing systems are defined and outlined in Table 7–3.

The choice of a nursing system is based on the answer to the question, who can or should perform self-care actions? The wholly compensatory nursing system is selected when the patient cannot or should not perform any self-care actions, and thus the nurse must perform them. The partly compensatory nursing system is selected when the patient can perform some, but not all, self-care actions. The supportive-educative nursing system is selected when the patient can and should perform all self-care actions.

The selection of the appropriate nursing system is followed by selection of appropriate method(s) of helping or assistance. Orem (1985) identified the following five methods that a person can use to give help or assistance to others:
   1. Acting for or doing for another
   2. Guiding another
   3. Supporting another physically or psychologically
   4. Providing an environment that promotes personal development
   5. Teaching another

The use of these methods of assistance in the nursing systems is shown in Table 7–3.

TABLE 7–3. Components of Nursing Systems

I. Wholly compensatory nursing systems
  A. Outcomes of nursing action
    1. Accomplishes patient's therapeutic self-care
    2. Compensates for patient's inability to engage in self-care
    3. Supports and protects the patient
  B. Subtype one
    1. Nursing systems for persons unable to engage in any form of deliberate action, including those who are:
      a. unable to control their position and movement in space
      b. unresponsive to stimuli or responsive to internal and external stimuli through hearing and feeling
      c. unable to monitor the environment and convey information to others because of loss of motor ability
    2. Method of helping
      a. acting for or doing for the patient
  C. Subtype two
    1. Nursing systems for persons who are aware and who may be able to make observations, judgments, and decisions about self-care and other matters but cannot or should not perform actions requiring ambulation and manipulative movements. This includes persons who are:
      a. aware of themselves and their immediate environment and able to communicate with others normally or in a restricted manner
      b. unable to move about and perform manipulative movements because of pathological processes or the effects or results of injury, immobilizing measures of medical treatment, or extreme weakness or debility
      c. under medical orders to restrict movement
    2. Methods of helping
      a. providing a developmental environment
      b. acting for or doing for the patient
      c. supporting the patient psychologically
      d. guiding the patient
      e. teaching the patient
  D. Subtype three
    1. Nursing systems for persons unable to attend to themselves and make reasoned judgments and decisions about self-care and other matters but who can be ambulatory and may be able to perform some measures of self-care with continuous guidance and supervision. This includes persons who:
      a. are conscious but unable to focus attention on themselves or others for purposes of self-care or care of others
      b. do not make rational or reasonable judgments and decisions about their own care and daily living without guidance
      c. can ambulate and perform some measures of self-care with continuous guidance and supervision
    2. Methods of helping
      a. providing a developmental environment
      b. guiding the patient
      c. providing support for the patient
      d. acting for or doing for the patient
II. Partly compensatory nursing system
  A. Outcomes

TABLE 7–3.   *Continued*

1. Nurse action
   a. performs some self-care measures for the patient
   b. compensates for self-care limitations of the patient
   c. assists the patient as required
   d. regulates self-care agency
2. Patient action
   a. performs some self-care measures
   b. regulates self-care agency
   c. accepts care and assistance from the nurse

B. Subtype one
   1. Patient performs universal measures of self-care; nurse performs medically prescribed measures and some universal self-care measures
   2. Methods of helping
      a. acting for or doing for the patient
      b. guiding the patient
      c. supporting the patient
      d. providing a developmental environment
      e. teaching the patient

C. Subtype two
   1. Patient learns to perform some new care measures
   2. Methods of helping
      a. acting for or doing for the patient
      b. guiding the patient
      c. supporting the patient
      d. providing a developmental environment
      e. teaching the patient

III. Supportive-educative nursing system
   A. Outcomes
      1. Nurse action
         a. regulates the exercise and development of self-care agency
      2. Patient action
         a. accomplishes self-care
         b. regulates the exercise and development of self-care agency
   B. Subtype one
      1. Patient can perform care measures
      2. Methods of helping
         a. guiding the patient
         b. supporting the patient
   C. Subtype two
      1. Patient can perform care measures
      2. Method of helping
         a. teaching the patient
   D. Subtype three
      1. Patient can perform care measures
      2. Method of helping
         a. providing a developmental environment
   E. Subtype four
      1. Patient is competent in self-care
      2. Method of helping
         a. guiding the patient periodically

Adapted from Orem, D.E. (1985). Nursing: Concepts of practice (3rd ed., pp. 154–157). New York: McGraw-Hill.

The planning component of the second step of the nursing process requires "specification of the time, place, environmental conditions, and equipment and supplies, [as well as] the number and qualifications of nurses or others necessary . . . to produce a designed nursing system or a portion thereof, to evaluate effects, and to make needed adjustments" (Orem, 1985, p. 237). The plan specifies the organization and timing of tasks to be performed, allocates task performance to nurse or patient, and identifies methods to be used by nurses to help the patient.

The final step of the nursing process encompasses the provision of direct nursing care and decisions regarding the continuing of direct care in its present form or changing the form. Regulatory nursing systems are produced "when nurses interact with patients and take consistent action to meet their prescribed therapeutic self-care demands and to regulate the exercise or development of their capabilities for self-care" (Orem, 1985, p. 237). Actions taken by nurses to accomplish this step are presented in Table 7–4.

Orem (1985) stated that nursing care may occur at three levels of prevention: primary, secondary, and tertiary. Universal self-care and developmental self-care, when therapeutic, constitute the primary level of prevention. Nursing care at this level includes assisting the patient to learn self-care practices that "maintain and promote health and development and [that] prevent specific diseases" (p. 192).

TABLE 7–4.   Nursing Actions for Production of Care to Regulate Therapeutic Self-Care Demand and Self-Care Agency

I. Direct nursing care actions
    A. Perform and regulate the self-care tasks for patients or assist patients with their performance of self-care tasks
    B. Coordinate self-care task performance so that a unified system of care is produced and coordinated with other components of health care
    C. Help patients, their families, and others bring about systems of daily living for patients that support the accomplishment of self-care and are, at the same time, satisfying in relation to patients' interests, talents, and goals
    D. Guide, direct, and support patients in their exercise of, or in the withholding the exercise of, their self-care agency
    E. Stimulate patients' interests in self-care by raising questions and promoting discussions of care problems and issues when conditions permit
    F. Support and guide patients in learning activities and provide cues for learning as well as instructional sessions
    G. Support and guide patients as they experience illness or disability and the effects of medical care measures and as they experience the need to engage in new measures of self-care or change their ways of meeting ongoing self-care requisites

TABLE 7–4. *Continued*

II. Decision making actions regarding direct nursing care
   A. Monitor patients and assist patients to monitor themselves to determine if self-care measures were performed and to determine the effects of self-care, the results of efforts to regulate the exercise or development of self-care agency, and the sufficiency and efficiency of nursing action directed to these ends
   B. Make characterizing judgments about the sufficiency and efficiency of self-care, the regulation of the exercise or development of self-care agency, and nursing assistance
   C. Make judgments about the meaning of the results derived from nurses' performance when monitoring patients and judging outcomes of self-care for the well-being of patients, and make or recommend adjustments in the nursing care system through changes in nurse and patient roles

Adapted from Orem, D.E. (1985). Nursing: Concepts of practice (3rd ed., p. 238). New York: McGraw-Hill.

Health-deviation self-care, when therapeutic, constitutes the secondary or tertiary level of prevention. Nursing care at these levels focuses on helping the patient learn self-care practices that "regulate and prevent adverse effects of the disease, prevent complicating diseases, prevent prolonged disability, or adapt or adjust functioning to overcome or compensate for the adverse effects of permanent or prolonged disfigurement or dysfunction" (p. 194).

Content of the Model: Propositions

The linkage of person, environment, and nursing is evident in the following statement regarding provision of a developmental environment as a method of assistance: "This method of asistance requires the helper to provide or help to provide environmental conditions that motivate the person being helped to establish appropriate goals and adjust behavior to achieve results specified by the goals" (Orem, 1985, pp. 140–141).

The linkage of person, health, and nursing is evident in the following proposition: "Nursing has as its special concern the individual's need for self-care action and the provision and management of it on a continuous basis in order to sustain life and health, recover from disease or injury, and cope with their effects" (Orem, 1985, p. 54). No statement linking person, environment, health, and nursing is evident in Orem's latest publications.

Areas of Concern

The major area of concern or problem in Orem's conceptual framework is the individual's capabilities regarding complete and effective self-care or dependent care. The source of this problem is any state or factor that imposes limitations on self-care or dependent care.

EVALUATION OF OREM'S SELF-CARE FRAMEWORK

This section presents an evaluation of Orem's conceptual framework. The evaluation is based on the results of the analysis, as well as publications and presentations by others who have used or commented on Orem's work.

Explication of Assumptions

Orem was explicit in articulating her assumptions and explicating her values and special points of emphasis. Taken together, the assumptions identified by Orem indicate that she values individuals' abilities to care for themselves without intervention from health care professionals except when actual or potential self-care deficits arise. Furthermore, Orem expects people to be responsible for themselves and to seek help when they cannot maintain therapeutic self-care or dependent-care.

Orem also values the person's perspective of his or her health status, as well as that of the physician. This indicates that she does not expect nursing care to be based solely on the nurse's view of the patient's situation.

The special points of emphasis in the conceptual framework are self-care requisites, self-care agency, and self-care deficits. Although Orem indicated that nursing is appropriate when the person experiences a self-care deficit, she noted that primary prevention also is appropriate, to help the person maintain self-care agency.

Comprehensiveness of Concepts and Propositions

Orem's descriptions of the person, the environment, health, and nursing are considerably well-refined for a conceptual model. The person is fully defined and described as he or she relates to nursing. Nursing also is fully defined and described in terms of scope and appropriate actions to be taken in relation to patients. However, the descriptions of environment and health could be clarified.

Although environment is mentioned repeatedly in the presentation of the model, its parameters are not identified. Moreover, environmental factors, elements, and conditions that affect self-care agency are not specified. The specification of these ideas would reduce confusion about the nature and extent of the environment of interest.

Moreover, although health and well-being are clearly defined, the relation of self-care agency to health is not fully explained in Orem's conceptual framework. The implication is that if the person is not able to engage in self-care, a state of illness prevails. What is not clear here is whether this means that illness occurs whenever a self-care deficit is apparent, regardless of the presence or absence of signs and symptoms of disease. For example, is a person considered ill when a developmental self-care requisite cannot be met without assistance but when he or she has no signs or symptoms of disease? Or, are self-care deficits separate from disease and illness?

Orem's description of the nursing process meets Walker and Nicholson's (1980) criteria. Nursing diagnoses and nursing actions are based on knowledge about the patient's therapeutic self-care demand and self-care or dependent-care agency. Orem noted that this knowledge should be grounded in scientifically valid theory. The nursing process is presented as a dynamic activity, with diagnosis viewed as ongoing and design of nursing systems tentative. The dynamic nature of the nursing process is further documented by the following statement:

> The degree to which designing nursing systems and planning their production can be separately performed in a block of time in between steps 1 and 3 of the nursing process varies. Factors that militate against this include (1) rapid and complex changes in the health status of patients, (2) needs for continuous adjustments in patients' therapeutic self-care demands, (3) insufficient amounts of valid and reliable factual information about patients and their environments, and (4) inability of the nurse to predict the future values of the patient variables (therapeutic self-care demand and self-care agency). (Orem, 1985, p. 231)

The applicability of Orem's nursing process in a variety of settings is well-established, as documented in the section on social utility and in the annotated bibliography at the end of this chapter. Orem's inclusion of the patient's perspective of health status reflects her concern with ethical standards. Furthermore, this criterion is documented by Orem's concern for obtaining enough information to make accurate diagnoses. She noted that "one danger to be avoided for the protection of patients and nurses is making nursing diagnoses and prescriptions on the basis of inadequate data about patients" (Orem, 1985, p. 226). Finally, the conceptual framework is essentially consistent with scientific findings about human behavior. In fact, Orem (1985) noted that nursing agency is based in large part on knowledge of nursing, sciences, arts, and humanities.

The criterion for the linkage of concepts requires that the propositions of the conceptual model link all four metaparadigm concepts. This criterion was not met, in that no statement linking person, environment, health, and nursing could be located in the third edition of

Orem's (1985) book or in the chapter by Orem and Taylor (1986). It should be noted, however, that the following statement, published in the second edition of Orem's (1980) book, does link the four metaparadigm concepts:

> Nursing is made or produced by nurses. It is a service, a mode of helping human beings. . . . Nursing's form or structure is derived from actions deliberately selected and performed by nurses to help individuals or groups under their care to maintain or change conditions in themselves or their environments. This may be done by individuals or groups through their own actions under the guidance of a nurse or through the actions of nurses when persons have health-derived or health-related limitations that cannot be immediately overcome. (Orem, 1980, p. 5)

Logical Congruence

World Views

Orem's conceptual framework reflects the organismic world view. The person is viewed as active in maintaining self-care and seeking health care when faced with a self-care deficit. Although Orem (1985) indicated that human beings have parts, she viewed the parts within the unity of human structure and functioning. She stated, "If there is acceptance of the real unity of individual human beings, there should be no difficulty in recognizing structural and functional differentiations within the unity" (p. 180). Thus, Orem clearly regarded the person as active and holistic.

Smith (1987) maintained that Orem's work "fits with the totality paradigm" (p. 97). To the extent that the totality paradigm reflects a mechanistic world view or even a bridge between mechanism and organicism, this classification seems inappropriate. Indeed, there is no evidence of a mechanistic view of the world in the content of Orem's conceptual framework.

Orem's emphasis on maintenance of self-care agency suggests a persistence world view. Stability of therapeutic self-care agency is the desired goal in the conceptual framework. Loss of self-care results from health-derived or health-related limitations and is not considered desirable. Although development is a major concept of this conceptual framework, the change inherent in this component does not present a logical inconsistency. Orem translated the two potentially competing views of persistence and change by emphasizing that maintenance of self-care agency is conditioned by age and developmental state. Thus, changes in self-care ability are necessary for survival as the person matures.

Classification of the Model

Orem's conceptual framework was classified as a systems model by Riehl and Roy (1980). No rationale for that classification was provided. Close examination of the conceptual framework failed to reveal any evidence of a match between its content and the characteristics of systems models. Although Orem used the term nursing system, she did not present this concept from a general system theory viewpoint, with its emphasis on input, output, and feedback.

Orem's conceptual framework is more appropriately classified as a developmental model. The characteristics of growth, development, and maturation are addressed by the developmental self-care requisites and by the consideration of self-care agency adjusted for age and developmental state.

The developmental model characteristic of change is addressed in terms of changes in self-care agency that occur throughout life. Direction of change is viewed as toward higher levels of integration and assumption of self-care and dependent care agency. This is reflected in the following statement of Orem's (1985) position about health and well-being:

> The point of view of human beings as persons is a moving rather than a static one. It is the view of personalization of the individual, that is, moving toward maturation and achievement of the individual's human potential. This process of coming to be a person involves individuals in communications with their worlds; in action; in the exercise of the human desire to know, to seek the truth; and in the giving of themselves in the doing of good for themselves and others. . . . Personalization proceeds as individuals live under conditions favorable or unfavorable to human developmental processes. . . . There is a striving by individuals to achieve the potential of their natural endowments for physical and rational functioning while living a life of faith with respect to things hoped for and to perfect themselves as responsible human beings who raise questions, seek answers, reflect, and come to awareness of the relationship between what they know and what they do. (p. 180)

Orem addressed the characteristic of identifiable state through her discussion of the differences in self-care agency throughout life. The child is viewed as being in a stage of dependent-care, and the healthy adult is in a stage of total self-care and dependent-care agency. Socially dependent adults, including ill and disabled persons, are in a stage of dependent-care. Orem (1985) explained:

> Infants and children require care from others because they are in the early stages of development physically, psychologically, and psychosocially. The aged person requires total care or assistance whenever

declining physical and mental abilities limit the selection or performance of self-care actions. The ill or disabled person requires partial
or total care from others (or assistance in the form of teaching or guidance) depending on his or her health state and immediate or future requirements for self-care. Self-care is an adult's continuous contribution
to his or her own continued existence, health, and well-being. Care of
others is an adult's contribution to the health and well-being of dependent members of the adult's social group. (p. 84)

Orem's conceptual framework addressed form of progression of
development as cycles of change in self-care agency. Although the
overall direction is toward increasing ability for self-care and dependent-care, loss of some agency does occur at various times throughout
life, such as when illness or disability imposes limitations on self-care
and dependent-care agency.

The characteristic of forces that produce growth and development
is viewed in Orem's conceptual framework as a natural component of
human development. That is, self-care and dependent-care agency
naturally increase as the person matures. Indeed, Orem assumed that
people have an inherent, overt potential for development of self-care
agency.

Meleis (1985) classified Orem's conceptual framework within the
needs category. Meleis apparently based her classification on the description of universal self-care requisites, which she labeled as "universal self-care needs" (p. 290). Marriner (1986) placed Orem's work
in her humanistic category. Stevens (1984) regarded Orem's conceptual framework as a good example of the substitution category of her
classification scheme.

Generation and Testing of Theory

The studies cited in the section on social utility and those listed
in the annotated bibliography are initial attempts to operationalize
and test the concepts of Orem's conceptual framework. In particular,
Kearney and Fleischer (1979), Denyes (1982), Hanson and Bickel
(1985), and Gulick (1987) have made important contributions to the
empirical measurement of self-care agency.

In addition to this work, three theories have been derived directly
from Orem's conceptual framework of nursing. These are the theory of
self-care deficit or dependent-care deficit, the theory of self-care, and
the theory of nursing systems. The central idea of the theory of self-
care or dependent-care deficit is that "people can benefit from nursing
because they are subject to health-related or health-derived limitations
that render them incapable of continuous self-care or dependent-care
or that result in ineffective or incomplete care" (Orem, 1985, pp. 34–
35). This theory is summarized in the following statement:

The self-care agency of mature or maturing individuals in its relations to their knowing and meeting their therapeutic self-care demands can be adversely affected by health-associated conditions and factors internal or external to such individuals that render their self-care agency wholly or partially nonoperational or qualitatively or quantitatively inadequate for knowing and meeting their therapeutic self-care demands and thus giving rise to legitimate requirements for nursing. (Orem & Taylor, 1986, p. 44)

The central idea of the theory of self-care is that "self-care and care of dependent family members are learned behaviors that purposely regulate human structural integrity, functioning, and human development" (Orem, 1985, p. 36). The theory is summarized in the following statement:

Mature or maturing persons contribute to the regulation of their own functioning and development and to the prevention, control, or amelioration of disease and injury and their effects by performing, within the context of their day-to-day living, learned actions directed to themselves or their environments that are known or assumed to have regulatory value with respect to human functioning and development. (Orem & Taylor, 1986, p. 44)

The central idea of the theory of nursing systems is that "nursing systems are formed when nurses use their abilities to prescribe, design, and provide nursing for legitimate patients (as individuals or groups) by performing discrete actions and systems of actions. These actions or systems regulate the value of or the exercise of individuals' capabilities to engage in self-care and meet the self-care requisites of the individual therapeutically" (Orem, 1985, p. 38). The theory of nursing systems is summarized in the following statement:

All action systems that are nursing systems are produced by nurses through the exercise of their nursing agency within the context of their contractual and interpersonal relations with individuals who are characterized by health associated self-care deficits for purposes of ensuring that their therapeutic self-care demands are known and met and their self-care agency is protected or its exercise or development is regulated. (Orem & Taylor, 1986, p. 44)

Orem and Taylor (1986) regarded the theory of nursing systems as the general theory of nursing, "because it explains the product made by nurses in nursing practice situations in relation to two conceptualized properties of individuals who need nursing, as these properties are expressed and related in the theory of self-care deficit" (p. 44). The theory of nursing systems, they explained, "is understood in its relationship to the theory of self-care deficit," which in turn "is understood in its relationship to the theory of self-care" (p. 44).

Orem (1985) presented the central ideas of the theories of self-care deficit, self-care, and nursing systems as well as a series of initial propositions or premises and presuppositions for each theory. The presuppositions serve as the basic assumptions underlying each theory and the propositions extend the central ideas. There is no evidence of empirical testing of the theories. However, the propositions of each theory are sound starting points for the generation of empirically testable hypotheses. The following example will illustrate this point. One proposition of the theory of self-care or dependent-care deficit is:

> The individual's abilities to engage in self-care or dependent care are conditioned by age, developmental state, life experience, sociocultural orientation, health, and available resources. (Orem, 1985, p. 35)

The concepts contained in this proposition are self-care (or dependent-care), age, developmental state, life experience, sociocultural orientation, health, and available resources. Each of these concepts must be operationally defined and measurement tools identified. Then, the proposition may be stated as an empirically testable hypothesis that can be supported or refuted by an appropriate empirical study.

Social Considerations

Social Congruence

Riehl-Sisca (1985b) noted that the self-care label associated with Orem's conceptual framework is appealing to nurses and to potential and actual patients. She pointed out that Orem's approach to nursing

> appeared on the scene when the general public was becoming more knowledgeable about medical treatment and disenchanted with physicians' care and motivation. . . . In some cases, the patient seems to know as much about his or her condition as does the physician. This encourages the taking care of oneself. (p. 308)

Orem's model is congruent with society's expectations that individuals should have decision-making responsibility regarding their health care. However, the emphasis on self-care agency during times of illness is not completely congruent with some people's expectations of nursing goals. Moreover, attention must be given to expectations of people of different socioeconomic and cultural groups. For example, Anna, Christensen, Hohon, Ord, and Wells (1978) found that the nursing goal of self-care agency for the patient was not well accepted by either patients or staff of a nursing home. In this situation, a more dependent sick role view, with the nurse doing for and acting for the patient, had been adopted by both patients and staff. Anna and his associates also noted that a Mexican-American patient in the nursing home "did not see the relevance of performing self-care activities, and he functioned with the expectation that the staff would do everything for him" (p. 11). Orem (1985) noted that when this occurs, the person must be helped to view himself or herself as a self-care agent. Elaborating, she stated:

> Self-care is performed largely out of habit, but individuals who have not thought about their self-care role may need to be helped to look at themselves as self-care agents in order to understand the values to which their habits commit them and to appraise the adequacy of their self-care abilities. (p. 107)

Furthermore, Behi (1986) discussed the constraints on use of Orem's conceptual framework of nursing in the United Kingdom. He stated, "Perhaps the most fundamental constraint in this country is society's attitude. Self-care as a concept, and more importantly, as a value, is stronger in American society where control of an individual's health is seen as that person's responsibility" (p. 35). Behi concluded, however, that Orem's conceptual framework could be used in general wards of the National Health Service in the United Kingdom.

The primary prevention aspect of Orem's conceptual framework is another area where attention to congruence with societal expectations must be given. Although consumers are becoming more aware of the value of health promotion and the nurse's role in promoting wellness, they still may need to be helped to accept this nursing role and utilize nursing services in this area.

Social Significance

It is not yet known with certainty whether Orem's conceptual framework leads to nursing actions that make important differences in the person's health status. However, Buckwalter and Kerfoot's (1982) work suggested that psychiatric patient discharge teaching that emphasizes self-care was effective in areas such as compliance with psychotropic medication regimens and appropriate use of community resources. Furthermore, Scherer (1988) reported that use of Orem's conceptual framework at the Newark, New Jersey, Beth Israel Medical Center is associated with enhanced patient satisfaction with nursing care, less staff turnover, and reduced costs.

The emphasis on self-care agency and recognition of the person's ability to care for self could lead to more efficient use of health care services. That is, if people can be helped to recognize and improve their own self-care abilities and to use health services only when they identify potential or actual self-care deficits, there may be less inappropriate use of the services. Furthermore, emphasis on self-care agency could reduce the length of time the person requires health care services. This may be especially important in the present era of cost containment.

Social Utility

The social utility of Orem's conceptual framework is extremely well-documented, as can be seen in the following discussion as well as in the annotated bibliography at the end of this chapter. The conceptual framework is being used by nurses throughout the United States and in Canada, Australia, Switzerland, Denmark, and Sweden (Orem, personal communication, August 6, 1987), as well as in Brazil (Beckmann, 1987). Books related to Orem's conceptual framework of nursing have been published by Munley and Sayers (1984) and Riehl-Sisca (1985a). Munley and Sayers (1986) also produced a series of slides designed for teaching the conceptual framework. The conceptual framework and the theories of self-care deficit, self-care, and nursing systems are the focus of an annual conference on their practical applications sponsored by the Newark, New Jersey, Beth Israel Medical Center and Nickle and Associates, as well as an annual self-care deficit theory of nursing conference, an annual self-care deficit theory of nursing institute, and research conferences sponsored by the University of Missouri-Columbia School of Nursing. This school also publishes the "Self-Care Deficit Theory Curriculum Network Newsletter." The newsletter, to which more than 200 individuals, schools, and clinical agencies subscribe, regularly lists schools of nursing, clinical agencies, and individual clinicians who use the conceptual framework. A directory of individuals and agencies who use the conceptual framework was begun in 1987 by faculty at the University of Missouri-Columbia School of Nursing. Another directory was begun in 1987 by the staff of the Self-Care Institute at George Mason University School of Nursing in Fairfax, Virginia. This organization was established to develop, compile, and maintain a database consisting of individuals and organizations united across disciplines by a common interest in self-care, and to promote self-care research. The interests of the Institute extend beyond Orem's approach to self-care to a consideration of self-care in a general manner.

The utility of Orem's conceptual framework as a guide for nursing research is apparent. Explict rules for research have not yet been developed, although Geden (1985) maintained that "at this time in the development of . . . self-care theory, all [research] approaches are appropriate and necessary" (p. 265). Many studies have been conducted within the context of Orem's conceptual framework and have been presented at various research conferences, including meetings devoted exclusively to Orem-based investigations such as those sponsored by the University of Missouri-Columbia School of Nursing, Georgetown University School of Nursing, and Wichita State University. Numerous master's theses and doctoral dissertations have used the conceptual framework as a guide. Smith (1979) cited two unpublished master's theses conducted by students at the University of Southern Mississippi based on Orem's conceptual framework. These were studies of therapeutic self-care demands of mentally retarded persons (Rachel, 1978) and of leadership effectiveness of head nurses (White, 1977). Hanson's (1981) and Bickel's (1982) master's theses at the University of Missouri-Columbia reported their work on development of an instrument to measure self-care agency. Flanagan's (1983) master's thesis, also at the University of Missouri-Columbia, focused on oxygen consumption required for bathing and being bathed in bed. Silva and Sorrell (1987) identified many doctoral dissertations related to Orem's conceptual framework, including those by Banks (1981), Barkauskas (1981), Brugge (1982), Clancy (1984), Denyes (1980), Dodd (1981), Eith (1983), Evans (1980), Fernsler (1984), Gast (1984), Hehn (1986), Kain (1986), Lantz (1982), Laurin (1979), Marten (1983), Michaels (1986), Musci (1984), Neves (1980), Olson (1986), Parker (1983), Pulliam (1986), Rieder (1982), Scheetz (1986), Schorfheide (1986), Sirles (1986), Stullenbarger (1985), Underwood (1979), and Wells-Biggs (1986). Pinkerton's (1983), Bliss-Holtz's (1986, 1988), Burns's (1986), Brawn's (1987), Harvey's (1987), and Stashinko's (1987) doctoral dissertations also were based on Orem's conceptual framework.

Several studies derived from Orem's conceptual framework have been published. Some of the investigations have focused on development of instruments to measure aspects of self-care agency. Kearney and Fleischer (1979) developed an instrument to measure exercise of self-care agency. They validated the instrument by comparing items to other instruments that measure various psychological characteristics of individuals. McBride (1987) reported additional research on the psychometric properties of this instrument. Denyes (1982) developed an instrument to measure the self-care agency of adolescents. Hanson and Bickel (1985) described their work to develop and determine the psychometric properties of a questionnaire designed to measure the adult's perception of his or her self-care agency. Questionnaire items reflected the 10 power components of Orem's conceptual framework. Hanson and Bickel noted that the perception of self-care agency instrument is being used by nursing students, faculty, and researchers in various settings to further determine its psychometric properties. Weaver (1987) examined the psychometric properties of the Hanson and Bickel questionnaire by means of factor analysis. He found that the factor structure of the instrument was significantly different from that proposed by Hanson and Bickel. Weaver concluded that his findings call into question the construct validity of Hanson and Bickel's instrument in non-institutionalized adults. Campbell (1986) developed the Danger Assessment instrument to measure the extent to which battered women are in danger of homicide. She stated that "within Orem's conceptual framework," the process of completing the Danger Assessment instrument "can be considered an instance of enhancing the woman's self-care agency or her ability to take deliberate action to perform self-care" (p. 37). Gulick (1987) used "Orem's self-care framework . . . to guide the development of a scale to measure activities of daily living (ADL) among persons diagnosed with multiple sclerosis" (p. 278). Compilation of a list of self-care instruments was begun in 1987 by the Office of Nursing Grants and Research at the University of Kansas School of Nursing in Kansas City.

Other studies have described patients' self-care practices. Allison (1971) explored the meaning of rest for patients. Brock and O'Sullivan (1985) identified factors that distinguish newly institutionalized elderly people from elderly people able to remain in the community within the context of Orem's conceptual framework. Chang and her associates (1984, 1985) studied factors affecting satisfaction with nursing care and adherence to health care regimens in elderly women. Crockett (1982) studied the self-care practices for coping used by adult psychiatric and non-psychiatric subjects. Dodd (1982, 1984b, 1988) described self-care behaviors of cancer patients who were receiving chemotherapy or radiation therapy. Geden (1985) placed her studies of oxygen consumption within the context of Orem's conceptual framework. She commented that the studies by Geden (1982), Hathaway and Geden (1983) and Flanagan (1983) "may be related to the universal self-care requisite of maintaining a balance between activity and rest and/or related to the power component of self-care agency" dealing with ability to control body position (p. 268). Hautman (1987) used Orem's definition of self-care in her study of self-care responses to respiratory illness in a sample of Vietnamese individuals residing in Texas. Kubricht (1984) described the therapeutic self-care demands of outpatients receiving radiation therapy. Miller (1982) identified categories of self-care needs for a sample of diabetics. Patterson and Hale (1985) described self-care practices related to menstruation. Rew (1987) compared the self-care behaviors of children with asthma before and after a one-week residential camping experience. Sandman, Norberg, Adolfsson, Axelsson, and Hedly (1986) used Orem's conceptual framework to guide their analysis of the behaviors of five patients with Alzheimer-type dementia and their nurses during morning care. Storm and Baumgartner (1987) presented a case study within the context of Orem's conceptual framework of a 41-year-old woman with multiple sclerosis who was discharged home with a mechanical ventilator. Woods (1985) and Maunz and Woods (1988) described self-care activities used by young adult women.

Still other studies have explored the effects of nursing intervention on self-care abilities. Blazek and McClellan (1983) examined the effect of an experimental treatment designed to help children become managers of their own health care on locus of control. Dodd (1983, 1984a) measured the effects of nursing interventions on self-care behavior in patients receiving cancer chemotherapy. Goodwin (1979) studied the effect of programmed instruction on recovery following pulmonary surgery. Harper (1984) investigated the effects of a medication program on medication knowledge, health locus of control, and self-care medication behaviors in a sample of elderly black women. Karl (1982) examined the effect of an exercise program on independence in self-care activities in a sample of elderly patients. Moore (1987) investigated the effects of different learning strategies on promotion of autonomy and self-care agency in school-aged children. Rothlis (1984) studied the effects of a self-help group on feelings of hopelessness and helplessness in a sample of patients with reactive depression. Stockdale-Woolley (1984) examined the effect of group education classes on the self-care agency of individuals with COPD. Toth (1980) used Orem's conceptual framework to guide her study of the effect of preparation for transfer from the coronary care unit on patient anxiety. Orem's conceptual framework also was used to guide Whetstone's (1986) study of the effect of social dramatics on social skills of chronically mentally ill patients.

Furthermore, Tompkins (1980) discussed her study findings in relation to a few conceptual models, including Orem's. There is, however, no evidence that this study was directly derived from Orem's conceptual framework of nursing.

The utility of Orem's conceptual framework of nursing for nursing practice is fully documented. Rules for nursing practice were identified by Orem (1985). She presented detailed lists of directives for nursing practice within the following five sets: (1) initial period of contact between nurse and patient, (2) continuing nurse-patient contacts, (3) the quality of interpersonal situations with patients, (4) the production of nursing, and (5) relationships of the nurse with other nurses and other health care providers. It is clear from these directives and the content of the conceptual framework that nursing practice is directed toward and contributes to facilitation of patients' self-care agency, and that the clinical problems of interest are the patients' self-care deficits. Nursing care is carried out in various settings and is directed toward persons who have deficits in self-care agency or dependent-care agency. The nursing process is clearly outlined, although a specific diagnostic taxonomy directly linked with Orem's conceptual framework has not yet been formulated.

Orem's conceptual framework has been used to guide nursing activities in various settings such as ambulatory clinics (Allison, 1973; Backscheider, 1974; Crews, 1972; Alford, 1985), obstetrical units (Wollery, 1983), a nursing home (Anna, et al., 1978), acute care units (Mullin, 1980), critical care units (Fawcett, et al., 1987), a college health program (Hedahl, 1983), psychiatric units (Moscovitz, 1984), rehabilitation units (Smith, 1977), and hospices (Murphy, 1981; Walborn, 1980). In these and other settings, the conceptual framework has been used to guide the nursing care of patients with conditions such as diabetes (Allison, 1973; Backscheider, 1974; Zach, 1982), congestive heart failure (Crews, 1972), coronary artery bypass surgery (Campuzano, 1982), cerebral vascular accidents (Anna, et al., 1978), gastroenteritis and upper respiratory infections (Facteau, 1980), neurological problems (Mitchell & Irving, 1977), end stage renal disease requiring peritoneal dialysis (Perras & Zappacosta, 1982), head and neck surgery (Dropkin, 1981), and terminal illness (Walborn, 1980). The conceptual framework also has been used to design nursing care for patients of various ages and with a variety of self-care requisites. For example, Facteau (1980) described the nursing care of hospitalized infants, toddlers, and preschool-age and school-age children. Gantz (1980) developed a health education program aimed at enhancing self-care agency for 10-year-old school children. Harrigan, Faro, VanPutte, and Stoler (1987) designed an educational program for juvenile diabetics that accounted for the children's locus of control orientation. Nursing care guidelines for adolescent alcohol abusers were presented by Michael and Sewall (1980). Harris (1980) used the model to design nursing care for patients having cesarean childbirth. Nursing care of the aged was described by Garvan, Lee, Lloyd, and Sullivan (1980) and Finnegan (1986). In each article, the concepts of the model were linked with relevant knowledge borrowed from other disciplines. Facteau (1980), for example, developed nursing interventions designed to increase the self-care agency of hospitalized children based on developmental theories. Crews (1972) used pharmacological knowledge of anticoagulants and knowledge of the pathophysiology of congestive heart failure to identify patients' self-care needs.

Orem's conceptual framework has been extended for use with the family (Chin, 1985; Orem, 1983a, 1983b, 1983c; Tadych, 1985) and in the community (Orem, 1984). Nowakowski (1980) described a community health education program developed at Georgetown University. Moreover, the conceptual framework has been adapted for use in diverse cultures (Branch, 1985; Chamorro, 1985; Hammonds, 1985; Isenberg, 1987).

The utility of Orem's Self-Care Framework for nursing education also is documented. Rules for nursing education are beginning to be formulated. Taylor (1985b) maintained that the conceptual framework of nursing provides the "structured body of knowledge essential for curriculum development" (p. 27). Her claim indicates that the focus of the curriculum is on components of self-care, self-care agency, self-care deficits, nursing agency, and nursing systems. Riehl-Sisca (1985c) and Taylor (1985b) identified content that should be included in a curriculum based on Orem's conceptual framework of nursing. In particular, Riehl-Sisca distinguished content for the undergraduate curriculum from that for the graduate curriculum. Taylor identified objectives and the curriculum pattern for an undergraduate baccalaureate program. Farnham and Fowler (1985) and Taylor (1985c) presented detailed discussions of teaching-learning strategies to be used when teaching Orem's conceptual framework of nursing. Taylor pointed out that the faculty "must have knowledge of self-care deficit theory and skill in its use in order to teach it to students" (p. 41).

Taylor (1985a) noted that Orem's conceptual framework is used by at least 45 schools of nursing but did not identify the schools by name. Orem (personal communication, August 6, 1987) listed several schools that use her conceptual framework, including the University of Missouri-Columbia; Palm Beach Atlantic College in West Palm Beach, Florida; Centennial College in Scarborough, Ontario, Canada; College de Bois-de-Boulogne in Montreal, Quebec, Canada; Catholic Education College in Melbourne, Australia; as well as the Open Learning Institute Refresher Program in British Columbia, Canada. Other schools of nursing that have used the conceptual framework include Elmhurst College in Elmhurst, Illinois; Olivet Nazarene College in Kankakee, Illinois; Wichita State University in Wichita, Kansas; College of St. Benedict in St. Joseph, Minnesota; the University of Southern Mississippi in Hattiesburg; Southwest Missouri State University in Springfield; Seton Hall University in South Orange, New Jersey; Mount Saint Mary College in Newburgh, New York; Queens College in Charlotte, North Carolina; the University of North Carolina at Greensboro; Medical College of Ohio in Toledo; Bethany Nazarene College in Bethany, Oklahoma; Edinboro University of Pennsylvania in Edinboro; Millersville University in Millersville, Pennsylvania; East Stroudsburg University in East Stroudsburg, Pennsylvania; Incarnate Word College in San Antonio, Texas; Stephen F. Austin State University in Nacogdoches, Texas; Georgetown University in Washington, D.C. (Asay & Ossler, 1984); Thornton Community College in South Holland, Illinois (Fenner, 1979); George Mason University in Fairfax, Virginia (Mullin & Weed, 1980); and the University of Ottawa in Ontario, Canada (Story & Ross, 1986).

Some descriptions of the use of Orem's conceptual framework in nursing education have been published. Fenner (1979) described use of the conceptual framework in the associate degree nursing program at Thornton Community College in South Holland, Illinois. Another publication described two clinical tools based on the nursing process of Orem's conceptual framework (Herrington & Houston, 1984).

The utility of Orem's conceptual framework for administration of nursing services also is documented. Although explicit rules for administration have not yet been formulated, implications for the rules are beginning to be developed by Orem (in press), who identified theories and hypotheses related to nursing administration, Nunn and Marriner (in press), who described the application of the conceptual framework to nursing administration situations, and Allison (1985) and Nickle-Gallagher (1985), who described strategies used to implement use of Orem's conceptual framework in rehabilitation settings.

Orem's conceptual framework of nursing is used to structure nursing practice in many clinical agencies. Taylor (1985a) indicated that approximately 18 clinical agencies use Orem's conceptual framework as a basis for nursing practice but did not list the agencies by name. Orem (personal communication, August 6, 1987) identified several clinical agencies that use her conceptual framework, including the Harry S. Truman Memorial Veterans Administration Hospital in Columbia, Missouri; Mississippi Methodist Rehabilitation Hospital in Jackson, Mississippi; Scarborough General Hospital in Scarborough, Ontario, Canada; Centre Hospitalier de Gatineau, Gatineau, Quebec, Canada; the Health Department in Vancouver, British Columbia, Canada; and the Geriatric Rehabilitation Center in Copenhagen, Denmark. Orem commented that her list included "only programs and agencies that I have personal awareness about through contact and communication within a two year period." P.A. Sayers (personal communication, September 18, 1987) indicated that Orem's conceptual framework is used at Beth Israel Medical Center in Newark, New Jersey; the Betty Bachrach Rehabilitation Center in Pomona, New Jersey; and in the psychiatric unit at the Atlantic City, New Jersey, Medical Center. Orem's conceptual framework also has been used to guide administration of nursing services at Binghamton General Hospital in Binghamton, New York (Feldsine, 1982); Georgetown University Hospital in Washington, D.C.; Children's Seashore House in Atlantic City, New Jersey; Deborah Heart and Lung Center in Browns Mills, New Jersey; St. Elizabeth's Hospital in Elizabeth, New Jersey; Phoenixville Hospital in Phoenixville, Pennsylvania; the Veterans Administration Hospital in Atlanta, Georgia; and Toronto General Hospital in Toronto, Ontario, Canada. Furthermore, the conceptual framework has been used as a guide for administration of nursing services at the Greater Southeast Community Center for the Aging Health Care Institute in Washington, D.C.

S. E. Allison (personal communication, June 24, 1982) reported that Orem's conceptual framework "has been the basis for structuring nursing practice and roles and functions of nurses" at the Mississippi Methodist Hospital and Rehabilitation Center since 1976. She explained that the conceptual framework "is incorporated within the philosophy and objectives of the nursing department and is operationalized through the organizational structure, nursing diagnostic and documentation tools, educational programs . . . and in planning for the production of nursing." Allison (1985) later published a detailed discussion of the process she used to implement use of the conceptual framework at the rehabilitation hospital. A. G. Teung (personal communication, May 17, 1982) reported that patient outcome criteria based on Orem's conceptual framework and Maslow's Hierarchy of Needs were developed by the Nursing Quality Assurance Committee at Deborah Heart and Lung Center in Browns Mills, New Jersey. According to Teung, "The criteria for assessment include dimensions of self-care categorized by physiological needs, skills, motivation, and knowledge. The outcome of assessment is the nursing diagnosis stated in terms of self-care deficits in health status, skill to do ADL, motivation, and knowledge." The criteria were developed for each major diagnostic category of patients treated at the hospital. The structure of nursing practice at the Deborah Heart and Lung Center is explained in a videotape produced by the Center (N. B. Kapeghian, personal communication, November 8, 1986). Use of Orem's conceptual framework at the Children's Seashore House in Atlantic City, New Jersey, is documented in a videotape produced at the University of Pennsylvania School of Nursing (Hale & Rhodes, 1985).

Descriptions of the use of Orem's conceptual framework in some clinical agencies have been published. Backscheider (1974), Crews (1972), and Allison (1973) described the organization provided by Orem's conceptual framework for the nurse-managed clinics at The Johns Hopkins Hospital in Baltimore, Maryland. Feldsine (1982) described a nursing process orientation program based on Orem's conceptual framework and biculturalism used at Binghamton General Hospital in Binghamton, New York. Beckmann (1987) described the influence of Orem's conceptual framework on the structure of nursing practice and the perinatal health-care delivery system in Brazil. Nickle-Gallagher (1985) explained the organization of nursing care based on Orem's conceptual framework in a rehabilitation setting and described her work as a mental health clinical nurse specialist in that setting. Hurst and Stullenbarger (1986) described the use of Orem's conceptual framework in a pediatric interdisciplinary phenylketonuria clinic.

Orem's conceptual framework has been used as a basis for patient classification systems and measures of the quality of nursing care. Coleman (1980) outlined a classification system for patients used at Augustana Hospital and Health Care Center in Chicago, Illinois. Clinton, Denyes, Goodwin, and Koto (1977) reported their work on development of patient outcome criteria derived from self-care requisites. Gallant and McLane (1979) described a process for validation of outcome criteria based on Orem's conceptual framework. Horn (1978) described the Horn and Swain (1977) measure of quality of nursing care. This instrument is based on the universal self-care requisites. Hageman and Ventura (1981) reported the results of their study of the use of an instrument designed to measure the quality of nursing care with regard to effects of medication teaching regimens. The instrument was adapted from medication-related items on the Horn and Swain instrument. Furthermore, Leatt and her colleagues (1981) used Orem's definition of self-care practices in their patient classification instrument.

Miller (1980) presented a model for dynamic nursing practice based on Orem's conceptual framework. The model emphasizes the changes in nursing strategies as the patient's health status changes.

P. A. Sayers (personal communication, December 12, 1986) has formed a corporation, Nursing Systems International, Inc., that is devoted to development of computer software based on Orem's conceptual framework of nursing. The software package will enable nurses to fully document nursing assessment and use of various nursing interventions and their outcomes.

Contributions to Nursing Knowledge

Orem's conceptual framework of nursing and her three theories represent a substantial contribution to nursing knowledge by providing an explicit and specific focus for nursing actions that is different from that of other health care professions. Orem has fulfilled her goal of identifying the domain and boundaries of nursing as a science and an art. Smith's (1979) elaboration of variables comprising nursing knowledge from the perspective of Orem's conceptual framework demonstrates the comprehensive scope of the model.

The emphasis on self-care agency in the conceptual framework and the consideration given to the patient's perspective of health status underscore the importance of the person in the nursing care situation. The wide acceptance of Orem's conceptual framework suggests that these features are especially attractive to nurses who view the person as capable of independent action. Moreover, the use of the model in many different settings and with different age groups suggests that this view of the person who is the patient may be an appropriate one for nursing.

The conceptual framework has an extensive and relatively unique vocabulary that requires mastery for full understanding of its content. Confusion about the meaning and measurement of each concept of the conceptual framework, which was noted by Anna and his associates (1978) and by Foster and Janssens (1985), should be lessened as tools are developed.

Orem (personal communication, August 6, 1987) continues to develop aspects of the conceptual framework and the theories of self-care deficit, self-care, and nursing systems. She stated that her current and future work focuses specifically on "development of practice models, development of rules for practice when certain conditions prevail, continued study of 'foundational capabilities and dispositions' in their relationship to action, and development of . . . models for each of the power components of self-care agency."

In conclusion, Orem's conceptual framework has been adopted enthusiastically by many nurses. Its utility for nursing practice, education, administration, and research is well-documented. In addition, the conceptual framework has generated three theories. These theories have not yet been empirically tested. The conceptual framework presents an optimistic view of patients' contributions to their health care that is in keeping with currently evolving social values. Despite these advantages, potential users are encouraged to continue to evaluate the effectiveness of the conceptual framework in nursing situations through systematic research so that its credibility may be determined.

REFERENCES

Alford, D.M. (1985). Self-care practices in ambulatory nursing clinics for older adults. In J. Riehl-Sisca. The science and art of self-care (pp. 253–261). Norwalk, CT: Appleton-Century-Crofts.

Allison, S.E. (1971). The meaning of rest: An exploratory nursing study. In ANA Clinical Sessions (pp. 191–205). New York: Appleton-Century-Crofts.

Allison, S.E. (1973). A framework for nursing action in a nurse-conducted diabetic management clinic. Journal of Nursing Administration, 3(4), 53–60.

Allison, S.E. (1985). Structuring nursing practice based on Orem's theory of nursing: A nurse administrator's perspective. In J. Riehl-Sisca, The science and art of self-care (pp. 225–235). Norwalk, CT: Appleton-Century-Crofts.

Anna, D.J., Christensen, D.G., Hohon, S.A., Ord, L., & Wells, S.R. (1978). Implementing Orem's conceptual framework. Journal of Nursing Administration, 8(11), 8–11.

Arnold, M.B. (1960). Deliberate action. In Emotion and Personality. Vol. II, Neurological and physiological aspects (pp. 193–204). New York: Columbia University Press.

Asay, M.K., & Ossler, C.C. (Eds.). (1984). Conceptual models of nursing. Applications in community health nursing. Proceedings of the Eighth Annual Community Health Nursing Conference. Chapel Hill: Department of Public Health Nursing, School of Public Health, University of North Carolina.

Backscheider, J.D. (1974). Self-care requirements, self-care capabilities and nursing systems in the diabetic nurse management clinic. American Journal of Public Health, 64, 1138–1146.

Banks, J. (1981). The effects of relaxation training and biofeedback on the weight of black, obese clients. Dissertation Abstracts International, 42, 965B.

Barkauskas, V.H. (1981). Effects of public health nursing interventions with primiparous mothers and their infants. Dissertation Abstracts International, 41, 338B.

Beckman, C.A. (1987). Maternal-child nursing in Brazil. Journal of Obstetric, Gynecologic, and Neonatal Nursing, 16, 238–241.

Behi, R. (1986). Look after yourself. Nursing Times, 82(37), 35–37.

Bickel, L. (1982). Factor structure of self-care agency questionnaire. Unpublished master's thesis, University of Missouri-Columbia.

Blazek, B., & McClellan, M. (1983). The effects of self-care instruction on locus of control in children. Journal of School Health, 53, 554–556.

Bliss-Holtz, V.J. (1986). Desire to learn infant care during the antepartal period: An exploratory study. Dissertation Abstracts International, 47, 991B.

Bliss-Holtz, V.J. (1988). Primiparas' prenatal concern for learning infant care. Nursing Research, 37, 20–24.

Branch, M. (1985). Self-care: Black perspectives. In J. Riehl-Sisca, The science and art of self-care (pp. 181–188). Norwalk, CT: Appleton-Century-Crofts.

Brawn, J.W. (1987). Self care agency and adult health promotion. Dissertation Abstracts International, 48, 1639B.

Brock, A.M., & O'Sullivan, P. (1985). A study to determine what variables predict institutionalization of elderly people. Journal of Advanced Nursing, 10, 533–537.

Brugge, P.A. (1982). The relationship between family as a social support system, health status, and exercise of self-care agency in the adult with a chronic illness. Dissertation Abstracts International, 42, 4361B.

Buckwalter, K.C., & Kerfoot, K.M. (1982). Teaching patients self care: A critical aspect of psychiatric discharge planning. Journal of Psychiatric Nursing and Mental Health Services, 20(5), 15–20.

Burns, M.A. (1986). The use of self-care agency to meet the need for solitude and social interaction by chronically ill individuals. Dissertation Abstracts International, 47, 992B–993B.

Campbell, J.C. (1986). Nursing assessment for risk of homicide with battered women. Advances in Nursing Science, 8(4), 36–51.

Campuzano, M. (1982). Self-care following coronery artery bypass surgery. Focus on Critical Care, 9 (2), 55–56.

Chamorro, L.C. (1985). Self-care in the Puerto Rican community. In J. Riehl-Sisca, The science and art of self-care (pp. 189–195). Norwalk, CT: Appleton-Century-Crofts.

Chang, B., Uman, G., Linn, L., Ware, J., & Kane, R. (1984). The effect of systematically varying components of nursing care on satisfaction in elderly ambulatory women. Western Journal of Nursing Research, 6, 367–386.

Chang, B., Uman, G., Linn, L., Ware, J., & Kane, R. (1985). Adherence to health care regimens among elderly women. Nursing Research, 34, 27–31.

Chin, S. (1985). Can self-care theory be applied to families? In J. Riehl-Sisca, The science and art of self-care (pp. 56–62). Norwalk, CT: Appleton-Century-Crofts.

Clancy, M.T. (1984). Complementarity defined and measured as a specific component of the nursing care process in comparisons made between nurse-patient and physician-patient interactions. Dissertation Abstracts International, 44, 3717B.

Clinton, J.F., Denyes, M.J., Goodwin, J.O., & Koto, E.M. (1977). Developing criterion measures of nursing care: Case study of a process. Journal of Nursing Administration, 7(7), 41–45.

Coleman, L.J. (1980). Orem's self-care concept of nursing. In J.P. Riehl & C. Roy. Conceptual models for nursing practice (2nd ed., pp. 315–328). New York: Appleton-Century-Crofts.

Crews, J. (1972). Nurse-managed cardiac clinics. Cardiovascular Nursing, 8, 15–18.

Crockett, M.S. (1982). Self-reported coping histories of adult psychiatric and nonpsychiatric subjects and controls. (Abstract). Nursing Research, 31, 122.

Denyes, M.J. (1980). Development of an instrument to measure self-care agency in adolescents. Dissertation Abstracts International, 41, 1716B.

Denyes, M.J. (1982). Measurement of self-care agency in adolescents. (Abstract). Nursing Research, 31, 63.

Dodd, M.J. (1981) Enhancing self-care behaviors through informational interventions in patients with cancer who are receiving chemotherapy. Dissertation Abstracts International, 42, 565B.

Dodd, M.J. (1982). Assessing patient self-care for side effects of cancer chemotherapy—Part 1. Cancer Nursing, 5, 447–451.

Dodd, M.J. (1983). Self-care for side effects in cancer chemotherapy. An assessment of nursing interventions—Part 2. Cancer Nursing, 6, 63–67.

Dodd, M.J. (1984a). Measuring informational intervention for chemotherapy knowledge and self-care behavior. Research in Nursing and Health, 7, 43–50.

Dodd, M.J. (1984b). Patterns of self-care in cancer patients receiving radiation therapy. Oncology Nursing Forum, 11, 23–27.

Dodd, M.J. (1988). Patterns of self-care in patients with breast cancer. Western Journal of Nursing Research, 10, 7–24.

Dropkin, M.J. (1981). Development of a self-care teaching program for postoperative head and neck patients. Cancer Nursing, 4, 103–106.

Eith, C.A. (1983). The nursing assessment of readiness for instruction of breast self-examination instrument (NARIB): Instrument development. Dissertation Abstracts International, 44, 1780B.

Evans, L.K. (1980). The relationship of needs awareness, locus of control, health state, and social support system to social interaction as a form of self-care behavior among elderly residents of public housing. Dissertation Abstracts International, 40, 3662B–3663B.

Facteau, L.M. (1980). Self-care concepts and the care of the hospitalized child. Nursing Clinics of North America, 15, 145–155.

Farnham, S., & Fowler, M. (1985). Demedicalization, bilingualization, and reconceptualization: Teaching Orem's self-care model to the RN-BSN student. In J. Riehl-Sisca, The science and art of self-care (pp. 35–40). Norwalk, CT: Appleton-Century-Crofts.

Fawcett, J., Cariello, F.P., Davis, D.A., Farley, J., Zimmaro, D., & Watts. R.J. (1987). Conceptual models of nursing: Application to critical care nursing practice. Dimensions of Critical Care Nursing, 6, 202–213.

Feldsine, F. (1982). Options for transition into practice: Nursing process orientation program. Journal of New York State Nurses' Association, 13, 11–16.

Fenner, K. (1979). Developing a conceptual framework. Nursing Outlook, 27, 122–126.

Fernsler, J.I. (1984). A comparison of patient and nurse perceptions of patients' self-care deficits associated with cancer chemotherapy. Dissertation Abstracts International, 45, 827B.

Finnegan, T. (1986). Self-care and the elderly. New Zealand Nursing Journal, 79(4), 10–13.

Flanagan, R. (1983). Energy expenditure of normal females during three bathing techniques. Unpublished master's thesis, University of Missouri-Columbia.

Foster, P.C., & Janssens, N.P. (1985). Dorothea E. Orem. In Nursing Theories Conference Group, Nursing theories. The base for professional nursing practice (2nd ed., pp. 124–139). Englewood Cliffs, NJ: Prentice-Hall.

Frederick, H.K., & Northam, E. (1938). A textbook of nursing practice (2nd ed.). New York: Macmillan.

Gallant, B.W., & McLane, A.M. (1979). Outcome criteria: A process for validation at the unit level. Journal of Nursing Administration, 9(1), 14–21.

Gantz, S.B. (1980). A fourth-grade adventure in self-directed learning. Topics in Clinical Nursing, 2(2), 29–38.

Garvan, P., Lee, M., Lloyd, K., & Sullivan, T.J. (1980). Self-care applied to the aged. New Jersey Nurse, 10(1), 3–5.

Gast, H.L. (1984). The relationship between stages of ego development and developmental stages of health self care operations. Dissertation Abstracts International, 44, 3039B.

Geden, E.A. (1982). Effects of lifting techniques on energy expenditures: A preliminary investigation. Nursing Research, 31, 214–218.

Geden, E.A. (1985). The relationship between self-care theory and empirical research. In J. Riehl-Sisca, The science and art of self-care (pp. 265–270). Norwalk, CT: Appleton-Century-Crofts.

Goodwin, J. (1979). Programmed instruction for self-care following pulmonary surgery. International Journal of Nursing Studies, 16, 29–40.

Gulick, E.E. (1987). Parsimony and model confirmation of the ADL self-care scale for multiple sclerosis persons. Nursing Research, 36, 278–283.

Hageman, P., & Ventura, M. (1981). Utilizing patient outcome criteria to measure the effects of a medication teaching regimen. Western Journal of Nursing Research, 3, 25–33.

Hale, M., & Rhodes, G. (1985). Care with a concept. Chapel Hill, NC: Health Sciences Consortium. (Videotape)

Hammonds, T.A. (1985). Self-care practices of Navajo indians. In J. Riehl-Sisca, The science and art of self-care (pp. 171–180). Norwalk, CT: Appleton-Century-Crofts.

Hanson, B.R. (1981). Development of a questionnaire measuring perception of self-care agency. Unpublished master's thesis, University of Missouri-Columbia.

Hanson, B.R., & Bickel, L. (1985). Development and testing of the questionnaire on perception of self-care agency. In J. Riehl-Sisca, The science and art of self-care (pp. 271–278). Norwalk, CT: Appleton-Century-Crofts.

Harper, D. (1984). Application of Orem's theoretical constructs to self-care medication behaviors in the elderly. Advances in Nursing Science, 6(3), 29–46.

Harrigan, J.F., Faro, B.Z., Van Putte, A., & Stoler, P. (1987). The application of locus of control to diabetes education in school-age children. Journal of Pediatric Nursing, 2, 236–243.

Harris, J.K. (1980). Self-care is possible after cesarean delivery. Nursing Clinics of North America, 15, 191–204.

Harvey, B.L. (1987). Self-care practices of industrial workers to prevent low back pain. Dissertation Abstracts International, 48, 89B.

Hathaway, D.K., & Geden, E.A. (1983). Energy expenditure during leg exercise programs. Nursing Research, 32, 147–150.

Hautman, M.A. (1987). Self-care responses to respiratory illnesses among Vietnamese. Western Journal of Nursing Research, 9, 223–243.

Hedahl, K. (1983). Assisting the adolescent with physical disabilities through a college health program. Nursing Clinics of North America, 18, 257–274.

Hehn, D.M. (1986). Hospice care: Critical role behaviors related to self-care and role supplementation. Dissertation Abstracts International, 46, 2623B.

Henderson, V. (1955). Textbook of the principles and practice of nursing (5th ed.). New York: Macmillan.

Herrington, J., & Houston, S. (1984). Using Orem's theory: A plan for all seasons. Nursing and Health Care, 5(1), 45–47.

Horn, B. (1978). Development of criterion measures of nursing care. (Abstract). In Communicating nursing research. Vol. 11: New approaches to communicating nursing research. Boulder, CO: Western Interstate Commission for Higher Education (pp. 87–89).

Horn, B., & Swain, M. (1977). Development of criterion measures of nursing care (Vols. 1 and 2). Ann Arbor, MI: University of Michigan. (NTIS Nos. PB-267 004 and PB–267 005).

Hurst, J.D., & Stullenbarger, B. (1986). Implementation of a self-care approach in a pediatric interdisciplinary phenylketonuria (PKU) clinic. Journal of Pediatric Nursing, 1, 159–163.

Isenberg, M.A. (Moderator). (1987). Testing of Orem's self-care deficit theory of nursing with diverse cultural groups. Symposium presented at American Nurses' Association Council of Nurse Researchers International Nursing Research Conference, Arlington, VA.

Kain, C.D. (1986). Dorothea E. Orem's Self-Care Model of Nursing: Implications for program development in associate degree nursing education. Dissertation Abstracts International, 47, 994B.

Karl, C. (1982). The effect of an exercise program on self-care activities for the institutionalized elderly. Journal of Gerontological Nursing, 8, 282–285.

Kearney, B., & Fleischer, B. (1979). Development of an instrument to measure exercise of self-care agency. Research in Nursing and Health, 2, 25–34.

Kubricht, D. (1984). Therapeutic self-care demands expressed by outpatients receiving external radiation therapy. Cancer Nursing, 7, 43–52.

Lantz, J.M. (1982). Self-actualization: An indicator of self-care practices among adults 65 years and over. Dissertation Abstracts International, 42, 4017B.

Laurin, J. (1979). Development of a nursing process-outcome model based on Orem's concepts of nursing practice for quality nursing care evaluation. Dissertation Abstracts International, 40, 1122B.

Leatt, P., Bay, K.S., & Stinson, S.M. (1981). An instrument for assessing and classifying patients by type of care. Nursing Research, 30, 145–150.

Lonergan, B.J.F. (1958). Insight: A study of human understanding. New York: Philosophical Library.

Marriner, A. (1986). Nursing theorists and their work. St. Louis: CV Mosby.

Marten, M.L.C. (1983). The relationship of level of depression to perceived decision making capabilities of institutionalized elderly women. Dissertation Abstracts International, 43, 2855B–2856B.

Maunz, E.R., & Woods, N.F. (1988). Self-care practices among young adult women: Influence of symptoms, employment, and sex-role orientation. Health Care for Women International, 9, 29–41.

McBride, S. (1987). Validation of an instrument to measure exercise of self-care agency. Research in Nursing and Health, 10, 311–316.

Meleis, A.I. (1985). Theoretical nursing: Development and progress. Philadelphia: Lippincott.

Michael, M.M., & Sewall, K.S. (1980). Use of the adolescent peer group to increase the self-care agency of adolescent alcohol abusers. Nursing Clinics of North America, 15, 157–176.

Michaels, C.L. (1986). Development of a self-care assessment tool for hospitalized chronic obstructive pulmonary disease patients: A methodological study. Dissertation Abstracts International, 46, 3783B.

Miller, J.F. (1980). The dynamic focus of nursing: A challenge to nursing administration. Journal of Nursing Administration, 10(1), 13–18.

Miller, J.F. (1982). Categories of self-care needs of ambulatory patients with diabetes. Journal of Advanced Nursing, 7, 25–31.

Mitchell, P., & Irvin, N. (1977). Neurological examination: Nursing assessment for nursing purposes. Journal of Neurosurgical Nursing, 9(1), 23–28.

Moore, J.B. (1987). Effects of assertion training and first aid instruction on children's autonomy and self-care agency. Research in Nursing and Health, 10, 101–109.

Moscovitz, A. (1984). Orem's theory as applied to psychiatric nursing. Perspectives in Psychiatric Care, 22(1), 36–38.

Mullin, V.I. (1980). Implementing the self-care concept in the acute care setting. Nursing Clinics of North America, 15, 177–190.

Mullin, V.I., & Weed, F. (1980, October). Orem's self-care concept as a conceptual framework for a nursing curriculum. Paper presented at Virginia Nurses' Association State Convention.

Munley, M.J., & Sayers, P.A. (1984). Self-care deficit theory of nursing. A primer for application of the concepts. North Brunswick, NJ: Personal and Family Health Associates.

Munley, M.J., & Sayers, P.A. (1986). Application of the self-care model for nursing practice. A series of slides designed for teaching Dorothea Orem's self-care framework for nursing practice (2nd ed.). North Brunswick, NJ: Personal and Family Health Associates.

Murphy, P.P. (1981). A hospice model and self-care theory. Oncology Nursing Forum, 8(2), 19–21.

Musci, E.C. (1984). Relationship between family coping strategies and self-care during cancer chemotherapy treatments. Dissertation Abstracts International, 44, 3712B.

Neves, E.P. (1980). The relationship of hospitalized individuals' cognitive structure regarding health to their health self-care behaviors. Dissertation Abstracts International, 41, 522B.

Nickle-Gallagher, L. (1985). Structuring nursing practice based on Orem's general theory. A practitioner's perspective. In J. Riehl-Sisca, The science and art of self-care (pp. 236–244). Norwalk, CT: Appleton-Century-Crofts.

Nowakowski, L. (1980). Health promotion/self-care programs for the community. Topics in Clinical Nursing, 2(2), 21–27.

Nunn, D., & Marriner, A. (in press). Applying Orem's model to nursing administration. In B. Henry, M. DiVincenti, C. Arndt, & A. Marriner (Eds.), Dimensions of nursing administration. Theory, research, education and practice. Boston: Blackwell Scientific Publications.

Nursing Development Conference Group. (1973). Concept formalization in nursing. Process and product. Boston: Little, Brown, and Co.

Nursing Development Conference Group. (1979). Concept formalization in nursing. Process and product (2nd ed.). Boston: Little, Brown, and Co.

Olson, G.P. (1986). Perceived opportunity for and preference in decision-making of hospitalized men and women. Dissertation Abstracts International, 47, 572B–573B.

Orem, D.E. (1956). Hospital nursing service: An analysis. Indianapolis: Division of Hospital and Institutional Services of the Indiana State Board of Health.

Orem, D.E. (1959). Guides for developing curriculum for the education of practical nurses. Washington, D.C.: U.S. Government Printing Office.

Orem, D.E. (1971). Nursing: Concepts of practice. New York: McGraw-Hill.

Orem, D.E. (1978, December). A general theory of nursing. Paper presented at the Second Annual Nurse Educator Conference, New York. (Cassette recording)

Orem, D.E. (1980). Nursing: Concepts of practice (2nd ed.). New York: McGraw-Hill.

Orem, D.E. (1983a). The self-care deficit theory of nursing: A general theory. In I.W. Clements & F.B. Roberts, Family health. A theoretical approach to nursing care (pp. 205–217). New York: John Wiley & Sons.

Orem, D.E. (1983b). The family coping with a medical illness. Analysis and application of Orem's theory. In I.W. Clements & F.B. Roberts, Family health. A theoretical approach to nursing care (pp. 385–386). New York: John Wiley & Sons.

Orem, D.E. (1983c). The family experiencing emotional crisis. Analysis and application of Orem's self-care deficit theory. In I.W. Clements & F.B. Roberts, Family health. A theoretical approach to nursing care (pp. 367–368). New York: John Wiley & Sons.

Orem, D.E. (1984). Orem's conceptual model and community health nursing. In M.K. Asay & C.C. Ossler, (Eds.), Conceptual models of nursing. Applications in community health nursing. Proceedings of the Eighth Annual Community Health Nursing Conference (pp. 35–50). Chapel Hill: Department of Public Health Nursing, School of Public Health, University of North Carolina.

Orem, D.E. (1985). Nursing: Concepts of practice (3rd ed.). New York: McGraw-Hill.

Orem, D.E. (in press). Theories and hypotheses for nursing administration. In B. Henry, M. DiVincenti, C. Arndt, & A. Marriner (Eds.), Dimensions of nursing administration. Theory, research, education and practice. Boston: Blackwell Scientific Publications.

Orem, D.E., & Taylor, S.G. (1986). Orem's general theory of nursing. In P. Winstead-Fry (Ed.), Case studies in nursing theory (pp. 37–71). New York: National League for Nursing.

Parker, M.E. (1983). The use of Orem's self-care concept of nursing in curricula of selected baccalaureate programs of nursing education. Dissertation Abstracts International, 43, 2224A.

Patterson, E.T., & Hale, E.S. (1985). Making sure: Integrating menstrual care practices into activities of daily living. Advances in Nursing Science, 7(3), 18–31.

Perras, S., & Zappacosta, A. (1982). The application of Orem's theory in promoting self-care in a peritoneal dialysis facility. American Association of Nephrology Nurses and Technicians Journal, 9(3), 37–39.

Phillips, J.R. (1977). Nursing systems and nursing models. Image, 9, 4–7.

Pinkerton, M. (1983). Self-care and burn-out in the professional nurse. Dissertation Abstracts International, 44, 1783B.

Pulliam, L.W. (1986). Relationship between social support and the nutritional status of patients receiving radiation therapy for cancer. Dissertation Abstracts International, 46, 262B.

Rachel, M. (1978). Therapeutic self-care demands of residents of an institution for the mentally retarded as perceived by the residents and by their direct-care givers. Unpublished master's thesis. University of Southern Mississippi.

Rew, L. (1987). The relationship between self-care behaviors and selected psychosocial variables in children with asthma. Journal of Pediatric Nursing, 2, 333–341.

Rieder, K.A. (1982). The relationship among attitudinal, perceptual, and behavioral factors as indicators of hospitalized patients' participation in care. Dissertation Abstracts International, 43, 1044B.

Riehl-Sisca, J. (1985a). The science and art of self-care. Norwalk, CT: Appleton-Century-Crofts.

Riehl-Sisca, J. (1985b). Epilogue: Future implications for the science and art of self-care. In J. Riehl-Sisca, The science and art of self-care (pp. 307–309). Norwalk, CT: Appleton-Century-Crofts.

Riehl-Sisca, J. (1985c). Determining criteria for graduate and undergraduate self-care curriculums. In J. Riehl-Sisca, The science and art of self-care (pp. 20–24). Norwalk, CT: Appleton-Century-Crofts.

Riehl, J.P., & Roy, C. (1980). Conceptual models for nursing practice (2nd ed.). New York: Appleton-Century-Crofts.

Rothlis, J. (1984). The effect of a self-help group on feelings of hopelessness and helplessness. Western Journal of Nursing Research, 6, 157–173.

Sandman, P.O., Norberg, A., Adolfsson, R., Axelsson, K., & Hedly, V. (1986). Morning care of patients with Alzheimer-type dementia. A theoretical model based on direct observations. Journal of Advanced Nursing, 11, 369–378.

Saucier, C. (1984). Self concept and self-care management in school-age children with diabetes. Pediatric Nursing, 10, 135–138.

Scheetz, S.L. (1986). The relationship of social network characteristics to the performance of self-care by the chronically mentally ill adult in the community. Dissertation Abstracts International, 47, 2377B.

Scherer, P. (1988). Hospitals that attract (and keep) nurses. American Journal of Nursing, 88, 34–40.

Schorfheide, A.M. (1986). The relationship of reported self-care practice, parental motivation for self-care, and health locus of control with insulin dependent diabetic children and their families. Dissertation Abstracts International, 46, 3008B–3009B.

Silva, M.C., & Sorrell, J.M. (1987, April). Doctoral dissertation research based on five nursing models: A select bibliography. January 1952 through February 1987. (Available from M.C. Silva, George Mason University School of Nursing, Fairfax, VA)

Sirles, A.T. (1986). The effect of a self-care health education program on parents' self-care knowledge, health locus of control and children's medical utilization rate. Dissertation Abstracts International, 46, 2628B.

Smith, M.C. (1977). Self-care: A conceptual framework for rehabilitation nursing. Rehabilitation Nursing, 2(2), 8–10.

Smith, M.C. (1979). Proposed metaparadigm for nursing research and theory development. An analysis of Orem's self-care theory. Image, 11, 75–79.

Smith, M.J. (1987). A critique of Orem's theory. In R.R. Parse, Nursing science. Major paradigms, theories, and critiques (pp. 91–105). Philadelphia: W.B. Saunders.

Stashinko, E. (1987). The relationship between self-perceptions of competence and self-care behaviors in third-grade children. Dissertation Abstracts International, 48, 1644B.

Stevens, B.J. (1984). Nursing theory. Analysis, application, evaluation (2nd ed.). Boston: Little, Brown and Co.

Stockdale-Woolley, R. (1984). The effects of education on self-care agency. Public Health Nursing, 1, 97–106.

Storm, D.S., & Baumgartner, R.G. (1987). Achieving self-care in the ventilator-dependent patient: A critical analysis of a case study. International Journal of Nursing Studies, 24, 95–106.

Story, E.L., & Ross, M.M. (1986). Family centered community health nursing and the Betty Neuman Systems Model. Nursing Papers, 18(2), 77–88.

Stullenbarger, N.E. (1985). A Q-analysis of the self-care abilities of young, schoolaged children. Dissertation Abstracts International, 45, 2872B–2873B.

Tadych, R. (1985). Nursing in multiperson units: The family. In J. Riehl-Sisca, The science and art of self-care (pp. 49–55). Norwalk, CT: Appleton-Century-Crofts.

Taylor, S.G. (1985a, August). Dorothea Orem's framework. Paper presented at conference on Nursing Theory in Action, Edmonton, Alberta, Canada. (Cassette recording)

Taylor, S.G. (1985b). Curriculum development for preservice programs using Orem's theory of nursing. In J. Riehl-Sisca, The science and art of self-care (pp. 25–32). Norwalk, CT: Appleton-Century-Crofts.

Taylor, S.G. (1985c). Teaching self-care deficit theory to generic students. In J. Riehl-Sisca, The science and art of self-care (pp. 41–46). Norwalk, CT: Appleton-Century-Crofts.

Tompkins, E.S. (1980). Effect of restricted mobility and dominance on perceived duration. Nursing Research, 29, 333–338.

Toth, J.C. (1980). Effect of structured preparation for transfer on patient anxiety on leaving coronary care unit. Nursing Research, 29, 28–34.

Underwood, P.R. (1979). Nursing care as a determinant in the development of self-care behavior by hospitalized adult schizophrenics. Dissertation Abstracts International, 40, 679B.

Walborn, K.A. (1980). A nursing model for the hospice: Primary and self-care nursing. Nursing Clinics of North America, 15, 205–217.

Walker, L.O., & Nicholson, R. (1980). Criteria for evaluating nursing process models. Nurse Educator, 5(5), 8–9.

Weaver, M.T. (1987). Perceived self-care agency: A LISREL factor analysis of Bickel and Hanson's questionnaire. Nursing Research, 36, 381–387.

Wells-Biggs, A.J. (1986). Hermeneutic interpretation of the work of Dorothea E. Orem: A nursing metaphor. Dissertation Abstracts International, 47, 576B.

Whetstone, W.R. (1986). Social dramatics: Social skills development for the chronically mentally ill. Journal of Advanced Nursing, 11, 67–74.

White, R. (1977). Relationship between leadership effectiveness and personality traits among head nurses. Unpublished master's thesis. University of Southern Mississippi.

Wollery, L. (1983). Self-care for the obstetrical patient. Journal of Obstetric, Gynecologic, and Neonatal Nursing, 12, 33–37.

Woods, N. (1985). Self-care practices among young adult married women. Research in Nursing and Health, 8, 227–233.

Zach, P. (1982). Self-care agency in diabetic ocular sequelae. Journal of Ophthalmic Nursing Techniques, 1(2), 21–31.

ANNOTATED BIBLIOGRAPHY

Aggleton, P., & Chalmers, H. (1985). Orem's self-care model. Nursing Times, 81(1), 36–39.

This article presents a brief overview of Orem's work and an explanation of how the conceptual framework can be applied in practice using the nursing process.

Allison, S.E. (1971). The meaning of rest: An exploratory nursing study. In ANA clinical sessions (pp. 191–205). New York: Appleton-Century-Crofts.

This paper presents a few of the major findings from a study designed to explore the meaning of rest. Data were collected from a group of businessmen who described their rest activities. The data collection instrument is included in the appendix to the report.

Allison, S.E. (1973). A framework for nursing action in a nurse-conducted diabetic management clinic. Journal of Nursing Administration, 3(4), 53–60.

Orem's concept of self-care is employed as the framework for development of a diabetic management clinic. The article describes the model-building process that preceded founding of the clinic. The responsibilities and roles of nursing and other staff are outlined. The model was found to be a useful framework in this clinical setting.

Anna, D.J., Christensen, D.G., Hohon, S.A., Ord, L., & Wells, S.R. (1978). Implementing Orem's conceptual framework. Journal of Nursing Administration, 8(11), 8–11.

Orem's conceptual framework is reviewed and related to practice in a nursing home setting. Reactions of patients and nurses to implementation of the conceptual framework are presented. The conceptual framework was found to be useful in the setting. The authors speculated on the cost effectiveness of nursing care based on this conceptual framework.

Backscheider, J.E. (1974). Self-care requirements, self-care capabilities and nursing systems in the diabetic nurse management clinic. American Journal of Public Health, 64, 1138–1146.

Use of Orem's conceptual framework in a diabetic management clinic is discussed. The article focuses on the patient capabilities necessary for therapeutic self-care of diabetes. An assessment tool designed to determine individual capabilities is presented. An example of use of the tool to assess a diabetic clinic patient is included.

Beckmann, C.A. (1987). Maternal-child health in Brazil. Journal of Obstetric, Gynecologic, and Neonatal Nursing, 16, 238–241.

The social and economic climates of Brazil are discussed in this article and their influence on the delivery of health care and nursing education are explained. An overview of perinatal care in the country is given. The author explains that the Brazilian philosophy of nursing is based on Orem's self-care framework.

Behi, R. (1986). Look after yourself. Nursing Times, 82(37), 35–37.

Orem's conceptual framework is discussed and its implications and appropriateness as a guide for nursing practice in the United Kingdom are outlined in this article.

Bennett, J.G. (Guest ed.) (1980). Symposium on the self-care concept of nursing. Nursing Clinics of North America, 15, 129–217.

This symposium includes several articles related to Orem's conceptual framework of nursing. Each article is described below.

Facteau, L.M. Self-care concepts and the care of the hospitalized child. Pp. 145–155.

The ability of children to engage in self-care is discussed. The potential for self-care at various ages and the role of substitute self-care agents are presented. Examples of nursing care of an infant, a toddler, a preschooler, and a school age child are included.

Harris, J.K. Self-care is possible after cesarean delivery, Pp. 191–204.

Use of the self-care concept in increasing the self-care agency of families experiencing cesarean deliveries is presented. Principles of family-centered care are discussed. An educational program for planned cesarean births is outlined and contrasted with general prepared childbirth classes. Unplanned cesarean deliveries are also discussed. Self-care needs during delivery, post-partum, and return to home are identified.

Joseph, L.S. Self-care and the nursing process. Pp. 131–143.

Orem's self-care conceptual framework is described. The concepts of the conceptual framework are operationalized within the nursing process. The conceptual framework was found to be useful as a guide for patient education.

Michael, M.M., & Sewall, K.S. Use of the adolescent peer group to increase the self-care agency of adolescent alcohol abusers. Pp. 157–176.

Developmental tasks and the significance of peer groups in adolescence are discussed. Reality therapy is combined with the nursing process, and with Orem's conceptual framework to guide nursing care. A group formed at an adolescent alcohol treatment center is described in detail, and a nursing care plan designed to promote group cohesion, to accomplish group goals, and to accomplish other nursing care goals is presented.

Mullin, V.I. Implementing the self-care concept in the acute care setting. Pp. 177–190.

Orem's conceptual framework is applied in an acute care, medical-surgical setting. Difficulties encountered in implementing nursing actions derived from the conceptual framework are presented. Methods for using the conceptual framework, despite the difficulties imposed by the setting, are outlined.

Walborn, K.A. A nursing model for the hospice: Primary and self-care nursing. Pp. 205–217.

The use of Orem's conceptual framework in a hospice setting is reported. A nursing model that focuses on the care of the patient and the family is presented. A partly compensatory nursing system for care of the family is outlined. Orem's conceptual framework is viewed as useful in this clinical situation.

Bilitski, J.S. (1981). Nursing science and the laws of health: The test of substance as a step in the process of theory development. Advances in Nursing Science, 4(1), 15–29.

Orem's conceptual framework is reviewed and combined with a nursing process model. The resultant framework was operationalized by use of instruments designed to measure family coping and self-care agency. A family case study using the instrument is presented.

Bliss-Holtz, V.J. (1988). Primiparas' prenatal concern for learning infant care. Nursing Research, 37, 20–24.

This article reports the findings of a study derived from Orem's conceptual framework that was designed to determine differences in pregnant women's desire to learn infant care skills during the antenatal period. Analysis of data obtained from interviews of 189 primiparous women revealed that there were differences in desire to learn infant care and infant care skills between the early and late and the middle and late stages of pregnancy. There were, however, no differences in desire to become a caring mother among the three stages of the antepartal period.

Blazek, B., & McClellan, M. (1983). The effects of self-care instruction on locus of control in children. Journal of School Health, 53, 554–556.

This article reports the findings of a study of the effects of self-care instruction on fifth graders. The experimental group participated in a program designed to show children how to become managers in their own health care; the control group attended a health discussion. Study results indicated that self-care instruction can increase the extent to which children view health event outcomes as being due to their own actions.

Brock, A.M., & O'Sullivan, P. (1985). A study to determine what variables predict institutionalization of elderly people. Journal of Advanced Nursing, 10, 533–537.

This article reports the results of a study designed to determine variables that distinguish newly institutionalized elderly individuals from those able to remain in the community. The investigators pointed out that Orem maintains that individuals have the right to be able to care for themselves and their dependents.

Bromley, B. (1980). Applying Orem's self-care theory in enterostomal therapy. American Journal of Nursing, 80, 245–249.

Orem's conceptual framework is applied to enterostomal therapy. Use of the conceptual framework to guide nursing care of a patient with a colostomy is described. Wholly compensatory, partly compensatory, and supportive-educative nursing systems are outlined for the patient.

Buckwalter, K.C., & Kerfoot, K.M. (1982). Teaching patients self care: A critical aspect of psychiatric discharge planning. Journal of Psychiatric Nursing and Mental Health Services, 20(5), 15–20.

Techniques that can be incorporated into inpatient and outpatient psychiatric mental health programs to decrease chances of rehospitalization are discussed in this article. The authors maintain that research findings and clinical experiences support the use of self-care strategies.

Butterfield, S. (1983). In search of commonalities: An analysis of two theoretical frameworks. International Journal of Nursing Studies, 20, 15–22.

This article presents the central assumptions and propositions of Orem's and Rogers's conceptual models. A framework for theory analysis is used to examine the work for the purpose of determining commonalities. Many similarities are discussed. The most apparent differences were in relative emphases and the explicitness of abstract concepts.

Calley, J.M., Dirksen, M., Engalla, M., & Hennrich, M.L. (1980). The Orem self-care nursing model. In J.P. Riehl & C. Roy, Conceptual models for nursing practice (2nd ed., pp. 302–314). New York: Appleton-Century-Crofts.

Orem's conceptual framework is reviewed, including historical development, definitions of major concepts, and central elements. The conceptual framework is applied to care of a psychiatric patient. The assessment is detailed and interventions are outlined. Use of the conceptual framework appeared to benefit the development and delivery of nursing care in this clinical situation.

Campbell, J.C. (1986). Nursing assessment for risk of homicide with battered women. Advances in Nursing Science, 8(4), 36–51.

This study report describes the development of the Danger Assessment, an instrument designed as a clinical and research instrument to help battered women assess their danger of homicide. The investigator maintained that completing the Danger Assessment with a nurse is a means of increasing the self-care agency of battered women.

Campuzano, M. (1982). Self-care following coronary artery bypass surgery. Focus on Critical Care, 9(2), 55–56.

The author describes the use of Orem's conceptual framework to guide nursing care of clients in a cardiac rehabilitation setting following coronary artery bypass surgery.

Chang, B.L. (1980). Evaluation of health care professionals in facilitating self-care: Review of the literature and a conceptual model. Advances in Nursing Science, 3(1), 43–58.
> Orem's conceptual framework is reviewed, as is the general literature dealing with self-care. The author presents a framework for evaluation of health care professionals' contributions to client self-care.

Chang, B., Uman, G., Linn, L., Ware, J., & Kane, R. (1984). The effect of systematically varying components of nursing care on satisfaction in elderly ambulatory women. Western Journal of Nursing Research, 6, 367–386.
> This article reports the findings of a study designed to determine the effects of four components of care (medical-technical, psychosocial, patient participation in planning care, and courtesy of care) on elderly women's evaluation of health care. Orem's concepts of nursing practice were used as a basis for the conceptual framework of the study.

Chang, B., Uman, G., Linn, L., Ware, J., & Kane, R. (1985). Adherence to health care regimens among elderly women. Nursing Research, 34, 27–31.
> This article reports the findings of a study designed to determine the effects of three components of care (technical quality, psychosocial care, and patient participation in planning care) and personal characteristics on elderly women's intent to adhere to a health care regimen. Orem's self-care concepts served as the basis of the conceptual framework of the study.

Clinton, J.F., Denyes, M.J., Goodwin, J.O., & Koto, E.M. (1977). Developing criterion measures of nursing care: Case study of a process. Journal of Nursing Administration, 7(7), 41–45.
> Orem's concepts of self-care, universal self-care requisites, and health-deviation self-care requisites are used to identify patient outcome criteria.

Coleman, L.J. (1980). Orem's self-care concept of nursing. In J.P. Riehl & C. Roy, Conceptual models for nursing practice (2nd ed., pp. 315–328). New York: Appleton-Century-Crofts.
> Concepts of Orem's conceptual framework that have utility for nursing service administration are reviewed. Use of the conceptual framework as a guide for a nursing service department in a medical hospital is described.

Crews, J. (1972). Nurse-managed cardiac clinics. Cardio-Vascular Nursing, 8, 15–18.
> The establishment of cardiac clinics based on Orem's conceptual framework is described. Self-care needs of clients resulting from anticoagulation therapy and symptoms of congestive heart failure are identified.

Dear, M.R., & Keen, M.F. (1982). Promotion of self-care in the employee with rheumatoid arthritis. Occupational Health Nursing, 30(1), 32–34.
> Orem's conceptual framework is used to guide care of the rheumatoid arthritic in the work setting. Nursing care during various stages of the disease is discussed. Use of the conceptual framework was found to facilitate delivery of dynamic nursing care based on mutual goal-setting.

Dickson, G., & Lee-Villasenor, H. (1982). Nursing theory and practice: A self-care approach. Advances in Nursing Science, 5(1), 29–40.
> This article reports the findings of a study designed to determine if nursing within the self-care framework makes a difference in the lives of others. The qualitative study was conducted by the authors, who are in independent practice. Study subjects were patients in their practice.

Dodd, M.J. (1982). Assessing patient self-care for side effects of cancer chemotherapy—Part 1. Cancer Nursing, 5, 447–451.
> The article reports the findings of a study of cancer patients' self-care behaviors related to side effects of chemotherapy. A large discrepancy was found between experienced side effects and initiated self-care behavior, which was attributed to lack of information from physicians and nurses and the patients' limited knowledge of self-care measures.

Dodd, M.J. (1983). Self-care for side effects in cancer chemotherapy: An assessment of nursing interventions—Part 2. Cancer Nursing, 6, 63–67.
> This article describes the effectiveness of nursing interventions designed to enhance self-care behaviors of cancer patients who were receiving chemotherapy.

Patients who were given information about side effect management techniques reported initiating more self-care behaviors with a higher degree of perceived effectiveness than did the patients who had not received the information.

Dodd, M.J. (1984). Measuring informational intervention for chemotherapy knowledge and self-care behavior. Research in Nursing and Health, 7, 43–50.
This article reports the findings of a study of the effects of information given to cancer patients receiving chemotherapy. Patients who received information on side effect management techniques alone or in combination with other information performed more self-care behaviors than those in a control group.

Dodd, M.J. (1984). Patterns of self-care in cancer patients receiving radiation therapy. Oncology Nursing Forum, 11, 23–27.
This article reports the results of a longitudinal descriptive study of self-care behaviors related to side effects from radiation therapy experienced by cancer patients. Patients exhibited little self-care activity for side effects. There was a significant association between patient knowledge of therapy and self-care, although patients cited themselves as the most frequent source of information for their self-care activities, the physician a frequent source, and the nurse, a less frequent source.

Dodd, M.J. (1988). Patterns of self-care in patients with breast cancer. Western Journal of Nursing Research, 10, 7–24.
This report focuses on the findings of a study of factors affecting self-care behaviors of breast cancer patients who experience the side effects of chemotherapy.

Dropkin, M.J. (1981). Development of a self-care teaching program for postoperative head and neck patients. Cancer Nursing, 4, 103–106.
A program based on Orem's conceptual framework and designed to facilitate rehabilitation of patients who have had major head and neck surgery is outlined in this article.

Eban, J.D., Nation, M.J., Marriner, A., & Nordmeyer, S.B. (1986). Dorothea E. Orem: Self-care deficit theory of nursing. In A. Marriner, Nursing theorists and their work (pp. 117–130). St. Louis: C.V. Mosby.
This book chapter presents an overview of Orem's work.

Edgar, L., Shamian, J., & Patterson, D. (1984). Factors affecting the nurse as a teacher and practicer of breast self-examination. International Journal of Nursing Studies, 21, 255–265.
This article reports the results of a study designed to explore factors associated with why nurses do not teach or practice breast self-examination. Orem's conceptual framework led to the proposition that nurses with knowledge, supportive attitudes, and confidence would engage in breast self-examination as a self-care activity. Study findings revealed significant differences in knowledge levels and confidence between the nurse and non-nurse groups, but extremely small differences in the frequency of practice of breast self-examination.

Eichelberger, K.M., Kaufman, D.N., Rundahl, M.E., & Schwartz, N.E. (1980). Self-care nursing plan: Helping children to help themselves. Pediatric Nursing, 6(3), 9–13.
Orem's conceptual framework is extended to nursing care of children. A general self-care nursing plan is presented for use with children. Use of the conceptual framework in the care of an 8-year-old child is described. The care plan for this child is included in the article.

Fawcett, J., Cariello, F.P., Davis, D.A., Farley, J., Zimmaro, D.M., & Watts, R.J. (1987). Conceptual models of nursing: Application to critical care nursing practice. Dimensions of Critical Care Nursing, 6, 202–213.
This article includes a brief analysis of Orem's conceptual framework and a nursing care plan based on the conceptual framework for a critically ill 62-year-old man.

Feldsine, F. (1982). Options for transition into practice: Nursing process orientation program. Journal of New York State Nurses' Association, 13, 11–16.
This article describes the Nursing Process Orientation Program at Binghamton General Hospital in New York. The program is based on Orem's conceptual framework and biculturalism.

Fenner, K. (1979). Developing a conceptual framework. Nursing Outlook, 27, 122–126.
Orem's conceptual framework is used as the framework for curriculum development in an associate degree program. The conceptual framework is interpreted in relation to technical education and illustrated by curriculum content. Implementation of the curriculum and plans for its future evaluation are described.

Finnegan, T. (1986). Self-care and the elderly. New Zealand Nursing Journal, 79(4), 10–13.
The author of this article presents an overview of aging and the aged and explains how Orem's conceptual framework can be used to guide care of the elderly.

Fitzgerald, S. (1980). Utilizing Orem's self-care nursing model in designing an educational program for the diabetic. Topics in Clinical Nursing, 2(2), 57–65.
Orem's conceptual framework is used as the framework for education of the diabetic patient. Specific areas for assessment, planning, implementation, and evaluation of the diabetic are delineated. The concept of self-care provides the central focus of this application of the conceptual framework.

Fitzpatrick, J.J., Whall, A., Johnston, R., & Floyd, J. (1982). Nursing models and their psychiatric mental health applications. Bowie, MD: Brady.
This book presents a brief analysis of Orem's conceptual framework, among others. Reformulated theoretical approaches consistent with Orem's conceptual framework in individual psychotherapy and family therapy are discussed.

Foster, P.C., & Janssens, N.P. (1980). Dorothea E. Orem. In Nursing Theories Conference Group, Nursing theories. The base for professional nursing practice (pp. 90–106). Englewood Cliffs, NJ: Prentice-Hall.

Foster, P.C., & Janssens, N.P. (1985). Dorothea E. Orem. In Nursing Theories Conference Group, Nursing theories. The base for professional nursing practice (2nd ed., pp. 124–139). Englewood Cliffs, NJ: Prentice-Hall.
Orem's conceptual framework is reviewed. Self-care is defined and the nursing process is delineated. Nursing systems are outlined. Analysis of the conceptual framework in terms of the concepts of man, learning, health, society, and nursing is presented. Strengths and weaknesses of the conceptual framework are discussed.

Gallant, B.W., & McLane, A.M. (1979). Outcome criteria: A process for validation at the unit level. Journal of Nursing Administration, 9(1), 14–21.
This article describes the development of a process for validation of outcome criteria derived from Orem's conceptual framework. The process was found to be useful at the unit level and to differentiate between valid and invalid nursing care outcomes for patients being discharged from a postoperative cardiovascular surgical unit.

Gantz, S.B. (1980). A fourth-grade adventure in self-directed learning. Topics in Clinical Nursing, 2(2), 29–38.
The author of this article describes a project designed to enhance the fourth graders' abilities to help themselves to better health.

Garvan, P., Lee, M., Lloyd K., & Sullivan, T.J. (1980). Self-care applied to the aged. New Jersey Nurse, 10(1), 3–5.
The self-care concept is applied to the aged population. Specific examples of use of the conceptual framework include medication use and remotivation therapy. Factors influencing self-care are identified.

Geden, E.A. (1982). Effects of lifting techniques on energy expenditure: A preliminary investigation. Nursing Research, 31, 214–218.
This report explains the findings of a study designed to determine the effects of different lifting techniques on oxygen consumption, heart rate, blood pressure, and respiratory rate.

Gibson, K.T. (1980). The type A personality: Implications for nursing practice. Cardio-Vascular Nursing, 16(5), 25–28.
This article presents a discussion of type A personality in patients with premature coronary heart disease and nursing practice implications for these patients based on Orem's conceptual framework.

Goldstein, N., Zink, M., Stevenson, L., Anderson, M., Wollery, L., & DePompolo, T.

(1983). Self-care: A framework for the future. In P.L. Chinn (Ed.), Advances in nursing theory development (pp. 107–121). Rockville, MD: Aspen.

The authors present their framework of nursing practice, derived from Orem's conceptual framework of nursing as well as other conceptualizations of self-care. The framework was designed specifically for a tertiary care center.

Goodwin, J.O. (1979). Programmed instruction for self-care following pulmonary surgery. International Journal of Nursing Studies, 16, 29–40.

This article reports the findings of a study of the effects of a programmed instruction booklet on the knowledge, self-care, recovery, and distress of patients who had had pulmonary surgery.

Goodwin, J.O. (1980). A cross-cultural approach to integrating nursing theory and practice. Nurse Educator, 5(6), 15–20.

A general model of the nursing process is outlined. Orem's conceptual framework is presented as one example of integration of a conceptual model with the general nursing process model. Use of the combined model in a French nursing school is described. Modifications in the model for the French culture and nursing practice are identified.

Gulick, E.E. (1987). Parsimony and model confirmation of the ADL self-care scale for multiple sclerosis persons. Nursing Research, 36, 278–283.

The investigator reports further development of a scale designed to assess activities of daily living for individuals with multiple sclerosis. Orem's conceptual framework served as the basis for scale items.

Hageman, P., & Ventura, M. (1981). Utilizing patient outcome criteria to measure the effects of a medication teaching regimen. Western Journal of Nursing Research, 3, 25–33.

The article reports the results of a study of interrater reliability of an outcome instrument and determination of the effectiveness of a special teaching regimen.

Harper, D. (1984). Application of Orem's theoretical constructs to self-care medication behaviors in the elderly. Advances in Nursing Science, 6(3), 29–46.

This article reports the findings of a study of the effectiveness of a self-care medication program on knowledge of medication, health locus of control, and self-care medication behaviors of elderly black patients with hypertension.

Harrigan, J.F., Faro, B.Z., VanPutte, A., & Stoler, P. (1987). The application of locus of control to diabetes education in school-aged children. Journal of Pediatric Nursing, 2, 236–243.

This article reports the findings of a study designed to investigate the relationships between locus of control and knowledge of diabetes in a sample of school-aged diabetic children. The investigators outline an educational program that emphasizes self-care.

Hartweg, D., & Metcalfe, S. (1986). Self-care attitude changes of nursing students enrolled in a self-care curriculum—A longitudinal study. Research in Nursing and Health, 9, 347–353.

The article reports the results of a study describing changes in nursing students' self-care attitudes after being socialized through a curriculum based on Orem's conceptual framework.

Hathaway, D.K., & Geden, E.A. (1983). Energy expenditure during leg exercise programs. Nursing Research, 32, 147–150.

The investigators report the findings of their study of the effects of three types of leg exercise programs on oxygen consumption, heart rate, respiratory rate, and blood pressure. Although Orem is not cited in the article, Geden linked this research to Orem's conceptual framework in her chapter in Riehl-Sisca's book on self-care.

Hedahl, K. (1983). Assisting the adolescent with physical disabilities through a college health program. Nursing Clinics of North America, 18, 257–274.

This article presents a description and results of an evaluation of a nursing care program for disabled students based on Orem's conceptual framework and concepts from a model of independent living.

Herrington, J., & Houston, S. (1984). Using Orem's theory: A plan for all seasons. Nursing and Health Care, 5(1), 45–47.
The article describes two clinical tools developed by faculty at the University of Southern Mississippi School of Nursing. The tools are based on Orem's nursing process format.

Horn, B.J., & Swain, M.A. (1976). An approach to development of criterion measures for quality patient care. In Issues in evaluation research (pp. 74–82). Kansas City: American Nurses Association.

Horn, B.J., & Swain, M.A. (1977). Development of criterion measures of nursing care (Vols. 1–2, NTIS Nos. PB–267 004 and PB–267 005). Ann Arbor, MI: University of Michigan,
The authors describe their project to develop, refine, and validate an instrument to measure the quality of the nursing care process. The instrument is based on Orem's conceptual framework and includes items designed to measure patients' physical and emotional status, the extent of their knowledge about how to monitor their health status and what measures they need to use to maintain or improve their health status, and their ability to perform activities of daily living.

Hurst, J.D., & Stullenbarger, B. (1986). Implementation of a self-care approach in a pediatric interdisciplinary phenylketonuria (PKU) clinic. Journal of Pediatric Nursing, 1, 159–163.
This article describes the implementation of nursing practice based on Orem's conceptual framework in a clinic for PKU patients.

Johnston, R.L. (1983). Orem self-care model of nursing. In J.J. Fitzpatrick & A.L. Whall, Conceptual models of nursing: Analysis and application (pp. 137–155). Bowie, MD: Brady.
This book chapter presents an analysis and evaluation of Orem's conceptual framework.

Karl, C. (1982). The effect of an exercise program on self-care activities for the institutionalized elderly. Journal of Gerontological Nursing. 8, 282–285.
This article reports the results of a study of the effects of a range of motion exercise program on independence in self-care activities of elderly patients.

Kearney, B.Y., & Fleischer, B.J. (1979). Development of an instrument to measure exercise of self-care agency. Research in Nursing and Health, 2, 25–34.
This article describes a study designed to develop an instrument to measure a person's exercise of self-care agency. Construct validity, content validity, and test-retest reliability were established using a sample of associate degree nursing students and psychology students.

Kruger, S., Shawver, M., & Jones, L. (1980). Reactions of families to the child with cystic fibrosis. Image, 12, 67–72.
Orem's conceptual framework is used as the framework for a descriptive study of behavior patterns of families, specifically well siblings, of children with cystic fibrosis. The study indicated that behavior patterns changed, especially in the universal self-care requisite for solitude and social interaction. Specific nursing interventions are offered to increase nurses' involvement with families of cystic fibrosis patients.

Kubricht, D. (1984). Therapeutic self-care demands expressed by outpatients receiving external radiation therapy. Cancer Nursing, 7, 43–52.
Orem's concept of self-care and Magoon's constructivist methodology were used to guide a descriptive study of participants' verbal expressions of changes that had occurred after beginning radiation treatments. Data were categorized according to universal self-care requisites.

Leatt, P., Bay, K.S., & Stinson, S.M. (1981). An instrument for assessing and classifying patients by type of care. Nursing Research, 30, 145–150.
This article reports the findings of a study designed to develop an instrument for assessing and classifying chronically ill patients who require long-term care. Orem's definition of therapeutic self-care practices was used.

Marten, L. (1978). Self-care nursing model for patients experiencing radical change in

body image. Journal of Obstetric, Gynecologic and Neonatal Nursing, 7(6), 9–13.
This article describes an approach to the emotional care of a woman recovering from a radical vulvectomy that linked Orem's conceptual framework with theoretical knowledge of self-concept and body image.

Maunz, E.R., & Woods, N.F. (1988). Self-care practices among young adult women: Influence of symptoms, employment, and sex-role orientation. Health Care for Women International, 9, 29–41.
The article reports the findings of a study designed to explore the influence of symptoms, employment, and sex-role orientation on illness-related self-care practices used by 96 young adult women.

McBride, S. (1987). Validation of an instrument to measure exercise of self-care agency. Research in Nursing and Health, 10, 311–316.
The author reports the findings of her study of the reliability and construct validity of Kearney and Fleischer's Exercise of Self-Care Agency Scale. Findings supported the test-retest and split-half reliability of the Scale for both post-basic nursing student and adult diabetic patient samples. Construct validity was supported only in the student sample.

McIntyre, K. (1980). The Perry model as a framework for self-care. Nurse Practitioner, 5(6), 34–38.
This article describes the utility of the Perry model of cognitive learning for evaluation of nursing care based on Orem's conceptual framework.

Melnyk, K. (1983). The process of theory analysis: An examination of the nursing theory of Dorothea E. Orem. Nursing Research, 32, 170–174.

Melnyk, K. (1983). Re: Nursing theory. (Letter to the editor). Nursing Research, 32, 318.

Melnyk, K. (1983). To the editor. (Letter to the editor). Nursing Research, 32, 383.

Allison, S. (1983). To the editor. (Letter to the editor). Nursing Research, 32, 381.

Burns, M., & Whelton, B. (1983). To the editor. (Letter to the editor). Nursing Research, 32, 381.

Geden, E. (1983). To the editor. (Letter to the editor). Nursing Research, 32, 381–382.

Orem, D. (1983). To the editor. (Letter to the editor). Nursing Research, 32, 382.

Pearson, B. (1983). To the editor. (Letter to the editor). Nursing Research, 32, 318.

Taylor, S. (1983). To the editor. (Letter to the editor). Nursing Research, 32, 382–383.
The article by Melnyk presents an examination of Orem's work using the analytic framework devised by B.J. Stevens. Orem's work is described, analyzed, and evaluated. Melnyk concluded that the physician provides the dynamic that drives Orem's theory of nursing and that should Orem's theory be implemented, nursing practice would focus solely on adults in acute care hospitals.
Letters to the editor from Allison, Burns & Whelton, Geden, Orem, Pearson, and Taylor identify inaccuracies in Melnyk's discussion and express their concerns regarding the publication of an article that misrepresented Orem's work.
Letters to the editor from Melnyk present her response to the criticisms of her article.

Miller, J.F. (1980). The dynamic focus of nursing: A challenge to nursing administration. Journal of Nursing Administration, 10(1), 13–18.
The article presents a model for nursing practice based on Orem's conceptual framework that takes the individual's progression on the illness-to-health continuum into account.

Miller, J.F. (1982). Categories of self-care needs of ambulatory patients with diabetes. Journal of Advanced Nursing, 7, 25–31.
The article reports the findings of a study of categorization of needs of ambulatory diabetic patients using a self-care framework. The investigator maintained that the categories may be used for ambulatory patients who have other chronic health problems.

Mitchell, P., & Irvin, N. (1977). Neurological examination: Nursing assessment for nursing purposes. Journal of Neurosurgical Nursing, 9(1), 23–28.
This article presents a modification of the traditional neurological examination that

focuses on determination of nervous system dysfunction and the effect of that dysfunction on individuals' self-care activities.

Moore, J.B. (1987). Effects of assertion training and first aid instruction on children's autonomy and self-care agency. Research in Nursing and Health, 10, 101–109.
This article reports the results of a study the effects of learning strategies for promoting autonomy and self-care agency in a sample of 92 fifth-grade students. The subjects were randomly assigned to four learning groups: assertion training, first aid instruction, assertion/first aid, and control. Findings indicated that autonomy was higher where either or both assertion training and first aid instruction had occurred and that self-care agency was higher where first aid instruction had occurred.

Moscovitz, A. (1984). Orem's theory as applied to psychiatric nursing. Perspectives in Psychiatric Care, 22(1), 36–38.
This article focuses on the application and limitations of Orem's conceptual framework in the psychiatric setting.

Munley, M.J., & Sayers, P.A. (1984). Self-care deficit theory of nursing. A primer for application of the concepts. North Brunswick, NJ: Personal and Family Health Associates.
This book presents the basic ideas of Orem's conceptual framework.

Murphy, P.P. (1981). A hospice model and self-care theory. Oncology Nursing Forum, 8(2), 19–21.
The author describes the use of Orem's conceptual framework as a guide for delivery of nursing services in the hospice at Overlook Hospital in Summit, New Jersey.

Nowakowski, L. (1980). Health promotion/self-care programs for the community. Topics in Clinical Nursing, 2(2), 21–27.
The article describes the development of health promotion programs for community members based on Orem's conceptual framework at Georgetown University in Washington, D.C. The program included a series of self-care programs and consultation services for community participants.

Nursing Development Conference Group. (1973). Concept formalization in nursing. Process and product. Boston: Little, Brown and Co.

Nursing Development Conference Group. (1979). Concept formalization in nursing. Process and product. Boston: Little, Brown and Co.
This book represents the efforts of 11 nurses to formalize a framework for nursing knowledge. The content includes concepts from the philosophy of science, descriptions of general nursing concepts, and documentation of the process of attempting to formalize nursing knowledge. Aspects of Orem's conceptual framework are included. The second edition presents further development in the study of the conceptual structure of nursing. Orem's conceptual framework is developed and presented in greater detail than in the first edition of the book.

Orem, D.E. (1959). Guides for developing curricula for the education of practical nurses. Washington, D.C.: U.S. Government Printing Office.
This book presents Orem's perspective of the central concepts of nursing and an application of these concepts to practical nurse education. Practical nursing is discussed and a framework to guide curriculum planning is provided.

Orem, D.E. (1971). Nursing: Concepts of practice. New York: McGraw-Hill.
Orem's self-care conceptual framework is presented and offered as a framework for structuring nursing knowledge.

Orem, D.E. (1980). Nursing: Concepts of practice (2nd ed.). New York: McGraw-Hill.
Refinements in Orem's conceptual framework are presented. Propositions for Orem's theories of self-care, self-care deficits, and nursing systems are listed.

Orem, D.E. (1981). Nursing: A triad of action systems. In G.E. Lasker (Ed.), Applied systems and cybernetics. Vol. IV. Systems research in health care, biocybernetics and ecology (pp. 1729–1733). New York: Pergamon Press.
Orem describes the nursing systems component of her conceptual framework.

Orem, D.E. (1983). The self-care deficit theory of nursing: A general theory. In I.W.

Clements & F.B. Roberts, Family Health. A theoretical approach to nursing care (pp. 205–217). New York: John Wiley & Sons.
This chapter presents a brief biography of Orem and a detailed description of the object of nursing, as well as a discussion of the theories of self-care, self-care deficits, and nursing systems.

Orem, D.E. (1983). The family coping with a medical illness. Analysis and application of Orem's theory. In I.W. Clements & F.B. Roberts, Family health. A theoretical approach to nursing care (pp. 385–386). New York: John Wiley & Sons.
This chapter presents Orem's analysis of a case study involving the reactions of a father and those in his family to his diagnosis of and treatment for leukemia.

Orem, D.E. (1983). The family experiencing emotional crisis. Analysis and application of Orem's self-care deficit theory. In I.W. Clements & F.B. Roberts, Family health. A theoretical approach to nursing care (pp. 367–368). New York: John Wiley & Sons.
This chapter presents Orem's analysis of a case study of a three-generation Mexican-American family whose care has been delegated to a mental health nurse following the discharge of both daughters from a state mental institution.

Orem, D.E. (1984). Orem's conceptual model and community health nursing. In M.K. Asay & C.C. Ossler (Ed.), Conceptual models of nursing. Applications in community health nursing. Proceedings of the Eighth Annual Community Health Nursing Conference (pp. 35–50). Chapel Hill: Department of Public Health Nursing, School of Public Health, University of North Carolina.
Orem explains the use of her work in community health nursing. She maintains that the unit of service is individuals.

Orem, D.E. (1985). Nursing: Concepts of practice (3rd ed.). New York: McGraw-Hill.
The most recent refinements in Orem's work are presented in this book.

Orem, D.E. (1987). Orem's general theory of nursing. In R.R. Parse, Nursing science. Major paradigms, theories, and critiques (pp. 67–89). Philadelphia: WB Saunders.
This chapter is the publication of Orem's presentation at the Nurse Theorist Conference held in Pittsburgh, Pennsylvania, in May 1985.

Orem, D.E. (in press). Theories and hypotheses for nursing administration. In B. Henry, M. DiVincenti, C. Arndt, & A. Marriner (Eds.), Dimensions of nursing administration. Theory, research, education and practice. Boston: Blackwell Scientific Publications.
This chapter is a presentation of Orem's ideas regarding the use of her work in administration of nursing services.

Orem, D.E., & Parker, K.S. (Eds.) (1963). Nurse education workshop proceedings. Washington, D.C.: Catholic University of America.
These proceedings report the faculty's attempt to identify a rationale for nursing content and clinical nursing experiences. Specific papers dealing with aspects of nursing education are presented. Summaries of discussion groups are included. Criteria for nursing content are identified.

Orem, D.E., & Taylor, S.G. (1986). Orem's general theory of nursing. In P. Winstead-Fry (Ed.), Case studies in nursing theory (pp. 37–71). New York: National League for Nursing.
This book chapter presents an historical overview of the development of Orem's conceptual framework and theories, a discussion of the conceptual framework and theories with clear and concise definitions of major concepts, review of research that has been derived from Orem's work, and a case study of a 34-year-old man with diabetes.

Patterson, E., & Hale, E. (1985). Making sure: Integrating menstrual care practices into activities of daily living. Advances in Nursing Science, 7(3), 18–31.
The qualitative research reported in this article focuses on the self-care process of "making sure." This recurring self-care process enables menstruating women to continue their activities of daily living.

Perras, S., & Zappacosta, A. (1982). The application of Orem's theory in promoting self-care in a peritoneal dialysis facility. American Association of Nephrology Nurses and Technicians Journal, 9(3), 37–39.
This article, co-authored by a nurse and a physician, suggests the use of Orem's conceptual framework as the basis for a self-care peritoneal dialysis program.

Orem's nursing process and nursing systems are described and related to end-stage renal disease patients requiring peritoneal dialysis.

Piemme, J.A., & Trainor, M.A. (1977). A first-year nursing course in a baccalaureate program. Nursing Outlook, 25, 184–187.
This article describes a freshman year non-clinical nursing course taught at Georgetown University School of Nursing. The curriculum of the school is based on Orem's conceptual framework. The course includes content on nursing as a practice discipline; role responsibilities related to practice, scholarship, research, and education needed to develop an organized body of nursing knowledge; the health and assisting dimensions of nursing; and the importance to society of nursing and nursing education.

Porter, D., & Shamian, J. (1983). Self-care in theory and practice. Canadian Nurse, 79(8), 21–23.
This article introduces the reader to Orem's conceptual framework. Application of Orem's work in a hospital setting is illustrated by a case study of a patient from admission through discharge.

Rew, L. (1987). The relationship between self-care behaviors and selected psychosocial variables in children with asthma. Pediatric Nursing, 2, 333–341.
This article reports the findings of a study of factors associated with self-care behaviors of 72 children with asthma who attended a one-week residential camp. Age, gender, and health locus of control were found to be associated with post-camp self-care behavior scores.

Riehl-Sisca, J. (1985). The science and art of self-care. Norwalk, CT: Appleton-Century-Crofts.
This book includes a discussion of Orem's conceptual framework and theories and many chapters describing application of Orem's work in nursing research, education, practice, and administration.

Romine, S. (1986). Applying Orem's theory of self-care to staff development. Journal of Nursing Staff Development, 2(2), 77–79.
This article presents an overview of Orem's work and definitions of the concepts of the framework in terms of the education setting. Examples of how staff development may be guided by Orem's work are included.

Rothlis, J. (1984). The effect of a self-help group on feelings of hopelessness and helplessness. Western Journal of Nursing Research, 6, 157–173.
This article reports the findings of a study of the effect of a self-help group on feelings of hopelessness and helplessness in patients with reactive depression. Orem's conceptual framework was used to bring the facilitation of a self-help group into the realm of nursing. The manuscript includes the research report, two commentaries, and a response by the investigator.

Rosenbaum, J. (1986). Comparison of two theorists on care: Orem and Leininger. Journal of Advanced Nursing, 11, 409–419.
This article presents a comparison of Orem's and Leininger's use of the concepts of care and self-care.

Sandman, P.O., Norberg, A., Adolfsson, R., Axelsson, K., & Hedly, V. Morning care of patients with Alzheimer-type dementia. A theoretical model based on direct observation. Journal of Advanced Nursing, 11, 369–378.
The article describes the use of Orem's conceptual framework as a frame of reference for compensation of patients' lack of self-care capabilities as well as an analysis of patients' and nurses' behaviors during morning care of patients with Alzheimer-type dementia.

Saucier, C. (1984). Self concept and self-care management in school-age children with diabetes. Pediatric Nursing, 10, 135–138.
This article reports the results of a study of the relationship between self-concept and participation in self-care activities of 10- to 12-year-old children with diabetes.

Scherer, P. (1988). Hospitals that attract (and keep) nurses. American Journal of Nursing, 88, 34–40.
The author reports the findings of a survey of strategies used by hospitals to reduce staff turnover. Included is a description of the use of Orem's conceptual framework at the Beth Israel Medical Center in Newark, New Jersey. The survey indicated that

the use of Orem's framework on three units in the hospital has enhanced patient satisfaction with care, reduced morbidity and infection rates, and virtually eliminated staff turnover. In addition, the units require lower budgets and fewer staff members.

Smith, M.C. (1977). Self-care: A conceptual framework for rehabilitation nursing. Rehabilitation Nursing, 2(2), 8–10.
The need for a conceptual framework for practice is discussed in this article, which also presents a description of the self-care perspective as well as suggestions for its use by individuals and departments of nursing.

Smith, M.C. (1979). Proposed metaparadigm for nursing research and theory development. An analysis of Orem's self-care theory. Image, 11, 75–79.
The author develops a classification scheme to analyze existing research derived from Orem's conceptual framework. Future directions for research related to the conceptual framework are identified. Orem's conceptual framework is proposed as a metaparadigm, and methods for use of the metaparadigm are outlined.

Smith, M.J. (1987). A critique of Orem's theory. In R.R. Parse, Nursing science. Major paradigms, theories, and critiques (pp. 91–105). Philadelphia: W.B. Saunders.
This chapter is the publication of a critique of Orem's work that was presented at the Nurse Theorist Conference held in Pittsburgh, Pennsylvania, in May 1985.

Smith, S.R. (1981). Sound off! "Oremization," the curse of nursing. RN, 44(10), 83.
The author criticizes Orem for making simple ideas complex. The basic premises of the conceptual framework are presented and deemed to be self-evident. The terminology of the conceptual framework, as well as other nursing models, is considered needlessly confusing.

Spangler, Z.S., & Spangler, W.D. (1983). Self-care: A testable model. In P.L. Chinn (Ed.), Advances in nursing theory development (pp. 89–105). Rockville, MD: Aspen.
The authors present a testable model composed of Orem's propositions of self-care and ideas from economics and social psychology.

Steiger, N., & Lipson, J. (1985). Self-care nursing: Theory and practice. Bowie, MD: Brady.
This book presents an exploration and discussion of various approaches to self-care, including Orem's work.

Stockdale-Woolley, R. (1984). The effects of education on self-care agency. Public Health Nursing, 1, 97–106.
The article presents a report of a study of the effect of group education classes on self-care agency of individuals with COPD.

Storm, D.S., & Baumgartner, R.G. (1987). Achieving self-care in the ventilator-dependent patient: A critical analysis of a case study. International Journal of Nursing Studies, 24, 95–106.
This article presents an analysis of a case study of a 41-year-old woman with multiple sclerosis who was discharged to her home with a mechanical ventilator and 24-hour nursing care after a 4-month hospitalization. Nursing care is discussed within the context of Orem's conceptual framework and diagnoses from the North American Nursing Diagnosis Association list.

Sullivan, T.J. (1980). Self-care model for nursing. In Directions for nursing in the 80s (pp. 57–68). Kansas City: American Nurses Association.
This study was designed to develop a model of nursing practice for care of the aged based on Orem's conceptual framework and theoretical knowledge from the gerontological, geriatric, and gerontological nursing literature. Four self-care systems levels were identified: independents, independents-threaded, independents-delegators, and dependents.

Taylor, S. (1978, December/1979, January). The unique object and system of nursing. Missouri Nurse, 3–5.
This article presents a discussion of the nursing system viewed as a system within the larger health care system. The self-care deficit concept of nursing is used to describe that which is uniquely nursing.

Thibodeau, J.A. (1983). Nursing models: Analysis and evaluation. Monterey, CA: Wadsworth.
This book includes a chapter that presents an analysis and evaluation of Orem's conceptual framework, using an early version of the framework for analysis and evaluation of conceptual models presented in Chapter 2 of the present book.

Toth, J.C. (1980). Effect of structured preparation for transfer on patient anxiety on leaving coronary care unit. Nursing Research, 29, 28–34.
This study compared the effect of structured and unstructured pretransfer information on manifestations of anxiety in 20 myocardial infarction patients after they were transferred from the coronary care unit. Orem's conceptual framework concept of self-care was used as the basis for the pretransfer information. Findings supported the hypothesis that structured information would reduce anxiety more than unstructured information.

Underwood, P.R. (1980). Facilitating self-care. In Pothier, P. (Ed.), Psychiatric nursing. A basic text (pp. 115–132). Boston: Little, Brown and Co.
Orem's conceptual framework is described in considerable detail and applied to the nursing care of psychiatric patients in a continual-care facility. A detailed nursing care plan is included.

Uys, L.R. (1987). Foundational studies in nursing. Journal of Advanced Nursing, 12, 275–280.
This article presents a brief discussion of Orem's conceptual framework within the context of foundationalist study with emphasis on evaluation of philosophical grounding for the framework.

Weaver, M.T. (1987). Perceived self-care agency: A LISREL factor analysis of Bickel and Hanson's questionnaire. Nursing Research, 36, 381–387.
This article presents the findings of a study designed to examine the psychometric properties of Bickel and Hanson's perceived self-care agency questionnaire. Results did not confirm the original factor structure of the questionnaire and raised questions regarding its construct validity as a measure of self-care agency in non-institutionalized adults. The investigator recommends extreme caution in the use of the questionnaire in the testing of propositions from Orem's conceptual framework and theories.

Whelen, E. (1984). Analysis and application of Dorothea Orem's self-care practice model. Journal of Nursing Education, 23, 342–345.
This article presents an overview of Orem's conceptual framework for the nurse educator. A brief discussion of the application of the framework to a clinical situation is included. The appendix includes an example of the assessment of a specific patient and the associated nursing elements and factors.

Whetstone, W.R. (1986). Social dramatics: Social skills development for the chronically mentally ill. Journal of Advanced Nursing, 11, 67–74.
This article reports the finding of a study of the effects of social dramatics as a clinical tool for teaching social skills to chronically mentally ill patients in a state hospital.

Wollery, L. (1983). Self-care for the obstetrical patient. Journal of Obstetric, Gynecologic, and Neonatal Nursing, 12, 33–37.
This article describes the use of Orem's conceptual framework for obstetrical nursing practice. A case study is presented.

Woods, N.F. (1985). Self-care practices among young adult married women. Research in Nursing and Health, 8, 227–233.
This study report presents data from a study of the universal and illness-related self-care activities employed by young adult women.

Zach, P. (1982). Self-care agency in diabetic ocular sequelae. Journal of Ophthalmic Nursing Techniques, 1(2), 21–31.
This article describes the assessment of self-care agency for diabetics experiencing ocular problems.

CHAPTER

8

Rogers's Science of Unitary Human Beings_____

This chapter presents an analysis and evaluation of Martha E. Rogers's conceptual model of nursing, which is referred to as the Science of Unitary Human Beings. Rogers (personal communication, June 17, 1987) regards her work as an abstract conceptual system that "is not of the same order as the other conceptual models, nor does it derive from the same world view. Rather, it derives from a different world view and deals with a different phenomenon." The Science of Unitary Human Beings does, however, fit the definition of a conceptual model used in this book.

The key terms of Rogers's Science of Unitary Human Beings are listed below. These terms were taken from two book chapters that present the most recent versions of her work. One chapter is Rogers's 1980 publication, "Nursing: A science of unitary man." The second chapter is Rogers's 1986 publication, "Science of unitary human beings."

KEY TERMS_____

Unitary Human Beings	Openness
Energy Fields	Pattern
Human Beings	Four Dimensionality
Environment	Resonancy

Helicy	Goal of Nursing
Integrality	To Help All People Achieve
Health	Maximum Well-Being
An Expression of the Life	Nursing Process
Process	Theory of Accelerating Evolution
Nursing	Theory of Paranormal
A Learned Profession	Phenomena
A Science and an Art	Theory of Rhythmical Correlates
	of Change

ANALYSIS OF ROGERS'S SCIENCE OF UNITARY HUMAN BEINGS

This section presents an analysis of Rogers's Science of Unitary Human Beings. The analysis draws from several of Rogers's publications, including her 1970 book, *An introduction to the theoretical basis of nursing;* her 1980 book chapter, "Nursing: A science of unitary man"; her 1986 book chapter, "Science of unitary human beings"; and her 1987a book chapter, "Nursing research in the future."

Development of the Model

Rogers first presented her conceptual model in her 1970 book, *An introduction to the theoretical basis of nursing.* Further development and refinement of the model was presented by Rogers (1978a) at the Second Annual Nurse Educator Conference. This presentation, with some further refinement, was later published in Riehl and Roy's (1980) book, *Conceptual models for nursing practice* (Rogers, 1980a). The two latter papers also introduced theoretical formulations derived from the model. An expanded explanation of the model, as well as a comprehensive discussion of the theories derived from the conceptual model, were presented in a series of video and audio tapes in 1980 (Rogers, 1980b–g). Further refinements of the conceptual model were published in Malinski's (1986a) book, *Explorations on Martha Rogers' Science of Unitary Human Beings* (Rogers, 1986). Rogers (personal communication, June 17, 1987) stated that her 1986 publication contains the most recent version of the Science of Unitary Human Beings. She also noted that the revisions and refinements of her conceptual model were undertaken in an attempt to clarify the meaning of essential ideas and to eliminate misinterpretation of certain terms. For example, the principles of reciprocy and synchrony have been eliminated and the principle of complementarity has been replaced by the principle of integrality because the terms reciprocy, synchrony, and complementarity lead to the false interpretation of separation between the human and environmental energy fields. Similarly, the term unidirectionality has been eliminated because it led to the false interpretation of human development as linear. And development, per se, has been dropped because it "implies certain kinds of linearity" (Rogers, cited in Malinski, 1986b, p. 11). Another example of refinement, undertaken to enhance clarity and to avoid charges of sexist language, has been the change from "man" to "unitary man" and finally to "unitary human beings" (Young, 1985).

Rogers (1978b) stated that she deliberately set out to develop her conceptual system when she realized that "there had to be a body of knowledge that was specific to and unique to nursing, or there was no need for higher education in nursing at all." Rogers's recognition of the need for an organized body of nursing knowledge was evident in her early writings on nursing education, especially in the books, *Educational revolution in nursing* (Rogers, 1961) and *Reveille in nursing* (Rogers, 1964).

Rogers was a pioneer in the development of unique nursing knowledge. She was one of the first modern nurse scholars to explicitly identify the central phenomenon of interest to the discipline of nursing as man (Newman, 1972a). Moreover, she focused attention on the environment as an equally important phenomenon for study. Rogers (1978a) traced the dual concern with people and their environments to Nightingale (1859).

Rogers (1978a) stated that she directed her efforts "to evolve a conceptual system that would give identity to nursing as a knowledgeable endeavor." The following assumptions provided the foundation for the model:

- Nursing is a learned profession.
- The explication of an organized body of abstract knowledge specific to nursing is indispensable to nursing's transition from pre-science to science.
- Nursing is both an empirical science and an art.
- Nursing science is an organized body of abstract knowledge arrived at by scientific research and logical analysis.
- The art of nursing is the utilization of scientific nursing knowledge for the betterment of people.
- People need knowledgeable nursing.
- The practice of nursing is the use of nursing knowledge in human service.
- The descriptive, explanatory, and predictive principles that direct nursing practice are derived from a conceptual system.
- Nursing's long-established concern is with human beings and their world.

- People have the capacity to participate knowingly and probabilistically in the process of change. (Rogers, 1970, 1978a, 1978b, 1980a, 1986)

Rogers used a deductive approach to develop her conceptual system. She stated that her conceptual system "does not derive from one or more of the basic sciences. Neither does it come out of a vacuum. A multiplicity of knowledges from many sources flows in novel ways to create a kaleidoscope of potentialities" (Rogers, 1986, p. 4). In the various presentations of the conceptual system, Rogers has cited many notable philosophers and scientists, including Bertalanffy (1960), Burr and Northrop (1935), Chardin (1961), Einstein (1961), Goldstein (1939), Herrick (1956), Lewin (1964), and Polanyi (1958), among others.

Rogers (1985a) implied that system theory was especially influential in the development and refinement of her conceptual model when she stated,

> The introduction of systems theories several decades ago set in motion new ways of perceiving people and their world. Science and technology escalated. Space exploration revised old views. New knowledge merged with new ways of thinking. The second industrial revolution was born—far more dramatic in its implications and potentials than the first. A pressing need to study people in ways that would enhance their humanness coordinate with accelerating technological advances forced a search for new models. (p. 16)

Rogers has always emphasized the uniqueness of nursing knowledge in general and her conceptual model in particular. In fact, she regards the model as an emergent, a new product synthesized from the work of many theoreticians and researchers. She explained,

> The development of a conceptual system is a process of the creative synthesis of facts and ideas out of which a new product emerges. . . . Certainly, the conceptual system and what comes out of it is not derived from any of the basic sciences of any other field. Nursing is not based on any of these; rather, it has its own unique irreducible mix. The parts cannot be removed or changed around or revised without altering the system. This conceptual system is the peculiar synthesis that has led to the product called the science of unitary human beings. (Rogers, 1987d, p. 141)

Content of the Model: Concepts

Person and Environment

Rogers (1986) identified unitary human beings and their environments as the central focus of her conceptual system. The relationship between unitary human beings and their environments is such that they must be discussed together.

Human beings and the environment are regarded as irreducible wholes that cannot be understood when they are reduced to their particulars. Rogers (1986) defined the unitary human being as "an irreducible four-dimensional energy field identified by pattern and manifesting characteristics that are different from those of the parts and cannot be predicted from knowledge of the parts" (p. 5). The environment was defined as "an irreducible, four-dimensional energy field identified by pattern and manifesting characteristics different from those of the parts" (p. 5). Rogers went on to explain that "each environmental field is specific to its given human field. Both change continuously, mutually, and creatively. The human and environmental fields are infinite and integral with one another" (p. 5).

The definitions of unitary human beings and their environments identify the four concepts of the Science of Unitary Human Beings as energy fields, openness, pattern, and four-dimensionality. Rogers (1986) pointed out that the concept of energy field represents "a means of perceiving people and their respective environments as irreducible wholes" (p. 4). Energy fields, according to Rogers,

> are postulated to constitute the fundamental unit of both the living and the nonliving. *Field* is a unifying concept. *Energy* signifies the dynamic nature of the field. *Energy fields* are infinite . . . human beings and environment *are* energy fields. They do not have them. (p. 4)

The distinctive nature of human and environmental energy fields was underscored by Rogers (1986) when she pointed out that

> human and environmental fields are *not* biological fields or physical fields, or social or psychological fields. Neither are human and environmental fields a summation of biological, physical, social, and psychological fields. This is not a denial of other fields. Rather, it is to make clear that human and environmental fields have their own identity and are not to be confused with parts. (pp. 4–5)

Rogers (1986) characterized unitary human beings and their environments as open systems. She maintained that there is no variance in the openness of the human and environmental energy fields, explaining that "energy fields are open—not a little bit or sometimes, but continuously" (p. 5).

Energy fields have pattern. Rogers (1986) defined pattern as "the distinguishing characteristic of an energy field perceived as a single wave" (p. 5). Elaborating on this concept, Rogers stated,

> Pattern is an abstraction. It gives identity to the field. The nature of the pattern changes continuously. Each human field pattern is unique and is integral with its own unique environmental field pattern. (p. 5)

Pattern is an abstraction that cannot be seen. Rather, "manifestations of field patterning are observable events in the real world. They are postulated to emerge out of the human-environmental field process" (Rogers, 1986, p. 6).

The pattern of an energy field is conceptualized as a wave phenomenon. Rogers (1970) noted, "A multiplicity of waves characterizes the universe. Light waves, sound waves, thermal waves, atomic waves, gravity waves flow in rhythmic patterns" (p. 101).

Energy field pattern changes continuously. The change, according to Rogers (1986), is relative, innovative, and increasingly diverse. This means there is no repetition in human life, no regression to former states or stages. Rather, the human and environmental field patterns change constantly, always evolving into other novel, innovative forms (Rogers, 1970). Although the direction of changes is invariant, the rate of change may vary for an individual over the course of life. Change also varies between individuals. Indeed, "individual differences point up the significance of relative diversity" (Rogers, 1986, p. 6).

Rogers (1986) described the human and environmental fields as four-dimensional. She defined four-dimensionality as "a nonlinear domain without spatial or temporal attributes. All reality is postulated to be four dimensional" (p. 5). Rogers explained that in a four-dimensional world, "the relative nature of change becomes explicit" (p. 5).

The four-dimensional (4-D) energy field, according to Rogers (1980a),

> is characterized by continuously fluctuating imaginary boundaries. The present as a point in time is not relevant to a 4-D model. Rather the four-dimensional human field is the 'relative present' for any individual. . . . Four-dimensional reality is perceived as a synthesis of nonlinear coordinates from which innovative change continuously and evolutionally emerges. (pp. 331–332)

Rogers (1986) formulated three mutually exclusive principles of homeodynamics to explicitly and concisely state her ideas about human and environmental energy field patterns. According to Rogers (1986), "pattern is the key concept in these principles" (p. 6).

The principle of resonancy delineates the direction of evolutionary change in energy field pattern. Resonancy is "the continuous change from lower to higher frequency wave patterns in human and environmental fields" (Rogers, 1986, p. 6).

The principle of helicy speaks to the continuous change that characterizes human and environmental field patterns. Helicy is "the continuous, innovative, probabilistic increasing diversity of human and environmental field patterns characterized by nonrepeating rhythmicities" (Rogers, 1986, p. 6).

The principle of integrality emphasizes the nature of the relationship between the human and environmental fields. Integrality is "the continuous mutual human field and environmental field process" (Rogers, 1986, p. 6).

Health

Rogers (1970) defined health as an expression of the life process. She referred to health and illness, ease and dis-ease, normal and pathological processes, and maximum well-being and sickness. Such dichotomous notions, Rogers (1970) maintained, "are arbitrarily defined, culturally infused, and value laden" (p. 85). She went on to explain,

> Health and sickness, however defined, are expressions of the process of life. Whatever meaning they may have is derived out of an understanding of the life process in its totality. Life's deviant course demands that it be viewed in all of its dimensions if valid explanations of its varied manifestations are to emerge. (p. 85)

Wellness and illness, then, are not differentiated within the context of this conceptual system. Rather, these are considered value terms imposed by society. As such, manifestations of human and environmental field pattern deemed to have high value are labeled wellness by the society, and those deemed to have low value are labeled illness (Rogers, 1980f). More specifically, within the Science of Unitary Human Beings,

> There are no absolute norms for health. There are patterns that emerge from the human process that may cause pain, happiness, illness, or any behavior. Society labels some of these behaviors "sick." What behaviors a society accepts as sick or well varies with culture and history. Families also have their own definitions of sick or well. . . . So there are no absolutes about what constitutes sickness or wellness. (Madrid & Winstead-Fry, 1986, p. 91)

Madrid and Winstead-Fry then defined health as "participation in the life process by choosing and executing behaviors that lead to the maximum fulfillment of a person's potential" (p. 91).

Despite her lack of differentiation of wellness and illness, Rogers (1970) viewed these health states in the form of a continuum. She explained,

> Health and illness are part of the same continuum. They are not dichotomous conditions. The multiple events taking place along life's axis denote the extent to which man is achieving his maximum health potential and vary in their expressions from greatest health to those conditions which are incompatible with maintaining life processes. (p. 125)

However, Rogers (1970) indicated that she thinks society views wellness and illness as dichotomous, discrete entities.

Nursing

Rogers (1987a) regards nursing as a learned profession that is both a science and an art. The science of nursing is "an organized body of abstract knowledge arrived at by scientific research and logical analysis" (p. 121). The art of nursing "is the imaginative and creative use of this knowledge in human service" (p. 121). Rogers went on to say, "Historically, the term nursing most often has been used as a verb signifying 'to do.' When nursing is perceived as a science the term nursing becomes a noun signifying 'a body of abstract knowledge'" (p. 121).

Rogers (1970) acknowledged the importance of technological tools and personal procedural activities used by nurses, but pointed out that

> it must be thoroughly understood that tools and procedures are adjuncts to practice and are safe and meaningful only to the extent that knowledgeable nursing judgments underwrite their selection and the ways in which they may be used. (p. 126)

Rogers (1970) described nursing's mission as social, stating,

> Nursing exists to serve people. Its direct and over-riding responsibility is to society . . . the safe practice of nursing depends on the nature and amount of scientific nursing knowledge the individual brings to practice and the imaginative, intellectual judgment with which such knowledge is made explicit in service to mankind. (p. 122)

> Nursing's abstract system is the outgrowth of concern for human health and welfare. The science of nursing aims to provide a growing body of theoretical knowledge whereby nursing practice can achieve new levels of meaningful service to man. (p. 88)

The social mission of nursing also is evident in Rogers's (1970) statement concerning the scope of nursing's service to people:

> The arenas of nursing's services extend into all areas where there are people: at home, at school, at work, at play; in hospital, nursing home, and clinic; on this planet and now moving into outer space. (p. 86)

The distinction between nursing and other disciplines, according to Rogers (1980b), lies in the phenomenon of central interest to each, in what is known rather than what is done in practice. From the perspective of Rogers's conceptual model, the phenomenon of central concern is unitary human beings and their environments. Rogers (1986) maintained that the uniqueness of nursing lies in this concern. She stated,

> Nursing's long-established concern with human beings and their world is a natural forerunner of an organized abstract system encompassing people and their environments. The irreducible nature of individuals

as energy fields, different from the sum of their parts and integral with their respective environmental fields, differentiates nursing from other sciences and identifies nursing's focus. (p. 3)

The goal of nursing identified by Rogers is predicated on a view of the practitioner as "an environmental component for the individual receiving services" (Rogers, 1970, pp. 124–125). The following quotes indicate that the goal of nursing focuses on promotion of health and on the integral relationship between the human and environmental energy fields:

The purpose of nursing is to help individuals and groups to achieve maximum well-being within the potential of each. (Rogers, 1978a)

The purpose of nursing is to help all people achieve maximum well-being within their potential, wherever they are. (Rogers, 1987a, p. 121)

Nurses participate in the process of change, to help people move toward what is deemed better health. (Rogers, 1980g)

Nursing is appropriate in all areas of health care, as is evident in the following statement: "Nursing is engaged in maintenance and promotion of health and rehabilitation of the sick and disabled from conception through dying" (Rogers, 1978a).

Although Rogers mentioned prevention of disease in her 1970 book, she later pointed out that prevention is a negative concept that is contradicted by the ideas comprising her conceptual model (Rogers, 1980g). She also pointed out that promotion of health is a more positive, optimistic concept and, therefore, is consistent with her conceptual system.

The nursing process, according to Rogers (1970), follows from the science of nursing. She explained,

Broad principles are put together in novel ways to help explain a wide range of events and multiplicity of individual differences. Action, based on predictions arising out of intellectual skill in the merging of scientific principles, becomes underwritten by intellectual judgments. (pp. 87–88)

Rogers (1970) maintained that the nursing process must focus on the person as a unified whole. Moreover, Rogers (1980f, 1980g) emphasized the need for individualized nursing care. She maintained that this is necessary to help people achieve their maximum potential in a positive fashion. The nurse must look at each individual and determine the range of behaviors that are normal for him or her. Diversity among individuals always must be taken into account, for it has distinct implications for what will be done and how it will be done. Thus, nursing intervention always is novel, because it is based on the needs of the individual. The novelty of nursing intervention is explained by Rogers (1970) in the following quotation:

> Judicious and wise identification of interventive measures consonant with the diagnostic pattern and the purposes to be achieved in any given situation requires the imaginative pulling together of nursing knowledges in new ways according to the particular needs of the individual or group. (p. 125)

Rogers (1985a, 1987b) noted that alternative forms of healing and non-invasive modalities, such as therapeutic touch, imagery, meditation, and humor are consistent with her conceptual system.

Rogers (1978b) regarded the nursing process as a modality for implementation of nursing knowledge but lacking in any substance of its own. She did not specify a particular nursing process format but did mention assessment, diagnosis, goal setting, intervention, and evaluation in her 1970 book. Although elements of each of these nursing process components can be extracted from Rogers's 1970 book (Fawcett, 1984), much of the detail is based on the early version of her conceptual model and, therefore, does not reflect the latest version of the Science of Unitary Human Beings. Rogers's recent publications and presentations do not address nursing process. Readers are referred to publications by Falco and Lobo (1985) and Madrid and Winstead-Fry (1986), who have developed nursing process guidelines that appear to be consistent with the Science of Unitary Human Beings.

Content of the Model: Propositions

Rogers repeatedly linked the metaparadigm concepts, person and environment. This linkage is most evident in the principle of integrality: "The continuous mutual human field and environmental field process" (Rogers, 1986, p. 6).

The linkage of the metaparadigm concepts, person, environment, and nursing, is evident in the following statement: "Nursing's long-established concern with human beings and their world is a natural forerunner of an organized abstract system encompassing people and their environments" (Rogers, 1986, p. 3)

No single statement linking all four metaparadigm concepts—person, environment, health, nursing—is evident in Rogers's recent publications. However, the linkage can be made by adding the purpose of nursing, as stated by Rogers, to a quote linking person, environment, and nursing. The statement would then read as follows: "Nursing's . . . concern is [with] human beings and the world they live in. . . . The purpose of nurses is to help all people achieve maximum well being" (Rogers, 1987a, p. 121).

Areas of Concern

Rogers's Science of Unitary Human Beings is concerned with "human beings and their world" (Rogers, 1986, p. 3). In particular, the human and environmental energy fields are areas of concern. More specifically, the conceptual system is concerned with those patterns of the human and environmental energy fields that are associated with maximum well-being, as well-being is defined by the society in which the human being is located. It is important to point out that this conceptual system does not deal with health problems, but rather is concerned with the "evolution of change in the direction of wherever human beings think they are going" (Rogers, 1987c).

EVALUATION OF ROGERS'S SCIENCE OF UNITARY HUMAN BEINGS

This section presents an evaluation of Rogers's Science of Unitary Human Beings. The evaluation is based on the results of the analysis as well as publications by others who have used or commented on Rogers's conceptual model.

Explication of Assumptions

Rogers explicitly identified the assumptions upon which her conceptual system is based. These assumptions indicate that Rogers views nursing as a legitimate science and an art that must base its practice on a body of knowledge that has been validated by empirical research.

The assumptions also indicate that Rogers values a unitary view of the person and the environment. Rogers pointed out that this perspective of the person identifies nursing as a unique discipline.

Rogers emphasized her view that health is socially defined. This suggests that she expects specific goals for nursing intervention to be based on the values of society, not those of the nurse alone. Moreover, Rogers's discussion of nursing intervention indicates that she values individualized care for each person. In fact, individualized care is mandated by this conceptual system due to the uniqueness of each human energy field.

Comprehensiveness of Concepts and Propositions

Rogers defined and described the four metaparadigm concepts—person, environment, health, nursing—sufficiently for a conceptual model. Person and environment were clearly defined, and the relationship between unitary human beings and their environments was explicitly identified. Health was defined through its relation to the life process, and determination of wellness and illness was considered a social value.

Furthermore, nursing was defined and emphasis was placed on its characteristics as a noun. The goal of nursing was clearly delineated. However, a particular nursing process was not presented in Rogers's recent publications. Despite the lack of an explicit nursing process, Rogers's view of nursing may be discussed in relation to Walker and Nicholson's (1980) criteria. Rogers repeatedly emphasized that nursing is an empirical science, such that any and all judgments must be based on scientific knowledge. The dynamic nature of nursing is evident in the following statement:

> The dynamic nature of life signifies continuous revision of the nature and meaning of diagnostic data and concomitant revision of interventional measures. (Rogers, 1970, p. 125)

Rogers intended that her conceptual system would be applicable to all nursing situations. Although conclusive evidence supporting achievement of this aim is not yet available, this conceptual system has been used to guide many nursing activities, several of which are described in the section on social utility.

Rogers's view of nursing is compatible with ethical standards for nursing practice and is consistent with scientific findings. This is evident in Rogers's insistence that nursing actions stem from an organized and valid knowledge base. This point is underscored by the following comment:

> The education of nurses has identity in the transmission of nursing's body of theoretical knowledge. The practice of nursing is the creative use of this knowledge for human betterment. (Rogers, 1986, p. 4)

Rogers clearly linked the metaparadigm concepts person and environment and also linked these concepts with nursing. However, the linkage between all four metaparadigm concepts had to be constructed from a series of statements.

Logical Congruence

World Views

Rogers's Science of Unitary Human Beings reflects an organismic view of the world. This conceptual system clearly reflects a holistic view of the person and environment. In fact, although Rogers (1986) noted that human and environmental energy fields manifest "characteristics that are different from those of the parts and cannot be predicted from knowledge of the parts" (p. 5), she never identified any parts. Rather, Rogers conceptualized the person and the environment as irreducible wholes. This emphasis on holism and expansionism is documented in the following statement:

> Human and environmental fields are not biological fields or physical fields, or social or psychological fields. Neither are human and environmental fields a summation of biological, physical, social, and psychological fields. (Rogers, 1986, pp. 4–5)

Although Rogers's conceptual system reflects a holistic view of the world, she does not use the term holistic because of its ambiguous and varied meanings. She pointed out, "The use of the term *unitary* human beings is not to be confused with current popular usage of the term *holistic*, generally signifying a summation of parts, whether few or many" (Rogers, 1986, p. 4).

This conceptual system views the person as an active organism that is integral with its environment. Rogers (1986) stated, "People's capacity to participate knowingly in the process of change is postulated" (p. 4). Moreover, Rogers viewed change as qualitative. She emphasized the continuous changes in human environmental energy field pattern and pointed out that these changes are relative and innovative.

There is no evidence of a mechanistic view of the world in this conceptual system. Rogers (1970) explicitly rejected the mechanistic tenet of reductionism, with its focus on parts, stating, "Reductionism, representative of an atomistic world view in which complex things are built up of simple elements, is contrary to a perception of wholeness" (p. 87). She also stated that her conceptual system "is humanistic, not mechanistic. Moreover, this is an optimistic model though not a utopian one" (Rogers, 1987d, p. 141). She also explicitly rejected mechanistic causality, stating, "In a universe of open systems, causality is not an option. Acausality had come in with quantum theory. . . . Causality is invalid" (Rogers, 1986, p. 5). Furthermore, Rogers rejected the mechanistic view of the person as reacting to environmental stimuli, as can be seen in the following comment:

> The all-too-common perception of man predominantly subjected to multiple negative environmental influences with pathological outcomes denies man's unity with nature and his evolutionary becoming. (Rogers, 1970, p. 85)

Parse (1987b) claimed that Rogers's work reflects the simultaneity paradigm. Rogers (1985b), however, stated that her work does not fit into either the totality or the simultaneity paradigm. Indeed, she claimed that the "Science of Unitary Human Beings . . . requires a new world view" (Rogers, 1986, p. 3).

Rogers's conceptual system clearly and explicitly reflects a change world view. She repeatedly referred to continuous change in human and environmental field patterns. She viewed change as natural and desirable, always in the direction of increasing diversity. Thus, the person is always progressing, always reaching toward his or her potential. This interpretation of the model is supported by the following quotation: "The nature of the pattern changes continuously. . . . Change is continuous, relative, and innovative. Increasing diversity of field patterning characterizes the process of change" (Rogers, 1986, pp. 5–6).

Classification of the Model

Careful review of the content of Rogers's conceptual system indicated that it reflects characteristics of both systems and developmental models. The basic characteristic of systems model, integration of parts, was addressed in Rogers's (1986) statement that the unitary human beings and their environments are irreducible energy fields that manifest "characteristics that are different from those of the parts and cannot be predicted from knowledge of the parts" (p. 5). The characteristic, system, was addressed in the discussion of the human and environmental energy fields as open systems. Rogers (1986) pointed out that from her perspective, this means that the systems are always open—"not a little bit or sometimes, but continuously" (p. 5). The characteristic, environment, was addressed explicitly and was defined as a four-dimensional energy field that is integral with the human four-dimensional energy field (Rogers, 1986).

Boundary was not addressed explicitly in the most recent version of Rogers's conceptual system. The lack of boundaries is implied in Rogers's (1986) statement that the "human and environmental fields are infinite and integral with one another" (p. 5). The characteristic of tension, stress, strain, and conflict also was not addressed in this conceptual system. Rogers clearly rejected the idea that any external force impinges on the human field. Rather, the human and environmental fields are integral.

Rogers (1986) regarded the characteristics of equilibrium and steady state as obsolete. Instead, she presented an innovative view of the relationship between human beings and their environments that goes beyond general system thinking. For Rogers, there is no fixed equilibrium point or even a dynamic equilibrium nor is there any feedback process of input and output. Rather, the principle of integrality postulates that the human and environmental energy fields engage in continuous mutual process.

Although Rogers addressed the characteristics of systems models, she placed major emphasis on human development in the form of changes in human field pattern. Rogers (cited in Malinski, 1986b), however, no longer uses the term human development "because development implies certain kinds of linearity" (p. 11).

The developmental model characteristics of growth, development, and maturation; change; and direction of change are addressed by the principles of helicy and resonancy. These principles postulate that field pattern is characterized by continuous change that is innovative, probabilistic, and increasing in diversity. The direction of change is always toward increasing diversity, from lower frequency to higher frequency wave patterns (Rogers, 1986).

Identifiable state is addressed by the concept of pattern. According to Rogers (1986), "pattern is the distinguishing characteristic of an energy field . . . it gives identity to the field" (p. 5).

The form of progression most clearly reflected by Rogers's conceptual system is the differentiated type. The principle of helicy postulates that human and environmental field patterns increase in diversity and are characterized by nonrepeating rhythmicities. Although the term helicy might imply a spiral, Chin's (1980) definition of this form as returning to former problems, but dealing with them at a higher level, is at odds with Rogers's (1980a) contention that "there is no going back, no repetition" (p. 333).

The developmental model characteristic of forces is not addressed. In fact, such an idea is rejected by Rogers. Rather, she posits that the nature of the energy field is to evolve. No special forces are required for this. Thus, the potentiality for development is overt.

There is no evidence of logical incompatibility in Rogers's conceptual system. The distinctive view of the person and the environment is carried through all components of the model. Characteristics of systems and developmental models are addressed in a logically congruent manner.

Meleis (1985) placed Rogers's work within the outcomes category of her classification scheme. Marriner (1986) placed Rogers's work in the energy fields category. Stevens (1984) regarded Rogers's work as an example of her enhancement category. No rationales were given by any of these authors for their categorizations of Rogers's conceptual system.

Generation and Testing of Theory

Rogers (1980a) has derived three rudimentary theories from her conceptual system. The theory of accelerating evolution posits that evolutionary change is speeding up and that the range of diversity of life processes is widening. More specifically, this theory postulates that change proceeds "in the direction of higher wave frequency field pattern . . . characterized by growing diversity" (p. 334). "Higher frequency wave patterns of growing diversity," Rogers (1986) explained, "portend new norms coordinate with accelerating change" (p. 6). An example of new norms offered by Rogers is the change in developmental norms. The theory provides an explanation for hyperactivity in children, regarding this manifestation of pattern as accelerating evolution of the human energy field (Rogers, 1986).

Rogers's theory of paranormal phenomena focuses on explanations for precognition, déjà vu, clairvoyance, and telepathy. Rogers (1980a) pointed out that "within this conceptual system such behaviors become 'normal' rather than 'paranormal' " (p. 335). This is because in a four-dimensional world, there is no linear time nor any separation of human and environmental fields, so the present is relative to the person. This theory also provides an explanation for the efficacy of noninvasive therapies, such as therapeutic touch, meditation, and imagery (Rogers, 1986).

The theory of rhythmical correlates of change focuses on human and environmental field rhythms, which "are not to be confused with biologic rhythms or psychologic rhythms or similar particulate phenomena" (Rogers, 1980a, p. 335). This theory deals with manifestations of field pattern such as changes in human sleep/wake patterns, indices of human field motion, perception of time passing, and other rhythmical developmental processes.

Correlates of patterning in unitary human beings were given by Malinski (1986b). The correlates "emerge out of the human-environmental field mutual process" (p. 10). The list of correlates presented by Malinski is given in Table 8–1.

Rogers (1980a, 1986) cited several examples of changes in human life that she claimed as support for her theories. For example, she noted that Toffler's (1970, 1980) work provides evidence of the increasing rate of change in many aspects of life. She also noted that sleep/wake patterns are changing, such that people of all ages sleep less now. More definitive empirical evidence supporting her theory of rhythmic correlates comes from work by Johnston, Fitzpatrick, and Donovan (1982), who found that developmental stage is related to past and future time orientation.

Other theories have been derived from Rogers's conceptual system. Newman (1979, 1986) has constructed a grand theory of health from the concepts of movement, space, time, and consciousness. The propositions interrelating these concepts are:

1. Time and space have a complementary relationship.
2. Movement is a means whereby space and time become a reality.
3. Movement is a reflection of consciousness.
4. Time is a function of movement.
5. Time is a measure of consciousness. (Newman, 1979, p. 60)

**TABLE 8–1.   Postulated Correlates of Patterning
in Unitary Human Beings**

Lower frequency	Higher frequency	Seem continuous
Longer rhythms	Shorter rhythms	Seem continuous
Slower motion	Faster motion	Seem continuous
Time drags	Time races	Timelessness
Sleeping	Waking	Beyond waking
Less diverse	More diverse	
Pragmatic	Imaginative	Visionary

From Malinski, V.M. (1986b). Further ideas from Martha Rogers, In V.M. Malinski (Ed.), Explorations on Martha Rogers' Science of Unitary Human Beings (p. 9). Norwalk, CT: Appleton-Century-Crofts, with permission.

Newman (1972b, 1976, 1982), Newman and Gaudiano (1984), Engle (1984), and Marchione (1986) have conducted research related to Newman's theory of health. The findings of these studies provide some support for the theory. Silva (1987), however, noted that instruments used in some of these studies lacked validity or reliability data and that statistically significant correlation coefficients were not high.

Parse (1981) has formulated a grand theory, called Man-Living-Health, that "synthesizes Martha E. Rogers's principles and concepts about man with major tenets and concepts from existential-phenomenological thought" (p. 4). In particular, Parse based her theory on Rogers's principles of helicy, complementarity (now integrality), and resonancy; and her concepts of energy field, openness, pattern and organization, and four-dimensionality; as well as on the existential phenomenological tenets of human subjectivity and intentionality and the concepts of coconstitution, coexistence, and situated freedom. The three major propositions of this theory are:

> Structuring meaning multidimensionally is cocreating reality through the languaging of valuing and imaging.
> Cocreating rhythmical patterns of relating is living the paradoxical unity of revealing-concealing and enabling-limiting while connecting-separating.
> Cotranscending with the possibles is powering unique ways of originating in the process of transforming. (Parse, 1981, p. 41)

Parse (1987a) stated that her theory has been supported by the findings of five studies. One phenomenological study focused on subjects' descriptions of situations in which they experienced health. Another phenomenological study dealt with persisting in change in terms of subjects' reordering of interrelationships with others when beginning new projects. An exploratory study focused on firefighters' lived experiences of being exposed to toxic chemicals. An ethnographic study dealt with aging and a case study, with retirement.

Fitzpatrick (1983) derived her life perspective rhythm model from Rogers's conceptual system and from the findings of research by Fitzpatrick (1980), Fitzpatrick and Donovan (1978), and Fitzpatrick, Donovan and Johnston (1980). The life perspective rhythm model, according to Fitzpatrick (1983),

> is a developmental model which proposes that the process of human development is characterized by rhythms. Human development occurs within the context of continuous person/environment interaction. Basic human rhythms that describe the development of persons include the identified indices of holistic human functioning, i.e., temporal patterns, motion patterns, consciousness patterns, and perceptual patterns. The rhythmic correlates developed by Rogers are consistent with this life perspective rhythm model. (p. 300)

Research that is explicitly derived from the life perspective rhythm model now is needed to determine its credibility.

Research based on Rogers's conceptual system has yielded mixed evidence for the principles of homeodynamics. Ference (1980) derived the concept of human field motion from Rogers's conceptual system. Her research findings provide some support for the principle of resonancy but called the principle of helicy into question. Barrett (1986) derived a theory of power from Rogers's principle of helicy. Her findings of the relationship between power and human field motion lend support to the principle of helicy.

Several other studies have been based on Rogers's conceptual system, but have used theories borrowed from other disciplines to guide development of hypotheses. These investigations, which are discussed in the section on social utility, provide mixed evidence for the credibility of the principles of Rogers's conceptual system. Obviously, much more research needs to be conducted before definitive conclusions regarding the credibility of Rogers's principles and theories may be drawn.

Social Considerations

Social Congruence

Rogers's emphasis on nursing care directed to all people, wherever they are, may exceed the expectations of some consumers of health care and some nurses. Furthermore, her emphasis on maintenance and promotion of health may not be congruent with some consumers' expectations. However, as more consumers recognize the value and cost effectiveness of wellness care, the nursing activities guided by this conceptual system should be more fully accepted and even anticipated.

The science of nursing depicted by Rogers's conceptual system is not congruent with some nurses' perspectives of nursing science. Moreover, Rogers's acceptance of nontraditional, noninvasive intervention modalities, such as therapeutic touch, is not congruent with many health care professionals' expectations of health care. The Science of Unitary Human Beings reflects a view of the world of people and their environments that requires a new way of thinking that not all people are willing or interested in undertaking.

Advocates of this conceptual system, of course, find it congruent with their views of nursing. For example, Blair (1979) commented, "Nursing science as conceptualized by Rogers provides a sound basis for achieving the goal of nursing—to serve man throughout the life process" (p. 302).

Social Significance

Rogers (1987a) maintained that the purpose of nursing is "to help all people achieve maximum well-being within their potential" (p. 121). Whelton (1979) speculated that use of Rogers's conceptual system could make differences in clients' health status. She stated, "By entering into a scientifically based therapeutic relationship with the patient, the nurse can make the difference between the patient continuing a life of inadvertent self-destruction or reaching for his optimum health potential" (p. 19). And Miller (1979, p. 286) noted, "If Rogers' [conceptual system] is followed, then perhaps nursing approaches would take into account a wider range of behavorial variability among individuals" (p. 286). There is, however, no published empirical evidence to support the social significance of this conceptual system.

Social Utility

The social utility of Rogers's conceptual system is documented by its use as a guide for nursing research, practice, education, and administration. National Rogerian Conferences, sponsored by New York University Division of Nursing, the Division of Nursing Alumni Association, and Upsilon Chapter of Sigma Theta Tau, have been held in New York City every two to three years since 1983. Malinski's (1986a) *Explorations on Martha Rogers' Science of Unitary Human Beings* is the first and only book published to date that is devoted exclusively to reports of and issues related to research derived from Rogers's conceptual system. In fact, Malinski's book is the only one that deals so extensively with research derived from any conceptual model of nursing.

The utility of Rogers's conceptual system for nursing research is well documented. Rules for nursing research are being formulated. "Research in nursing," Rogers (1987a) stated, "is the study of unitary human beings and their environments" (p. 121). Rogers (1987a) also stated, "The future of research in nursing is based on a commitment to nursing as a science in its own right. The science of nursing is identified as the science of unitary human beings" (p. 123). These statements clearly identify the purpose of nursing research and the phenomena to be studied. Rogers (1987a) also has begun to specify research approaches that are consistent with her conceptual system, noting that both basic and applied research are needed to continue to develop nursing knowledge. Basic research, according to Rogers (1987a), "is directed toward an increase in knowledge in a given science" whereas applied research "investigates the practical application of knowledge already available" (p. 122). Rogers (1987a) rejected the label clinical research, stating,

> Applied research should replace the use of the phrase "clinical research." According to dictionaries the term clinical means "investigation of a disease in the living subject by observation as distinguished from controlled study," "something done at the bedside." These definitions are inappropriate and inadequate for the scope and purposes of nursing. (p.122)

Rogers (1987a, 1987b) supported the use of both qualitative and quantitative methods of empirical research as well as philosophical inquiry. She did, however, note that "there are incongruities and contradictions between holistic directions in nursing and the forms of inquiry used by nurses. . . . There is a critical need for new tools of measurement appropriate to new paradigms" (1987a, p. 122). Reeder (1986) maintained that Husserlian phenomenology is an appropriate approach to basic research derived from Rogers's conceptual system. Cowling (1986) noted that existentialism, ecological thinking, and dialectical thinking are appropriate modes of inquiry for studies based on Rogers's work, as are historical and philosophical inquiries, as well as methods that focus on the uniqueness of each person, such as imagery, direct questioning, personal structural analysis, and the Q-sort. He also noted that although descriptive and correlational designs are consistent with Rogers's conceptual system, strict experimental designs are of "questionable value," given the fact that "the unitary system is a noncausal model of reality" (p. 73). However, Cowling went on to say that quasi-experimental and experimental designs "may be appropriate to specific theoretical propositions because they provide a mechanism for testing probabilistic change manifested from human-environmental process" (p. 73). Fawcett and Downs (1986) maintained that longitudinal research designs are more appropriate than cross-sectional studies, given Rogers's emphasis on the uniqueness of energy field patterns.

Given Rogers's emphasis on nursing as a service to all people, wherever they may be, virtually any setting and any person would be appropriate for study, with the proviso that both person and environment are taken into account. Data analysis techniques must take the integrality of person and environment into account, as well as the emphasis on unitary human beings. This view, according to Fawcett and Downs (1986), "precludes the use of standard data analysis techniques that employ the components of variance model of statistics, for this statistical model is logically inconsistent with the assumption of holism stating that the whole is greater than the sum of parts" (p. 87). Cowling (1986) indicated that "multivariate analysis procedures, particularly canonical correlation, can be useful methods for generating a constellation of variables representing human field pattern properties" (p. 73). The emphasis of Rogerian thought on the integrality of human and environmental energy fields indicates that research conducted within the context of this conceptual system will enhance understanding of the continuous mutual process of person and environment and changes in energy field patterns.

Rogers's conceptual system has guided many studies. Ference (1986) traced the evolution of research that has been guided by Rogers's conceptual system. She noted that the early studies "were based upon some guiding assumptions and a philosophy that the nurse cares for the whole person" (p. 37). Her retrospective analysis of these studies yielded groupings of research. In the mid 1960s, studies focused on human development, such as Porter's (1967) work, and on man-environment interaction, exemplified by Mathwig's (1967) study. Research conducted from the late 1960s to the late 1970s focused on body image, exemplified by Chodil's (1978) and Fawcett's (1976) studies. Several studies completed in the early to mid-1970s focused on the variable of time, such as the research by Newman (1971) and Fitzpatrick (1975). Studies conducted during the early 1970s also focused on locus of control, field independence, and differentiation, exemplified by works by Barnard (1973), Miller (1974), and Swanson (1975). Ference (1986) pointed out that much of the early work only mentioned Rogers's work and used theories borrowed from other disciplines as a basis for hypotheses. Research conducted during the late 1970s and into the 1980s used Rogers's conceptual system in a more comprehensive manner, often identifying a particular principle of homeodynamics as the focus of study. This research focus is exemplified by the many doctoral dissertations identified by Silva and Sorrell (1987), including those by Barrett (1984), Branum (1986), Brouse (1984), Conner (1986), Cora (1986), Cowling (1984), Ference (1980), Floyd (1983a), Fry (1985), Gueldner (1983), Johnston (1981), Kutlenios (1986), Macrae (1983), Malinski (1981), McDonald (1981), Miller (1985), Moore (1982), Quillin (1984), Quinn (1982), Raile (1983), Rankin (1985), Rawnsley (1977), Reeder (1985), Sanchez (1987), Sarter (1987), and Yaros (1986). Other examples are Bilitski's (1986), Chandler's (1987), Dzurec's (1987), Ludomirski-Kalmanson's (1985), McCanse's (1988), McEvoy's (1988), and Smith's (1987) doctoral dissertations and Lindley's (1981) master's thesis. Most of these studies used theories borrowed from other disciplines to support hypotheses but explicitly linked the theories to elements of Rogers's conceptual system. Ference's and Barrett's investigations are noteworthy in that a purpose of each study was to develop and test an instrument that was based directly on Rogers's conceptual system. Ference's

Human Field Motion Test was designed to measure the person's perception of the frequency of energy field motion. Barrett's Power as Knowing Participation in Change Test was designed to measure the person's capacity to participate knowingly in change, that is, the person's awareness of what he or she is choosing to do, feeling free to do it, and doing it intentionally.

The studies by Barrett, Cowling, Ference, Gueldner, Malinski, McDonald, Alligood (nee Raile), and Rawnsley were published in Malinski's (1986a) book. It is noteworthy that each of these published reports was accompanied by one or two critiques of the research and responses by the investigators.

Several other reports of research based on Rogers's conceptual system have been published. Goldberg and Fitzpatrick's (1980) study of the effect of movement therapy on morale and self-esteem reflected Rogers's assumptions about human beings. Gill and Atwood (1981) studied the effects of epidermal growth factor on wound healing from the perspective of Rogers's homeodynamic principles. Floyd (1983b, 1984) derived her studies of sleep-wake cycles of rotating shift workers and of the interactions between individual circadian rhythms of sleep and wakefulness and the rest-activity schedule in a psychiatric hospital from Rogers's conceptual system. Quinn (1984) based her study of the effect of therapeutic touch on anxiety in a sample of cardiovascular patients on Rogers's conceptual system. Keller and Bzdek (1986) also used Rogers's conceptual system to guide their study of the effects of therapeutic touch on tension headache pain. Smith (1984, 1986) used the principle of integrality to guide her studies of the relationships between diverse environmental conditions, temporal experience, and perception of restfulness. Boyd (1985) analyzed the concept of mother-daughter identification within the context of Rogers's conceptual system. Brouse (1985) reformulated theories of socialization, life span development, self-concept, and gender role identity within Rogers's conceptual system to guide her longitudinal study of the relationship of gender role identity to femininity and self-concept during pregnancy and the postpartum. Laffrey (1985) based her study of the relationships of self-actualization, conception of health, and choices about health practices on Rogers's conceptual system and theoretical notions of self-actualization. Clarke (1986) derived her study of the relationships between perceived body size, conversational distance, body weight, and self-actualization directly from Rogers's conceptual system. Sarter's (1987, 1988) philosophical inquiry explored the congruence of Rogers's work with the notion of evolutionary idealism. The extension of Rogers's conceptual system to the family is evident in Fawcett's (in press) report of a program of research designed to examine similarities in wives and husbands' pregnancy-related experiences, including body image changes and physical and psychological symptoms.

Other published research reports have cited Rogers's work, but present no evidence that their studies were directly derived from this conceptual system. Lum and her associates (1978) used Rogers's (1970) definition of nursing in their study of the effects of nursing activities on outcomes for oncology patients receiving chemotherapy. Reed (1987) noted that her study of the relationship between spirituality and well-being in terminally ill persons is within the context of the concept of transcendence, which is an aspect of various models, including Rogers's. Tompkins (1980) referred to Rogers's work, as well as to other conceptual models, in her discussion of the study findings. And Smith (1983) noted that the view of family used in her study of family development when a teenage mother and her infant are incorporated into the household was consistent with Rogers's work.

The utility of Rogers's conceptual system for nursing practice is evident. Rogers has always maintained that nursing practice must be theory-based. She stated,

> Nursing practice must be flexible and creative, individualized and socially oriented, compassionate and skillful. Professional practitioners in nursing must be continuously translating theoretical knowledge into human service. . . . Nursing's conceptual system provides the foundation for nursing practice. (Rogers, 1970, p. 128)

She also stated, "For nurses to fulfill their social and professional responsibilities in the days ahead demands that their practice be based upon a substantive theoretical base specific to nursing. . . . The practice of nurses is the use of this knowledge in service to people" (Rogers, 1987a, pp. 121–122). Furthermore, Rogers (1980a) commented, "Broad principles to guide practice must replace rule-of-thumb" (p. 337).

Rules for nursing practice may be extracted from publications by Rogers and others who have studied her work. The purpose of nursing "is to help all people achieve maximum well-being within their potential, wherever they are" (Rogers, 1987a, p. 121). Clinical problems of interest are those conditions that nursing as a discipline and society as a whole identify as relevant for nursing. Furthermore, "disease conditions can no longer be considered as entities unto themselves but must be regarded as manifestations of the total pattern of the individual in interaction with the environment" (Newman, 1979, p. 21). Nursing may be practiced in any setting in which nurses encounter patients, and all people are legitimate recipients of nursing care. Nursing processes, according to Rogers (1970, 1980f, 1980fg), must focus on the person as a unified whole and care must be individualized.

Nursing assessment may extend beyond physical assessment to non-physical assessment of the human energy field, "using therapeutic touch to assess the rhythms and flow of energy. [Furthermore], because patterning is a dynamic process, assessments need to be performed on an ongoing basis in the context of field interactions" (Malinski, 1986c, p. 30). Nursing interventions include noninvasive modalities such as therapeutic touch, imagery, and meditation, as well as "wave modalities such as light, color, music, and movement" (Malinski, 1986c, p. 29). Nursing practice contributes to the maximum well-being of people. Moreover, nursing practice guided by the Science of Unitary Human Beings can assist both patient and nurse "to become aware of their own rhythms and to make choices among a range of options congruent with their perceptions of well-being" (Malinski, 1986c, p. 29). Nursing guided by this conceptual system also leads to acceptance of diversity as the norm and of the integral connectedness of human beings and their environments, as well as viewing change as positive (Malinski, 1986c).

Falco and Lobo's (1985) work provides further specification of the rule regarding nursing process. They suggested that nursing assessment, diagnosis, intervention, and evaluation be guided by the principles of integrality, resonancy, and helicy. Assessment in terms of the principle of helicy, for example, focuses on the rhythmic life patterns of the person and the environment, life goals, and the growing complexity of the human being.

Madrid and Winstead-Fry's (1986) work also provides further specification of the nursing process rule. They proposed that assessment encompasses six parameters derived from the correlates of patterning, including consideration of the person's (1) awareness of the relative present, (2) verbal and nonverbal communication, (3) sense of rhythm, (4) connection to the environment, (5) beliefs about self, and (6) sense of integrity as a unique system.

Rogers (1987a) maintained that "the practical implications [of the Science of Unitary Human Beings] for human health and well-being are already demonstrable" (p. 123). Indeed, the utility of Rogers's conceptual system for creative nursing care of people of various ages and with diverse medical conditions is documented in the literature. Blair (1979) and Rogers (1986) discussed care of the hyperactive child. Katch (1983) and Rogers (1986) discussed the utility of the conceptual system for nursing care of the aged. Rogers (1986) also discussed the utility of her conceptual system for nursing care of persons with hypertension and for the dying person. And Madrid and Winstead-Fry (1986) used their assessment format to determine the energy field pattern for a 35-year-old man with a cerebral aneurysm and then described the planning, intervention, and evaluation phases of the nursing process for this patient.

Levine (1976) derived a theoretical explanation of the experience of pregnancy and implications for practice from Rogers's conceptual system. She stated,

> Pregnancy illustrates how needs arising within the female's field cause an inner-directed, contracted field experience that persists and intensifies throughout the 9 months, diminishes severely during labor and delivery, and reexpands around lactation. Implications for family and health personnel during these stages are knowledge, acceptance, and support of the female. . . . It becomes important to minimize environmental factors that could present or arrest the female's field contraction and expansion at the various states of pregnancy. (p. 15)

Whelton (1979) combined Rogers's model with a nursing process format and knowledge from physiology, psychology, and sociology to outline nursing care plans for patients with decreased cardiac output and those with impaired neurological function. She then applied the resultant conceptual-theoretical system to the care of a non-compliant patient with decreased cardiac output and a history of diabetes and hypertension, and a patient with total disability due to recurrent meningioma.

Hanchett (1979) developed several assessment tools based on Rogers's model and general system theory. These tools were designed specifically for assessment of the energy, individuality, and pattern and organization of communities.

Krieger (1975) introduced the healing method of therapeutic touch into the nursing literature. Miller (1979) placed this intervention within the context of Rogers's conceptual system. She stated, "The . . . science of unitary man as formulated by Rogers, may be used to account for the phenomenon of the therapeutic touch in healing, a phenomenon that other theories have failed to explain" (p. 279). Miller went on to explain that therapeutic touch is an instance of mutual interaction between nurse and patient. Boguslawski (1979) noted that therapeutic touch is thought to involve a transfer of energy from nurse to patient, with resultant change in the energy field pattern.

Other publications have addressed the use of Rogers's conceptual system for the family. Whall (1981) constructed a logically congruent conceptual-theoretical system of nursing knowledge from Rogers's conceptual system, Fawcett's (1975) extension of Rogers's model to the family system, and theories of family functioning. She then developed a guide for assessment of families, organized according to individual sub-system considerations, interactional patterns, unique characteristics of the whole family system, and environmental interface synchrony. Rogers (1983a, 1983b) extended the conceptual system to the family system and presented a discussion of the use of the extension of her conceptual system in specific family situations. Johnston (1986) and Reed (1986) derived family therapy protocols from Rogers's work.

Further documentation of the utility of Rogers's conceptual system for nursing practice is anticipated. Rogers (personal communication, June 11, 1987) stated that a book describing the practice implications of her work is being prepared.

The utility of Rogers's conceptual system for nursing education is documented and rules for nursing education are evident in Rogers's publications. The focus of the curriculum and the purposes of nursing education are identified in the following quotations:

> The education of professional practitioners in nursing requires the transmission of a body of scientific knowledge specific to nursing. This body of knowledge determines the safety and scope of nursing practice. The imaginative and creative use of knowledge for the betterment of man finds expression in the art of nursing. Education opens the doorway to developing the art of practice. The purpose of professional education is to provide the knowledge and tools whereby an individual may become an artist in his field. (Rogers, 1970, p. 88)

> The education of nurses has identity in transmission of nursing's body of theoretical knowledge. (Rogers, 1987a, p. 121)

"The liberal arts and sciences including extraterrestrial matters," according to Rogers (1987a, p. 121), are part of the content of professional nursing education programs. Young (1985) indicated that the principles of resonancy, helicy, and integrality are the "major integrating concepts of the curriculum" (p. 60) and outlined a sequence of content at one school of nursing. Further specification of content is implied in Rogers's (1987a) discussion of the focus of baccalaureate, master's, and doctoral education. She explained,

> Baccalaureate degree graduates in nursing properly possess beginning tools of inquiry and are able to exploit knowledge for the improvement of practice. Master's degree graduates in nursing possess more sophisticated tools of study, identify more complex problems, and design and implement applied research. Basic research requires doctoral study in nursing with a high level of scholarly sophistication and the ability to push back frontiers of knowledge. (p. 122)

Rogers's discussion indicates that education for professional nursing occurs at the baccalaureate, master's, and doctoral levels. Thus, nursing education occurs in college and university settings and students are those who meet the requirements for matriculation in nursing programs in these settings. The rule dealing with teaching-learning strategies is not yet explicit.

Rogers (cited in Safier, 1977) commented, "I know that many schools are using my book (*An introduction to the theoretical basis of nursing*), and also that many students are being oriented to this sort of thinking" (p. 328). Riehl's (1980) finding that Rogers's model was "being taught, practiced by students, and implemented by faculty" (p. 398) provided empirical evidence to support that statement. Riehl did not, however, provide the names of schools using Rogers's conceptual system.

More specific evidence of the use of Rogers's conceptual system as a curriculum guide is available. This conceptual system has been used to guide the development of the curriculum for the baccalaureate, master's, and doctoral programs at New York University Division of Nursing in New York City. Rogers (1978b) outlined the sequence of nursing courses in the baccalaureate program, which is structured according to stages of human development in a chronological fashion starting with the neonate. Young (1985) presented a detailed discussion of use of Rogers's conceptual system at Washburn University School of Nursing in Topeka, Kansas. This conceptual system also has been used to develop nursing curricula at Duquesne University in Pittsburgh, Pennsylvania; the College of Mount St. Vincent in Riverdale, New York; Fairleigh Dickinson University in Rutherford, New Jersey; Troy State University in Troy, Alabama; Olivet Nazarene College in Kankakee, Illinois; Bethany Nazarene College in Bethany, Oklahoma; Messiah College in Grantham, Pennsylvania; East Stroudsburg University in East Stroudsburg, Pennsylvania; and the University of Tennessee in Knoxville (Asay & Ossler, 1984; Winstead-Fry, cited in Meleis, 1985).

The utility of Rogers's conceptual system for nursing administration is beginning to be documented. Rules for nursing administration are not yet explicit, although implications are evident in Alligood's (in press) and Gueldner's (in press) applications of Rogers's conceptual system to nursing administration. Nursing practice at the Veterans Administration Hospital in San Diego, California, is being guided by Rogers's conceptual system. Other clinical agencies have expressed an interest in this conceptual system. Implications for use of the model by clinical agencies are evident. For example, the goal of nursing put forth in the conceptual system suggests standards for nursing care that could be used to develop quality assurance programs. Furthermore, Falco and Lobo's (1985) and Madrid and Winstead-Fry's (1986) nursing process formats could be used to develop nursing care plans for patients with various health problems.

Contributions to Nursing Knowledge

Rogers was one of the first nurse scholars to explicitly identify the person as the central phenomenon of nursing's concern. Summarizing the significance of this contribution to nursing knowledge, Newman (1972a) stated:

> Much of the confusion about what we should be studying was eliminated, in my opinion, when Rogers identified the phenomenon which is the center of nursing's purpose: MAN. . . . The clear-cut delineation of man as the focus of nursing gave direction for the development of theory that is not just relevant to nursing, but basic to nursing. (pp. 451–452)

Although other conceptual models consider the person in a holistic manner, Rogers's view of the person as a unitary human being is distinctive in that no parts or components or subsystems of the person are delineated—the person is a unified whole. Furthermore, although other conceptual models consider the environment and its relationship with the person, Rogers's view of person and environment as integral energy fields is unique and visionary.

Commenting on the contributions of her model, Rogers (cited in Safier, 1977) stated:

> The conceptual system . . . provides for a substantive body of knowledge in nursing that will have relevance for all workers concerned with people, but with special relevance for nurses, not because it matters to nurses per se, but because it matters to human beings, and consequently to nurses. (p. 320)

Moreover, Rogers (1986) pointed out that "the Science of Unitary Human Beings identifies nursing's uniqueness and signifies the potential of nurses to fulfill their social responsibility in human service" (p. 8).

Whall (1987) noted that Rogers's conceptual system has advanced the discipline of nursing through the many debates it has sparked. She pointed out that this conceptual system

> has generated lively debates and seems to have raised more questions than it answers. It has explained disparate views while engendering debate regarding techniques that may be used to measure concepts and relationships. The debates engendered by her model have in a sense forced nursing to move on. In a sense, it forced nurse scholars to question and seek answers again and again. If this . . . is in essence the value of a [conceptual system], Rogers's framework will stand as a milestone. (p. 158)

Rogers's conception of the person as a unitary human being and the presentation of her conceptual system in just four concepts and three principles might be considered elegant in its simplicity, yet as Newman (1972) noted, "many a graduate student will attest to the difficulty of reorganizing one's thinking about [the person] in order to consider [him or her] a unified being and not as a composite of organs and systems and various psychosocial components." Although the same thing might be said about any conceptual model that puts forth a holistic view of the person, some nurses seem to find it especially so for Rogers's model. Perhaps this is due to the fact that viewing the world from the perspective of the Science of Unitary Human Beings "requires a new synthesis, a creative leap and inculcation of new attitudes and values" (Rogers, 1987c, p. 146). Or it may be due to the fact that Rogers's conceptual system is made up of terms and ideas that are unfamiliar to some people. But Rogers (1970, 1978a, 1980b, 1986) has repeatedly defended her terminology, pointing out that she selected terms that are in the general language and initially defined these terms according to the dictionary. As the model evolved, Rogers recognized the need for more specific definitions to facilitate uniformity of usage and precision. She noted that this procedure is common in all sciences. Nevertheless, use of this model must be preceded by mastery of a vocabulary that may be new to many nurses. This task can be aided by use of the glossary of terms that was published in Malinski's (1986a) book, *Explorations on Martha Rogers' Science of Unitary Human Beings*.

Rogers, along with most other authors of nursing models, has continued to refine her conceptual system. Speaking to the need for continued evolution of her model, Rogers (1970) stated:

> The emergence of a science of nursing demands a clear, unequivocal conceptual frame of reference. This is not to propose that nursing's conceptual system is either static or inflexible. Quite the contrary. In its evolution it is properly subject to reformulation and change as empirical knowledge grows, as conceptual data achieve greater clarity, and as the interconnectedness between ideas takes on new dimensions. (p. 84)

Certainly the many revisions and refinements in what is now called the Science of Unitary Human Beings attest to Rogers's concern for precision in language as well as her desire to advance the discipline of nursing through development of a unique and substantive body of knowledge. Commenting on her concern and desire, Rogers (1987a) noted:

> The future of nursing is based on a commitment to nursing as a science in its own right. The science of nursing is identified as the science of unitary human beings. The research potentials of nursing's abstract system are multiple. It is logically and scientifically tenable, it is flexible and open-ended. The practice implications for human health and well-being are already demonstrable. (p. 123)

Rogers (1987c) has pointed out that her perspective of nursing is humanistic and optimistic but not utopian. Rogers's humanistic and scholarly approach to nursing has been cited as "a model for emulation" by Hugh R. K. Barber (1987, p. 12), a physician. He pointed out that "the new orientation of the nursing profession is achieving in a more sophisticated manner what physicians have been striving to achieve. However, while nursing is drawing closer to this goal, physicians seem to be slowly moving in the opposite direction" (p. 15).

Rogers's conceptual system has been adopted enthusiastically by some nurses. In fact, for many of its adherents, Rogers's conceptual system and its related theories and research comprise THE nursing science. Conversely, this conceptual system "will not be accepted if a nurse cannot perceive [energy] fields and resonating waves as the 'real world' of nursing" (Stevens, 1984, p. 36).

The utility of Rogers's conceptual system as a guide for nursing theory development and research is well documented, it has documented utility for education and practice, and its utility for nursing service administration is beginning to be documented. Potential users of the conceptual system are urged to consider its strengths and its limitations and work to systematically evaluate its credibility as a guide for the plethora of nursing activities for which it was developed.

REFERENCES

Alligood, M.R. (in press). Applying Rogers' model to nursing administration: Emphasis on environment, health. In B. Henry, M. DiVincenti, C. Arndt, & A. Marriner (Eds.), Dimensions of nursing administration. Theory, research, education, and practice. Boston: Blackwell Scientific Publications.

Asay, M.K., & Ossler, C.C. (Eds.). (1984). Conceptual models of nursing. Applications in community health nursing. Proceedings of the Eighth Annual Community Health Nursing Conference. Chapel Hill: Department of Public Health Nursing, School of Public Health, University of North Carolina.

Barber, H.R.K. (1987). Editorial: Trends in nursing: A model for emulation. The Female Patient, 12(3), 12, 14.

Barnard, R. (1973). Field independence-dependence and selected motor abilities. Unpublished doctoral dissertation, New York University.

Barrett, E.A.M. (1984). An empirical investigation of Martha E. Rogers' principle of helicy: The relationship of human field motion and power. Dissertation Abstracts International, 45, 615A.

Barrett, E.A.M. (1986). Investigation of the principle of helicy: The relationship of human field motion and power. In V.M. Malinski (Ed.), Explorations on Martha Rogers' Science of Unitary Human Beings (pp. 173–188). Norwalk, CT: Appleton-Century-Crofts.

Bertalanffy, L. (1960). Problems of life. New York: Harper Torchbooks.

Bilitski, J.S. (1986). Assessment of adult day care program and client health characteristics in U.S. Region III. Dissertation Abstracts International, 46, 3460A.

Blair, C. (1979). Hyperactivity in children: Viewed within the framework of synergistic man. Nursing Forum. 18, 293–303.

Boguslawski, M. (1979). The use of therapeutic touch in nursing. Journal of Continuing Education in Nursing, 10(4), 9–15.

Boyd, C. (1985). Toward an understanding of mother-daughter identification using concept analysis. Advances in Nursing Science, 7(3), 78–86.

Branum, Q.K. (1986). Power as knowing participation in change. A model for nursing intervention. Dissertation Abstracts International, 46, 3780B.

Brouse, S.H. (1984). Patterns of feminine and self concept scores of pregnant women from the third trimester to six weeks postpartum. Dissertation Abstracts International, 45, 827B.

Brouse, S.H. (1985). Effect of gender role identity on patterns of feminine and self-concept scores from late pregnancy to early postpartum. Advances in Nursing Science, 7(3), 32–48.

Burr, H.S., & Northrop, F.S.C. (1935). The electro-dynamic theory of life. Quarterly Review of Biology, 10, 322–333.

Chandler, G.E. (1987). The relationship of nursing work environment to empowerment and powerlessness. Dissertation Abstracts International, 47, 4822B.

Chardin, T. (1961). The phenomenon of man. New York: Harper Torchbooks.

Chin, R. (1980). The utility of systems models and developmental models for practitioners. In J.P. Riehl & C. Roy, Conceptual models for nursing practice (2nd ed., pp. 21–37). New York: Appleton-Century-Crofts.

Chodil, J. (1978). An investigation of the relation between perceived body space, actual body space, body image boundary, and self-esteem. Unpublished doctoral dissertation, New York University.

Clarke, P.N. (1986). Theoretical and measurement issues in the study of field phenomena. Advances in Nursing Science, 9(1), 29–39.

Conner, G.K. (1986). The manifestations of human field motion, creativity, and time experience patterns of female and male parents. Dissertation Abstracts International, 47, 1926B.

Cora, V.L. (1986). Family life process of intergenerational families with functionally dependent elders. Dissertation Abstracts International, 47, 568B.

Cowling, W.R., III. (1984). The relationship of mystical experience, differentiation, and creativity in college students: An empirical investigation of the principle of helicy in Rogers' Science of Unitary Man. Dissertation Abstracts International, 45, 458A.

Cowling, W.R., III. (1986). The Science of Unitary Human Beings: Theoretical issues, methodological challenges, and research realities. In V.M. Malinski (Ed.), Explorations on Martha Rogers' Science of Unitary Human Beings (pp. 65–77). Norwalk, CT: Appleton-Century-Crofts.

Dzurec, L.C. (1987). The nature of power experienced by individuals manifesting patterning labeled schizophrenic: An investigation of the principle of helicy. Dissertation Abstracts International, 47, 4467B.

Einstein, A. (1961). Relativity. New York: Crown.

Engle, V.F. (1984). Newman's conceptual framework and the measurement of older adults' health. Advances in Nursing Science, 7(1), 24–36.

Falco, S.M., & Lobo, M.L. (1985). Martha E. Rogers. In Nursing Theories Conference Group, Nursing theories. The base for professional nursing practice (2nd ed., pp. 214–234). Englewood Cliffs, NJ: Prentice-Hall.

Fawcett, J. (1975). The family as a living open system: An emerging conceptual framework for nursing. International Nursing Review, 22, 113–116.

Fawcett, J. (1976). The relationship between spouses' strength of identification and their patterns of change in perceived body space and articulation of body concept during and after pregnancy. Unpublished doctoral dissertation, New York University.

Fawcett, J. (1984). Analysis and evaluation of conceptual models of nursing. Philadelphia: FA Davis.

Fawcett, J. (in press). Spouses' experiences during pregnancy and the postpartum: A program of research and theory development. Applied Nursing Research.

Fawcett, J., & Downs, F.S. (1986). The relationship of theory and research. Norwalk, CT: Appleton-Century-Crofts.

Ference, H.M. (1980). The relationship of time experience, creativity traits, differentiation and human field motion. An empirical investigation of Rogers' correlates of synergistic human development. Dissertation Abstracts International, 40, 5206B.

Ference, H.M. (1986). Foundations of a nursing science and its evolution: A perspective. In V.M. Malinski (Ed.), Explorations on Martha Rogers' Science of Unitary Human Beings (pp. 25–32). Norwalk, CT: Appleton-Century-Crofts.

Fitzpatrick, J.J. (1975). An investigation of the relationship between temporal orientation, temporal extension, and time perception. Unpublished doctoral dissertation, New York University.

Fitzpatrick, J.J. (1980). Patients' perceptions of time: Current research. International Nursing Review, 27, 148–153, 160.

Fitzpatrick, J.J. (1983). Life perspective rhythm model. In J.J. Fitzpatrick & A.L. Whall, Conceptual models of nursing: Analysis and evaluation (pp. 295–302). Bowie, MD: Brady.

Fitzpatrick, J.J., & Donovan, M.J. (1978). Temporal experience and motor behavior among the aging. Research in Nursing and Health, 1, 60–68.

Fitzpatrick, J.J., Donovan, M.J., & Johnston, R.L. (1980). Experience of time during the crisis of cancer. Cancer Nursing, 3, 191–194.

Floyd, J.A. (1983a). Hospitalization, sleep-wake patterns, and circadian type of psychiatric patients. Dissertation Abstracts International, 43, 3535B–3536B.

Floyd, J.A. (1983b). Research using Rogers' conceptual system: Development of a testable theorem. Advances in Nursing Science, 5(2), 37–48.

Floyd, J.A. (1984). Interaction between personal sleep-wake rhythms and psychiatric hospital rest-activity schedule. Nursing Research, 33, 255–259.

Fry, J.E. (1985). Reciprocity in mother-child interaction, correlates of attachment, and family environment in three-year-old children with congenital heart disease. Dissertation Abstracts International, 46, 113B.

Gill, B.P., & Atwood, J.R. (1981). Reciprocy and helicy used to relate mEGF and wound healing. Nursing Research, 30, 68–72.

Goldberg, W.G., & Fitzpatrick, J.J. (1980). Movement therapy with the aged. Nursing Research, 29, 339–346.

Goldstein, K. (1939). The organism. New York: American Book Company.

Gueldner, S.H. (1983). A study of the relationship between imposed motion and human field motion in elderly individuals living in nursing homes. Dissertation Abstracts International, 44, 1411B.

Gueldner, S.H. (in press). Applying Rogers' model to nursing administration: Emphasis on client and nursing. In B. Henry, M. DiVincenti, C. Arndt, & A. Marriner (Eds.), Dimensions of nursing administration. Theory, research, education, and practice. Boston: Blackwell Scientific Publications.

Hanchett, E.S. (1979). Community health assessment: A conceptual tool kit. New York: John Wiley & Sons.

Herrick, J. (1956). The evolution of human nature. Austin: University of Texas Press.

Johnston, R.L. (1981). Temporality as a measure of unidirectionality with the Rogerian conceptual framework of nursing science. Dissertation Abstracts International, 41, 3740B.

Johnston, R.L. (1986). Approaching family intervention through Rogers' conceptual model. In A.L. Whall, Family therapy theory for nursing. Four approaches (pp. 11–32). Norwalk, CT: Appleton-Century-Crofts.

Johnston, R.L., Fitzpatrick, J.J., & Donovan, M.J. (1982). Developmental stage: Relationship to temporal dimensions. (Abstract). Nursing Research, 31, 120.

Katch, M.P. (1983). A negentropic view of the aged. Journal of Gerontological Nursing, 9, 656–660.

Keller, E., & Bzdek, V.M. (1986). Effects of therapeutic touch on tension headache pain. Nursing Research, 35, 101–106.

Krieger, D. (1975). Therapeutic touch: The imprimatur of nursing. American Journal of Nursing, 75, 784–787.

Kutlenios, R.M. (1986). A comparison of holistic, mental and physical health nursing interventions with the elderly. Dissertation Abstracts International, 47, 995B.

Laffrey, S.C. (1985). Health behavior choice as related to self-actualization and health conception. Western Journal of Nursing Research, 7, 279–295.

Levine, N.H. (1976). A conceptual model for obstetric nursing. Journal of Obstetric, Gynecologic, and Neonatal Nursing, 5(2), 9–15.

Lewin, K. (1964). Field theory in the social sciences. (D. Cartwright, Ed.) New York: Harper Torchbooks.

Lindley, P.A. (1981). An empirical study of the relationship of sensation seeking to the human energy field motion within Rogers' Science of Unitary Human Beings. Unpublished master's thesis, University of Rochester.

Ludomirski-Kalmanson, B. (1985). The relationship between the environmental energy wave frequency pattern manifest in red light and blue light and human field motion in adult individuals with visual sensory perception and those with total blindness. Dissertation Abstracts International, 45, 2094B.

Lum, J.J., Chase, M., Cole, S.M., Johnson, A., Johnson, J.A., & Link, M.R. (1978). Nursing care of oncology patients receiving chemotherapy. Nursing Research, 27, 340–346.

Macrae, J.A. (1983). A comparison between meditating subjects and non-meditating subjects on time experience and human field motion. Dissertation Abstracts International, 43, 3537B.

Madrid, M., & Winstead-Fry, P. (1986). Rogers's conceptual model. In P. Winstead-Fry (Ed.), Case studies in nursing theory (pp. 73–102). New York: National League for Nursing.

Malinski, V.M. (1981). The relationship between hyperactivity in children and perception of short wavelength light: An investigation into the conceptual system proposed by Dr. Martha E. Rogers. Dissertation Abstracts International, 41, 4459B.

Malinski, V.M. (Ed.). (1986a). Explorations on Martha Rogers' Science of Unitary Human Beings. Norwalk, CT: Appleton-Century-Crofts.

Malinski, V.M. (1986b). Further ideas from Martha Rogers. In V.M. Malinski (Ed.), Explorations on Martha Rogers' Science of Unitary Human Beings (pp. 9–14). Norwalk, CT: Appleton-Century-Crofts.

Malinski, V.M. (1986c). Nursing practice with the Science of Unitary Human Beings. In V.M. Malinski (Ed.), Explorations on Martha Rogers' Science of Unitary Human Beings (pp. 25–32). Norwalk, CT: Appleton-Century-Crofts.

Marchione, J.M. (1986). Pattern as methodology for assessing family health: Newman's theory of health. In P. Winstead-Fry (Ed.), Case studies in nursing theory (pp. 215–240). New York: National League for Nursing.

Marriner, A. (1986). Nursing theorists and their work. St. Louis: CV Mosby.

Mathwig, G. (1967). Living open systems, reciprocal adaptations and the life process. Unpublished doctoral dissertation, New York University.

McCanse, R.L. (1988). Healthy death readiness: Development of a measurement instrument. Dissertation Abstracts International, 48, 2606B.

McDonald, S.F. (1981). A study of the relationship between visible lightwaves and the experience of pain. Dissertation Abstracts International, 42, 569B.

McEvoy, M.D. (1988). The relationship among the experience of dying, the experience of paranormal events, and creativity in adults. Dissertation Abstracts International, 48, 2264B.

Meleis, A.I. (1985). Theoretical nursing: Development and progress. Philadelphia: JB Lippincott.

Miller, F.A. (1985). The relationship of sleep, wakefulness, and beyond waking experiences: A descriptive study of M. Rogers' concept of sleep-wake rhythm. Dissertation Abstracts International, 46, 116B.

Miller, L.A. (1979). An explanation of therapeutic touch using the science of unitary man. Nursing Forum, 18, 278–287.

Miller, S. (1974). An investigation of the relationship between mothers' general fearfulness, their daughters' locus of control, and general fearfulness in the daughter. Unpublished doctoral dissertation, New York University.

Moore, G. (1982). Perceptual complexity, memory and human duration experience. Dissertation Abstracts International, 42, 4363B.

Newman, M.A. (1971). An investigation of the relationship between gait tempo and time perception. Unpublished doctoral dissertation, New York University.

Newman, M.A. (1972a). Nursing's theoretical evolution. Nursing Outlook, 20, 449–453.

Newman, M.A. (1972b). Time estimation in relation to gait tempo. Perceptual and Motor Skills, 34, 359–366.

Newman, M.A. (1976). Movement tempo and the experience of time. Nursing Research, 25, 273–279.

Newman, M.A. (1979). Theory development in nursing. Philadelphia: FA Davis.

Newman, M.A. (1982). Time as an index of expanding consciousness with age. Nursing Research, 31, 290–293.

Newman, M.A. (1986). Health as expanding consciousness. St. Louis: CV Mosby.

Newman, M.A., & Gaudiano, J.K. (1984). Depression as an explanation for decreased subjective time in the elderly. Nursing Research, 33, 137–139.

Nightingale, F. (1859). Notes on nursing: What it is, and what it is not. London: Harrison. (Reprinted by JB Lippincott, 1946).

Parse, R.R. (1981). Man-living-health. A theory of nursing. New York: John Wiley & Sons.

Parse, R.R. (1987a). Man-living-health theory of nursing. In R.R. Parse, Nursing science.

Major paradigms, theories, and critiques (pp. 159–180). Philadelphia: WB Saunders.

Parse, R.R. (1987b). Nursing science. Major paradigms, theories, and critiques. Philadelphia: WB Saunders.

Polanyi, M. (1958). Personal knowledge. Chicago: University of Chicago Press.

Porter, L. (1967). Physical-physiological activity and infants' growth and development. Unpublished doctoral dissertation, New York University.

Quillin, S.I.M. (1984). Growth and development of infant and mother and mother-infant synchrony. Dissertation Abstracts International, 44, 3718B.

Quinn, J.F. (1982). An investigation of the effects of therapeutic touch done without physical contact on state anxiety of hospitalized cardiovascular patients. Dissertation Abstracts International, 43, 1797B.

Quinn, J.F. (1984). Therapeutic touch as energy exchange: Testing the theory. Advances in Nursing Science, 6(2), 42–49.

Raile, M.M. (1983). The relationship of creativity, actualization and empathy in unitary human development: A descriptive study of M. Rogers' principle of helicy. Dissertation Abstracts International, 44, 449B.

Rankin, M.K. (1985). Effect of sound wave repatterning on symptoms of menopausal women. Dissertation Abstracts International, 46, 796B–797B.

Rawnsley, M.M. (1977). Perceptions of the speed of time in aging and in dying. An empirical investigation of the holistic theory of nursing proposed by Martha Rogers. Dissertation Abstracts International, 38, 1652B.

Reed, P.G. (1986). The developmental conceptual framework: Nursing reformulations and applications for family therapy. In A.L. Whall, Family therapy theory for nursing. Four approaches (pp. 69–91). Norwalk, CT: Appleton-Century-Crofts.

Reed, P.G. (1987). Spirituality and well-being in terminally ill hospitalized adults. Research in Nursing and Health, 10, 335–344.

Reeder, F. (1985). Nursing research, holism and philosophies of science: Points of congruence between E. Husserl and M.E. Rogers. Dissertation Abstracts International, 44, 2498B–2499B.

Reeder, F. (1986). Basic theoretical research in the conceptual system of unitary human beings. In V.M. Malinski (Ed), Explorations on Martha Rogers' Science of Unitary Human Beings (pp. 45–64). Norwalk, CT: Appleton-Century-Crofts.

Riehl, J.P. (1980). Nursing models in current use. In J.P. Riehl & C. Roy, Conceptual models for nursing practice (2nd ed. pp. 393–398). New York: Appleton-Century-Crofts.

Riehl, J.P., & Roy, C. (1980). Conceptual models for nursing practice (2nd ed). New York: Appleton-Century-Crofts.

Rogers, M.E. (1961). Educational revolution in nursing. New York: Macmillan.

Rogers, M.E. (1964). Reveille in nursing. Philadelphia: FA Davis.

Rogers, M.E. (1970). An introduction to the theoretical basis of nursing. Philadelphia: FA Davis.

Rogers, M.E. (1978a, December). Nursing science: A science of unitary man. Paper presented at Second Annual Nurse Educator Conference, New York. (Cassette recording)

Rogers, M.E. (1978b, December). Application of theory in education and service. Paper presented at Second Annual Nurse Educator Conference, New York. (Cassette recording)

Rogers, M.E. (1980a). Nursing: A science of unitary man. In J.P. Riehl & C. Roy, Conceptual models for nursing practice (2nd ed., pp. 329–337). New York: Appleton-Century-Crofts.

Rogers, M.E. (1980b). Science of unitary man. Tape I. Unitary man and his world: A paradigm for nursing. New York: Media for Nursing. (Cassette recording)

Rogers, M.E. (1980c). Science of unitary man. Tape II. Developing an organized abstract system: Synthesis of facts and ideas for a new product. New York: Media for Nursing. (Cassette recording)

Rogers, M.E. (1980d). Science of unitary man. Tape III. Principles and theories: Directions for description, explanation and prediction. New York: Media for Nursing. (Cassette recording)

Rogers, M.E. (1980e). Science of unitary man. Tape IV. Theories of accelerating evolution, paranormal phenomena and other events. New York: Media for Nursing. (Cassette recording)

Rogers, M.E. (1980f). Science of unitary man. Tape V. Health and illness: New perspectives. New York: Media for Nursing. (Cassette recording)

Rogers, M.E. (1980g). Science of unitary man. Tape VI. Interventive modalities: Translating theories into practice. New York: Media for Nursing. (Cassette recording)

Rogers, M.E. (1983a). The family coping with a surgical crisis. Analysis and application of Rogers' theory of nursing. In I.W. Clements & F.B. Roberts, Family health. A theoretical approach to nursing care (pp. 390–391). New York: John Wiley & Sons.

Rogers, M.E. (1983b). Science of unitary human beings: A paradigm for nursing. In I.W. Clements and F.B. Roberts, Family Health. A theoretical approach to nursing care (pp. 219–227). New York: John Wiley & Sons.

Rogers, M.E. (1985a). A paradigm for nursing. In R. Wood & J. Kekahbah (Eds.), Examining the cultural implications of Martha E. Rogers' Science of Unitary Human Beings (pp. 13–23). Lecompton, KS: Wood-Kekahbah Associates.

Rogers, M.E. (1985b, May). Panel discussion with theorists. Discussion at Nurse Theorist Conference, Pittsburgh, PA. (Cassette recording)

Rogers, M.E. (1986). Science of unitary human beings. In V.M. Malinski (Ed), Explorations on Martha Rogers' Science of Unitary Human Beings (pp. 3–8). Norwalk, CT: Appleton-Century-Crofts.

Rogers, M.E. (1987a). Nursing research in the future. In J. Roode (Ed), Changing patterns in nursing education (pp. 121–123). New York: National League for Nursing.

Rogers, M.E. (1987b, May). Rogers' framework. Paper presented at Nurse Theorist Conference, Pittsburgh, PA. (Cassette recording)

Rogers, M.E. (1987c, May). Small group D. Discussion at Nurse Theorist Conference, Pittsburgh PA. (Cassette recording)

Rogers, M.E. (1987d). Rogers' Science of Unitary Human Beings. In R.R. Parse, Nursing science. Major paradigms, theories, and critiques (pp. 139–146). Philadelphia: WB Saunders.

Safier, G. (1977). Contemporary American leaders: An oral history. New York: McGraw-Hill.

Sanchez, R.O. (1987). The relationship of empathy, diversity, and telepathy in mother-daughter dyads. Dissertation Abstracts International, 47, 3297B.

Sarter, B. (1985). The stream of becoming: A metaphysical analysis of Rogers' Model of Unitary Man. Dissertation Abstracts International, 45, 2106B.

Sarter, B. (1987). Evolutionary idealism: A philosophical foundation for holistic nursing theory. Advances in Nursing Science, 9(2), 1–9.

Sarter, B. (1988). The stream of becoming: A study of Martha Rogers's theory. New York: National League for Nursing.

Silva, M.C. (1987). Conceptual models of nursing. In J.J. Fitzpatrick & R.L. Taunton (Eds), Annual review of nursing research (Vol. 5, pp. 229–246). New York: Springer.

Silva, M.C., & Sorrell, J.M. (1987, April). Doctoral dissertation research based on five nursing models: A select bibliography. January 1952 through February 1987. (Available from M.C. Silva, George Mason University School of Nursing, Fairfax, VA)

Smith, L. (1983). A conceptual model of families incorporating an adolescent mother and child into the household. Advances in Nursing Science, 6(1), 45–60.

Smith, M.C. (1987). An investigation of the effects of different sound frequencies on vividness and creativity of imagery. Dissertation Abstracts International, 47, 3708B.

Smith, M.J. (1984). Temporal experience and bed rest: Replication and refinement. Nursing Research, 33, 298–302.

Smith, M.J. (1986). Human-environment process: A test of Rogers' principle of integrality. Advances in Nursing Science, 9(1), 21–28.

Stevens, B.J. (1984). Nursing theory. Analysis, application, evaluation (2nd ed). Boston: Little, Brown and Co.

Swanson, A. (1975). An investigation of the relationship between a child's general fearfulness and the child's mother's anxiety, self differentiation, and accuracy of perception of her child's general fearfulness. Unpublished doctoral dissertation, New York University.

Toffler, A. (1970). Future shock. New York: Random House.

Toffler, A. (1980). The third wave. New York: William Morrow.

Tompkins, E.S. (1980). Effect of restricted mobility and dominance on perceived duration. Nursing Research, 29, 333–338.

Walker, L.O., & Nicholson, R. (1980). Criteria for evaluating nursing process models. Nurse Educator, 5(5), 8–9.

Whall, A.L. (1981). Nursing theory and the assessment of families. Journal of Psychiatric Nursing and Mental Health Services, 19(1), 30–36.

Whall, A.L. (1987). A critique of Rogers's framework. In R.R. Parse, Nursing science. Major paradigms, theories, and critiques (pp. 147–158). Philadelphia: WB Saunders.

Whelton, B.J. (1979). An operationalization of Martha Rogers' theory throughout the nursing process. International Journal of Nursing Studies, 16, 7–20.

Yaros, P.S. (1986). The relationship of maternal rhythmic behavior and infant interactional attention. Dissertation Abstracts International, 47, 136B.

Young, A.A. (1985). The Rogerian conceptual system: A framework for nursing education and service. In R. Wood & J. Kekehbah (Eds.), Examining the cultural implications of Martha E. Rogers' Science of Unitary Human Beings (pp. 53–69). Lecompton, KS: Wood-Kekahbah Associates.

ANNOTATED BIBLIOGRAPHY

Aggleton, P., & Chalmers, H. (1984). Rogers' unitary field model. Nursing Times, 80(50), 35–39.
This article presents a discussion of some of the traditional healing methods that focus on the holism of the individual and compares these methods to concepts of Rogers's conceptual model. An overview of Rogers's conceptual model is given with emphasis on therapeutic touch.

Allanach, E.J. (1988). Perceived supportive behaviors and nursing occupational stress: An evolution of consciousness. Advances in Nursing Science, 10(2), 73–82.
The author presents a holistic, noncausal formulation of the relationship between perception of support and occupational stress based on Rogers's conceptual framework and Sarter's extrapolations of evolutionary idealism. Implications for research are discussed, with emphasis on qualitative methodology.

Alligood, M.R. (in press). Applying Rogers' model to nursing administration: Emphasis on environment, health. In B. Henry, M. DiVincenti, C. Arndt, & A. Marriner (Eds.), Dimensions of nursing administration. Theory, research, education, and practice. Boston: Blackwell Scientific Publications.
The author discusses the implications of Rogers's conceptual model for administration of nursing services.

Barber, H.R.K. (1987). Editorial: Trends in nursing: A model for emulation. The Female Patient 12(3), 12, 14.
The author, who is a physician, comments on the insights into nursing and medicine that he had after reading Rogers's 1970 book. He decries contemporary medicine's shift from a humanistic focus.

Blair, C. (1979). Hyperactivity in children: Viewed within the framework of synergistic man. Nursing Forum, 18, 293–303.
The hyperactive child's behavior is examined within the context of Rogers's conceptual model.

Boyd, C. (1985). Toward an understanding of mother-daughter identification using concept analysis. Advances in Nursing Science, 7(3), 78–86.
This article presents an analysis of the concept of mother-daughter identification. Rogers's conceptual model is used to provide a nursing perspective for the concept.

Brouse, S.H. (1985). Effect of gender role identity on patterns of feminine and self-concept scores from late pregnancy to early postpartum. Advances in Nursing Science, 7(3), 32–40.
This article reports the results of a study that describes the relationship among gender role identity, femininity scores, self-concept, and perception of comfort in the mothering role. Rogers's concepts of energy fields and unidirectionality were used as part of the framework for the study.

Butterfield, S.E. (1983). In search of commonalities: An analysis of two theoretical frameworks. International Journal of Nursing Studies, 20, 15–22.
This article presents the central assumptions and propositions of Orem's and Rogers's conceptual models. A framework for theory analysis is used to examine the work for the purpose of determining commonalities. Many similarities are discussed. The most apparent differences were in relative emphases and the explicitness of abstract concepts.

Clarke, P.N. (1986). Theoretical and measurement issues in the study of field phenomena. Advances in Nursing Science, 9(1), 29–39.
The study reported in this article explored the relationships among indicators of the human field, including perceived body space, conversational distance, body weight, and self-actualization in a sample of healthy women.

Crawford, G. (1982). The concept of pattern in nursing: Conceptual development and measurement. Advances in Nursing Science, 5(1), 1–6.
The concept of pattern is discussed from the perspectives of different conceptual models of nursing. Rogers's conceptualization of pattern is examined and critiqued. The author presents approaches to the empirical study of pattern.

Crawford, G. (1985). A theoretical model of support network conflict experienced by new mothers. Nursing Research, 34, 100–102.
Rogers's concepts of integrality and helicy were used to provide a nursing perspective for a theoretical model of support network conflict experienced by new mothers. The author notes that research designed to test the theoretical model is in progress.

Daily, J.S., Maupin, J.S., & Satterly, M.C. (1986). Martha E. Rogers. Unitary human beings. In A. Marriner, Nursing theorists and their work (pp. 345–360). St. Louis: CV Mosby.
This book chapter presents a brief review of Rogers's work.

Falco, S.M., & Lobo, M.L. (1980). Martha E. Rogers. In Nursing Theories Conference Group, Nursing theories. The base for professional nursing practice (pp. 164–183). Englewood Cliffs, NJ: Prentice-Hall.

Falco, S.M., & Lobo, M.L. (1985). Martha E. Rogers. In Nursing Theories Conference Group, Nursing theories. The base for professional nursing practice (2nd ed., pp. 214–234). Englewood Cliffs, NJ: Prentice-Hall.
Rogers's conceptual model is reviewed. Included are an historical overview, definition of nursing, and Rogers's five basic assumptions. The principles of homeodynamics are outlined and the model is compared with other nursing models. The relationship between Rogers's model and the nursing process is explored. Limitations of the model are outlined.

Fawcett, J. (1975). The family as a living open system: An emerging conceptual framework for nursing. International Nursing Review, 22, 113–116.

Fawcett, J. (1977). The relationship between identification and patterns of change in spouses' body images during and after pregnancy. International Journal of Nursing Studies, 14, 199–213.

Fawcett, J. (1978). Body image and the pregnant couple. American Journal of Maternal Child Nursing, 3, 227–233.

Fawcett, J., Bliss-Holtz, V.J., Haas, M.B., Leventhal, M., & Rubin, M. (1986). Spouses' body image changes during and after pregnancy: A replication and extension. Nursing Research, 35, 220–223.

Drake, M.L., Verhulst, D., Fawcett, J., & Barger, D.F. (in press). Spouses' body image changes during and after pregnancy. Image. Journal of Nursing Scholarship.

Fawcett, J., & York, R. (1986). Spouses' physical and psychological symptoms during pregnancy and the postpartum. Nursing Research, 35, 144–148.

Fawcett, J., & York, R. (1987). Spouses' strength of identification and reports of symptoms during pregnancy and the postpartum. Florida Nursing Review, 2(2), 1–10.

Drake, M.L., Verhulst, D., & Fawcett, J. (in press). Physical and psychological symptoms experienced by Canadian women and their husbands during pregnancy and the postpartum. Journal of Advanced Nursing.

Fawcett, J. (in press). Spouses' experiences during pregnancy and the postpartum: A program of research and theory development. Applied Nursing Research.
   Fawcett presents a conceptual framework that extended the 1970 version of Rogers's conceptual model to the family. The concept of the family as an open system is developed. Implications of the framework for research, education, and practice are discussed.
   The conceptual framework was used to guide studies of similarities in wives' and husbands' body image changes and reports of symptoms during pregnancy and the postpartum. The findings of the studies raise serious questions about the credibility of the conceptual framework.

Fitzpatrick, J.J. (1980). Patients' perceptions of time: Current research. International Nursing Review, 27, 148–153, 160.
   Temporal experiences as indicators of the rhythmic nature of man are examined. The literature related to temporal experiences is reviewed. A series of studies that link the concept of temporality to the Rogerian model is described.

Fitzpatrick, J.J. (1983). Life perspective rhythm model. In J.J. Fitzpatrick & A.L. Whall, Conceptual models of nursing: Analysis and evaluation (pp. 295–302). Bowie, MD: Brady.
   The author presents her life perspective rhythm model and traces its origins from Rogers's conceptual model and the findings of empirical research.

Fitzpatrick, J.J., Whall, A.L., Johnston, R.L., & Floyd, J.A. (1982). Nursing models and their psychiatric mental health applications. Bowie, MD: Brady.
   The book presents a brief analysis of Rogers's conceptual model, among others. Reformulated theoretical approaches, consistent with Rogers's model, in individual psychotherapy and family therapy are discussed.

Floyd, J.A. (1983). Research using Rogers's conceptual system: Development of a testable theorem. Advances in Nursing Science, 5(2), 37–48.
   The author describes the development of empirical testing of a theorem of sleep-wakefulness patterns derived from Rogers's conceptual model. Findings from a study of rotating shift workers and from a study of hospitalized adult psychiatric patients yielded conflicting evidence.

Floyd, J.A. (1984). Interaction between personal sleep-wake rhythms and psychiatric hospital rest-activity schedule. Nursing Research, 33, 255–259.
   The article reports the findings of a study that explored the interactions between circadian rhythms of sleep and wakefulness and the hospital's rest-activity schedule. Rogers's conceptual model served as a guide to the research questions.

Gill, B.P., & Atwood, J.R. (1981). Reciprocy and helicy used to relate mEFG and wound healing. Nursing Research, 30, 68–72.

Kim, H.S. (1983). Use of Rogers' conceptual system in research: Comments. Nursing Research, 32, 89–91.

Atwood, J.R., & Gill-Rogers, B. (1984). Metatheory, methodology and practicality: Issues in research uses of Rogers' science of unitary man. Nursing Research, 33, 88–91.
   Gill and Atwood report the findings of their study of the relationship between epidermal growth factor (EGF) and wound healing in a sample of domestic pigs. The theoretical structure for the study linked Rogers's principles of helicy and reciprocy with knowledge regarding wound healing. Findings lend support to the two Rogerian principles.
   Kim presents a critique of the use of Rogers's conceptual model as the frame-

work for Gill and Atwood's study, questioning whether the research hypotheses and methodology are congruent with Rogers's model and discusses the difficulties in resolving the congruency problem.

Atwood and Gill-Rogers reply to Kim's critique of their study. They offer counterpoints to Kim's argument, present mathematical formulas to exemplify Rogers's work, and discuss the difficulty in testing a four-dimensional model.

Goldberg, W.G., & Fitzpatrick, J.J. (1980). Movement therapy with the aged. Nursing Research, 29, 339–346.

Rogers's conceptual model guided development of this study of the effect of participation in a movement therapy group on morale and self-esteem in a sample of 30 residents of a nursing home. Findings indicated that movement therapy group members (N = 15) demonstrated greater improvement in morale and attitudes toward their own aging than the control group (N = 15).

Gueldner, S.H. (in press). Applying Rogers' model to nursing administration: Emphasis on client and nursing. In B. Henry, M. DiVincenti, C. Arndt, & A. Marriner (Eds.), Dimensions of nursing administration. Theory, research, education, and practice. Boston: Blackwell Scientific Publications.

The author discusses the implications of Rogers's conceptual model for administration of nursing services.

Hanchett, E.S. (1979). Community health assessment: A conceptual tool kit. New York: John Wiley & Sons.

General system theory and the Rogerian model provide the framework for the assessment of community health. Chapters focus on assessment of the energy, individuality, organization, and pattern of communities through the use of a variety of tools, which are included in the book.

Johnston, R.L. (1986). Approaching family intervention through Rogers' conceptual model. In A.L. Whall, Family therapy theory for nursing. Four approaches (pp. 11–32). Norwalk, CT: Appleton-Century-Crofts.

Rogers's conceptual model and her views of family are presented, along with Fawcett's and Whall's work dealing with Rogers's model and the family system. A nursing process format for use with families that is consistent with Rogers's model is presented and a case study is described.

Katch, M.P. (1983). A negentropic view of the aged. Journal of Gerontological Nursing, 9, 656–660.

This article presents Rogers's science of unitary human beings as it applies to the aging process. The principles of resonancy, helicy, and integrality are used to describe aging.

Keller, E., & Bzdek, V.M. (1986). Effects of therapeutic touch on tension headache pain. Nursing Research, 35, 101–106.

The article reports a study of the effects of therapeutic touch versus a mimic form of therapeutic touch on tension headache pain. The study has its origins in Rogers's conceptual model and earlier work on therapeutic touch.

Krieger, D. (1974). The relationship of touch, in intent to help or heal to subjects' in-vivo hemoglobin values: A study in personalized interaction. In American Nurses' Association, Ninth Nursing Research Conference (pp. 39–58). Kansas City, MO: American Nurses' Association.

The investigator reports her study of the effect of touch with intent to heal on hemoglobin values of 43 experimental and 33 control subjects. Significant differences were found between the two groups. Rogers's conceptual model served as a general guide for the study. The study is one of the earliest reports dealing with what now is called therapeutic touch.

Laffrey, S.C. (1985). Health behavior choice as related to self-actualization and health conception. Western Journal of Nursing Research, 7, 279–295.

The study reported in this article was designed to investigate the relationship of self-actualization to health conception and health behavior choice. Concepts and propositions from Rogers's conceptual model are linked to theoretical notions of self-actualization.

Levine, N.H. (1976). A conceptual model for obstetric nursing. Journal of Obstetric, Gynecologic, and Neonatal Nursing, 5(2), 9–15.

The author describes the experience of pregnancy, labor and delivery, and the postpartum in terms of expansion and contraction of the human energy field. Implications for nursing care are presented in brief.

Madrid, M., & Winstead-Fry, P. (1986). Rogers's conceptual model. In P. Winstead-Fry (Ed.), Case studies in nursing theory (pp. 73–102). New York: National League for Nursing.

This book chapter presents a review of Rogers's conceptual model and a nursing process format that is consistent with the model. The nursing process format is used to describe the care of a 35-year-old man who had been admitted to an intensive care unit with elevated blood pressure, photophobia, and severe headaches. A few studies derived from Rogers's work are reviewed.

Malinski, V.M. (Ed.). (1986). Explorations on Martha Rogers' Science of Unitary Human Beings. Norwalk, CT: Appleton-Century-Crofts.

This landmark book presents chapters dealing with the most recent refinements in Rogers's conceptual model, issues related to research based on this model, and reports and critiques of several studies based on Rogers's work. Included are brief reports of the doctoral dissertations by Alligood (nee Raile), Barrett, Cowling, Ference, Gueldner, Malinski, McDonald, and Rawnsley. Each study is followed by at least one critique and a response by the investigator. Nursing practice within the context of the Science of Unitary Human Beings is discussed.

Miller, L.A. (1979). An explanation of therapeutic touch using the science of unitary man. Nursing Forum, 18, 278–287.

Therapeutic touch is explained within the context of Rogers's conceptual model.

Newman, M.A. (1979). Theory development in nursing. Philadelphia: FA Davis.

Newman describes a theory of health derived from Rogers's conceptual model of nursing. Major concepts of the theory are movement, time, space, and consciousness.

Newman, M.A. (1986). Health as expanding consciousness. St. Louis: CV Mosby.

This book presents refinements in Newman's theory of health.

Parse, R.R. (1981). Man-Living-Health. A theory of nursing. New York: John Wiley & Sons.

Parse describes her theory, Man-Living-Health, and explains its connections with Rogers's conceptual model and with existential-phenomenological tenets.

Porter, L.S. (1972). The impact of physical-physiological activity on infants' growth and development. Nursing Research, 21, 210–219.

Porter, L.S. (1972). Physical-physiological activity and infants' growth and development. In American Nurses' Association, Seventh Nursing Research Conference (pp. 1–43). New York: American Nurses' Association.

These papers present reports of a study of the relationship between physical activity and growth and development in infants. Activity was given in the form of passive cycling exercises. Rogers's early work was used to guide the study.

Quillin, S.I.M., & Runk, J.A. (1983). Martha Rogers' model. In J.J. Fitzpatrick & A.L. Whall, Conceptual models of nursing: Analysis and application (pp. 245–261). Bowie, MD: Brady.

This book chapter presents an overview of Rogers's conceptual model.

Quinn, J.F. (1984). Therapeutic touch as energy exchange: Testing the theory. Advances in Nursing Science, 6(2), 42–49.

The author reports the findings of her study of the effect of non-contact therapeutic touch on state anxiety in a sample of patients with cardiovascular problems.

Reed, P.G. (1986). The developmental conceptual framework: Nursing reformulations and applications for family therapy. In A.L. Whall, Family therapy for nursing. Four approaches (pp. 69–91). Norwalk, CT: Appleton-Century-Crofts.

This book chapter presents a reformulation of the family developmental framework and its application to nursing practice within the context of Rogers's conceptual model.

Reeder, F. (1984). Philosophical issues in the Rogerian science of unitary human beings. Advances in Nursing Science, 6(2), 14–23.
This article presents a discussion of the basic Rogerian assumptions and their relationship to logical-empiricism, phenomenological philosophy, and micro-physics.
The author recommends that some of the rules and assumptions of science be scru-
tinized and not accepted as the only truth.

Rogers, M.E. (1961). Educational revolution in nursing. New York: Macmillan.
This book presents an exploration of the changing nature of nursing and nursing
education. Rogers advocates higher education for nursing. The need for theoretical
content in nursing is discussed. The development of theory and subsequent nursing curricula are considered.

Rogers, M.E. (1963). Building a strong educational foundation. American Journal of
Nursing, 63(6), 94–95.
Rogers presents her ideas regarding nursing education at the undergraduate and
graduate levels.

Rogers, M.E. (1963). Some comments on the theoretical basis of nursing practice. Nursing Science, 1(1), 11–13, 60–61.
This article presents rudimentary ideas for Rogers's conceptual model.

Rogers, M.E. (1964). Reveille in nursing. Philadelphia: FA Davis.
This book presents a discussion of professional nursing education. Principles of
higher education are considered and a plan is formulated for implementing a professional curriculum in nursing. Areas of difference between actual and ideal education are delineated.

Rogers, M.E. (1970). An introduction to the theoretical basis of nursing. Philadelphia:
FA Davis.
Rogers presents her conceptual model in detail.

Rogers, M.E. (1980). Nursing: A science of unitary man. In J.P. Riehl & C. Roy, Conceptual models for nursing practice (2nd ed., pp. 329–337). New York: Appleton-
Century-Crofts.
Rogers presents her conceptual model with refinements. The theories of accelerating evolution, paranormal phenomena, and rhythmical correlates of change are described.

Rogers, M.E. (1981). Science of unitary man. A paradigm for nursing. In G.E. Lasker
(Ed.), Applied systems and cybernetics. Vol. 4. Systems research in health care,
biocybernetics and ecology (pp. 1719–1722). New York: Pergamon Press.
Rogers reviews the major concepts and propositions of her conceptual model of
nursing.

Rogers, M.E. (1983). Science of unitary human beings: A paradigm for nursing. In I.W.
Clements & F.B. Roberts, Family health. A theoretical approach to nursing care (pp.
219–227). New York: John Wiley & Sons.
This book chapter presents definitions of terms used by Rogers in her conceptual
model and a discussion of the principles of homeodynamics and theories derived
from the model.

Rogers, M.E. (1983). The family coping with a surgical crisis. Analysis and application
of Rogers' theory of nursing. In I.W. Clements & F.B. Roberts, Family health. A theoretical approach to nursing care (pp. 390–391). New York: John Wiley & Sons.
Rogers presents an analysis of a case study involving a woman who underwent a
mastectomy within the context of her work.

Rogers, M.E. (1987). Nursing research in the future. In J. Roode (Ed.), Changing patterns
in nursing education (pp. 121–123). New York: National League for Nursing.
Rogers discusses the implications of her conceptual model for nursing research,
practice, and education.

Rogers, M.E. (1987). Rogers' Science of Unitary Human Beings. In R.R. Parse, Nursing
science. Major paradigms, theories, and critiques (pp. 139–146). Philadelphia: WB
Saunders.
This book chapter is the publication of Rogers's presentation of her work at the
Nurse Theorist Conference held in Pittsburgh, Pennsylvania, in May 1985.

Roy, C. (1974). Rogers' theoretical basis of nursing. In J.P. Riehl & C. Roy, Conceptual models for nursing practice (pp. 96–99). New York: Appleton-Century-Crofts.
Roy presents the major components of Rogers's conceptual model.

Safier, G. (1977). Contemporary American leaders: An oral history. New York: McGraw-Hill.
Safier presents an interview with Rogers, among other leaders in nursing. The interview focuses on Rogers's beginnings in nursing, her contributions to nursing, and her conceptual model. In addition, Rogers responds to questions about nursing education and the profession of nursing.

Sarter, B. (1987). Evolutionary idealism: A philosophical foundation for holistic nursing theory. Advances in Nursing Science, 9(2), 1–9.
This article presents a discussion of the philosophical tradition of evolutionary idealism. The author maintains that this tradition is an appropriate foundation for nursing theory development based on a holistic view of people, with emphasis on Rogers's work.

Sarter, B. (1988). The stream of becoming: A study of Martha Rogers's theory. New York: National League for Nursing.
Sarter presents an analysis of the role of philosophical research in nursing and the history of evolutionary philosophy and different views of evolution, with discussion of the philosophies of Monod and Chardin. She also evaluates the metaphysics of Rogers's work and presents implications for theory development.

Schorr, J.A. Manifestations of consciousness and the developmental phenomenon of death. Advances in Nursing Science, 6(1), 26–35.
The author explores Rogers's conceptualization of the life process and links Rogers's work with theoretical ideas about consciousness and death.

Smith, M.J. (1975). Changes in judgement of duration with different patterns of auditory information for individuals confined to bed. Nursing Research, 24, 93–98.

Smith, M.J. (1979). Duration experience for bed-confined subjects: A replication and refinement. Nursing Research, 28, 139–144.

Smith, M.J. (1984). Temporal experience and bed rest: Replication and refinement. Nursing Research, 33, 298–302.

Smith, M.J. (1986). Human-environment process: A test of Rogers' principle of integrality. Advances in Nursing Science, 9(1), 21–28.
Smith reports the findings of a series of studies designed to determine the effect of auditory inputs on subjects' perceptions of time passing and restfulness. The research program was guided by Rogers's conceptual model.

Uys, L.R. (1987). Foundational studies in nursing. Journal of Advanced Nursing, 12, 275–280.
This article presents a brief discussion of Rogers's work within the context of a philosophical analysis, with emphasis on discussion of Rogers's philosophical view of the person as a unitary being.

Whall, A.L. (1981). Nursing theory and the assessment of families. Journal of Psychiatric Nursing and Mental Health Services, 19(1), 30–36.
A nursing model for family assessment is presented. The model is derived from Rogers's conceptual model and Fawcett's extension of that model to the family, as well as theories of family functioning. A tool for family assessment is included.

Whall, A.L. (1987). A critique of Rogers's framework. In R.R. Parse, Nursing science. Major paradigms, theories, and critiques (pp. 147–158). Philadelphia: WB Saunders.
This book chapter is the publication of the critique of Rogers's work that was presented at the Nurse Theorist Conference held in Pittsburgh, Pennsylvania, in May 1985.

Whelton, B.J. (1979). An operationalization of Martha Rogers' theory throughout the nursing process. International Journal of Nursing Studies, 16, 7–20.
The author combines Rogers's conceptual model with the nursing process and identifies general areas of assessment. In addition, assessment plans for neurological and cardiac patients are outlined and comprehensive nursing care plans for a

patient with decreased cardiac output and a patient with recurrent meningioma are presented.

Wilson, L.M., & Fitzpatrick, J.J. (1984). Dialectic thinking as a means of understanding systems-in-development: Relevance to Rogers's principles. Advances in Nursing Science, 6(2), 24–41.

Moccia, P. (1985). A further investigation of "Dialectical thinking as a means of understanding systems-in-development: Relevance to Rogers's principles." Advances in Nursing Science, 7(4), 33–38.

Wilson and Fitzpatrick discuss the concepts of determinism, lawfulness, and causality as a background for their description of Rogers's concepts of complementarity, resonancy, and helicy within the context of dialectic logic. Moccia argues that the dialectic approach used by Wilson and Fitzpatrick is based on a dualistic universe viewpoint and is, therefore, not congruent with Rogers's ideas. Another approach to dialectic logic that Moccia claims is congruent with Rogers's ideas is offered.

Wood, R., & Kekahbah, J. (Eds.). (1985). Examining the cultural implications of Martha E. Rogers's Science of Unitary Human Beings. Lecompton, KS: Wood-Kekahbah Associates.

This monograph contains the papers presented at an educational symposium sponsored by the American Indian/Alaska Native Nurses' Association in July 1984. Included are chapters dealing with Rogers's work, and implications of Rogers's work for various cultural groups and for nursing education.

Roy's Adaptation Model_____

This chapter presents an analysis and evaluation of Sister Callista Roy's Adaptation Model of Nursing. Roy's work clearly fits the definition of conceptual model used in this book. In fact, Roy has always referred to her work as a model.

The key terms of Roy's conceptual model are listed below. These terms were taken from the second edition of Roy's (1984a) book, *Introduction to nursing. An adaptation model,* and from the Andrews and Roy (1986) book, *Essentials of the Roy Adaptation Model.*

KEY TERMS_____

Adaptive System
  Cognator Mechanism
  Regulator Mechanism
Adaptive Modes
  Physiological
  Self-Concept
  Role Function
  Interdependence
Environment
  Internal
  External
Stimuli

Stimuli—*Cont.*
  Focal
  Contextual
  Residual
Adaptation
Adaptation Level
Adaptation Zone
Adaptive Response
Ineffective Response
Goal of Nursing
    To Promote Adaptation
Nursing Process

Nursing Process—*Cont.*	Nursing Process—*Cont.*
Assessment of Behavior	Intervention
Assessment of Influencing	Evaluation
Factors (Stimuli)	Theory of the Person as an
Nursing Diagnosis	Adaptive System
Goal Setting	Theories of the Adaptive Modes

ANALYSIS OF ROY'S ADAPTATION MODEL

This section presents an analysis of Roy's Adaptation Model. The analysis draws heavily from the second edition of Roy's (1984a) book, *Introduction to nursing. An adaptation model,* and from Andrews and Roy's (1986) book, *Essentials of the Roy Adaptation Model.*

Development of the Model

Roy first published the basic ideas comprising her conceptual model in 1970 in an article entitled, "Adaptation: A conceptual framework for nursing." She went on to publish additional elements of the model and implications for practice and education in 1971 and 1973. The model was explicated more fully in the 1974 edition of the Riehl and Roy book, *Conceptual models for nursing practice.* A major expansion of the model was presented in Roy's 1976 text, *Introduction to nursing. An adaptation model.* Refinements of the model then were presented in Roy's 1978 speech at the Second Annual Nurse Educator Conference, in the 1980 edition of Riehl and Roy's book, and in Roy and Roberts's 1981 text, *Theory construction in nursing, An adaptation model.* Further refinements and revisions in the model were published in the second edition of Roy's (1984a) text, *Introduction to nursing. An adaptation model,* and in the Andrews and Roy (1986) book, *Essentials of the Roy Adaptation Model.*

Andrews and Roy (1986) explained that "the roots of the model lie in Roy's own personal and professional background. Roy is committed to a philosophical belief in the innate capabilities, purpose, and worth of the human person. Her clinical practice in pediatric nursing provided experience with the resiliency of the human body and spirit" (p. 6). Roy (1978a) acknowledged the contributions to her thinking made by her mentor, Dorothy Johnson; her colleagues at Mount Saint Mary's College; nursing students across the country; and other nurse theorists. In particular, she cited the influences of Dorothy Johnson's focus on behavior, Martha Rogers's concern with holistic man, and Dorothea Orem's notion of self-care. The social sciences also have influenced Roy's thinking (Andrews & Roy, 1986).

In tracing the historical development of her conceptual model, Roy (1980) stated:

The Roy model had its beginning in 1964 when the author was challenged to develop a conceptual model for nursing in a seminar with Dorothy E. Johnson, at the University of California, Los Angeles. The adaptation concept, presented in psychology class, had impressed the author as an appropriate conceptual framework for nursing. The work on adaptation by the physiologic psychologist, Harry Helson, was added to the beginning concept and the model's present form began to take shape. In subsequent years the model was developed as a framework for nursing practice, research, and education. In 1968 work began on operationalizing the model in the baccalaureate nursing curriculum at Mount Saint Mary's College in Los Angeles. The first class of students to study with the model began their nursing major in the spring of 1970 and were graduated in June, 1972. Use of the model in nursing practice led to further clarification and refinement. In the summer of 1971 a pilot research study was conducted and in 1976–77 a survey research study was done that led to some tentative confirmations of the model. (pp. 179–180)

Development of the model continued during the 1970s, according to Andrews and Roy (1986), as "more than 1500 faculty and students at Mount St. Mary's College helped to clarify, refine, and extend the basic concepts of the Roy Adaptation Model for Nursing" (p. 6).

By accepting Johnson's challenge to develop a conceptual model, Roy joined the group of nurse scholars who recognized the need to explicate a body of nursing knowledge. Indeed, she stated:

As nursing education moves more and more into institutions of higher learning, the nurse educator needs a basis for developing a body of nursing knowledge. And as the general public becomes more sophisticated in knowing the meaning of good health, it expects the nurse to provide care based on scientific knowledge. It is from the theoretical conceptual framework of any discipline that its area of practice, its body of knowledge, and its scientific basis are developed. (Roy, 1970, p. 42)

Roy (1987a) explained that her conceptual model is based on scientific and philosophical asumptions reflecting "holism, mutuality, control processes, activity, creativity, purpose, and value" (p. 43). The scientific assumptions were drawn from systems theory and Helson's adaptation level theory. Elaborating, Roy stated,

The systems theory assumptions focus primarily on holism, interdependence, control processes, information feedback, and, most importantly, the highly complex nature of living systems. Helson focused on all behavior as adaptive. He believed that this behavior is the function of both the stimulus coming in, how light or dark it is, how hot the room is, and the adaptation level. The process of responding positively as well as very actively is also significant from Helson's view. (p. 37)

The following specific scientific assumptions were explicated by Roy (1980):

1. The person is a bio-psycho-social being.
2. The person is in constant interaction with a changing environment.
3. To cope with a changing world, the person uses both innate and acquired mechanisms, which are biologic, psychologic, and social in origin.
4. Health and illness are one inevitable dimension of the person's life.
5. To respond positively to environmental changes, the person must adapt.
6. The person's adaptation is a function of the stimulus he is exposed to and his adaptation level.
7. The person's adaptation level is such that it comprises a zone indicating the range of stimulation that will lead to a positive response.
8. The person is conceptualized as having four modes of adaptation: physiologic needs, self-concept, role function, and interdependence relations. (pp. 180–182)

The philosophic assumptions upon which Roy's conceptual model was based encompass several values and beliefs associated with the general principles of humanism and veritivity. Humanism, according to Roy (1988), refers to "a broad movement in philosophy and psychology that recognizes the person and subjective dimensions of human experience as central to knowing and valuing (p. 29)." The tenets of humanism that are relevant to Roy's conceptual model are creative power, purposefulness, holism, subjectivity, and interpersonal relationships. In particular, Roy (1988) believes that the individual "(a) shares in creative power, (b) behaves purposefully, not in a sequence of cause and effect, (c) possesses intrinsic holism, and (d) strives to maintain integrity and to realize the need for relationships (p. 32)."

Roy (1984a) pointed out that nursing has always "been concerned about the value of the human person" (p. 36). She then described the linkage between humanism and her conceptual model. She stated,

> As humanistic nurses, we believe in the person's own creative power. Roy places emphasis on the person's own coping abilities. Nurses see processes moving purposefully and not merely as chains of cause and effect. Roy views adaptation as an ongoing purposive process. Nursing's holistic approach is rooted in humanism. Roy's theoretical work is attempting to describe persons' functioning holistically and to point out holistic approaches to nursing care of persons. Nursing accepts the humanistic approach of valuing other persons' opinions and viewpoints. . . . Nursing has long recognized the significance of interpersonal relationships. This humanistic value also is basic to the Roy Adaptation Model's nursing process. (p. 36)

Veritivity is a philosophical premise that asserts that "there is an absolute truth" (Roy, 1988, p. 29). Roy (1987a) explained,

> On a more global level, the primacy of the notion of integration re-
> flecting on holism, mutuality and control processes of the system,
> leads to the principle of "verativity," [sic] a term coined recently when
> speaking of values for science. It comes from the Latin word *veritas*,
> meaning truth. In the adaptive person, verativity [sic] reflects activity,
> creativity, unity, purpose, and value. (p. 45)

As a principle of human nature, veritivity "affirms a common purposefulness of human existence" (Roy, 1988, p. 30). More specifically,
Roy (1988) believes that "the individual in society is viewed in the
context of the (a) purposefulness of human existence, (b) unity of purpose of humankind, (c) activity and creativity for the common good,
and (d) value and meaning of life (p. 32)."

Roy (1970) stated that her conceptual model drew heavily from
the work of Helson (1964). She also drew from Levine (1966) and compared the concepts of her model with ideas put forth by Henderson
(1960), Nightingale (1859), and Peplau (1952). Many other scholars in
several disciplines were cited by Roy as she continued the development and refinement of her conceptual model. The numerous citations to existing works indicate that Roy used a deductive approach
to develop her model.

There are indications that Roy also used an inductive approach.
In particular, the identification of the adaptive modes, a major component of Roy's conceptual model, was accomplished through classification of "about 500 samples of behavior of patients collected by
nursing students over a period of several months in all clinical settings" (Roy, 1971, p. 255). The classification was based in part on
Strickler and LaSor's (1970) work on threats in crisis situations. The
modes were then compared with the typologies developed by Abdellah, Beland, Martin, and Matheney (1960) and McCain (1965).

Content of the Model: Concepts

Person

"Nursing," according to Roy (1984a), "may focus on an individual
person, the family or group, a community, or society" (p. 28). Recipients of nursing care may be sick or well and may or may not be adapting positively (Roy, 1980; Andrews & Roy, 1986).

The recipient of nursing care was specifically identified as an
adaptive system. System is defined as "a set of parts connected to
function as a whole for some purpose and does so by virtue of the interdependence of its parts" (Andrews & Roy, 1986, p. 18). Adaptive
"means that the human system has the capacity to adjust effectively
to changes in the environment and, in turn, affects the environment"
(Andrews & Roy, 1986, p. 22). The adaptive system is regarded as a
holistic system. "Holistic pertains to the idea that the human system

functions as a whole and is more than the mere sum of its parts" (Andrews & Roy, 1986, pp. 21–22). The holistic adaptive system is regarded as an open system (Roy, 1984a).

The adaptive system has two major internal control processes, called the regulator and the cognator subsystems (Roy, 1984a). These subsystems are viewed as innate or acquired coping mechanisms used by the adaptive system to respond to changing internal and external environmental stimuli. Andrews and Roy (1986) explained that "innate coping mechanisms are genetically determined or common to a species whereas acquired coping mechanisms are developed through processes such as learning" (p. 21). The regulator subsystem "receives input from the external environment and from changes in the person's internal state. It then processes the changes through neural-chemical-endocrine channels to produce responses" (Roy, 1984a, p. 31). More specifically,

> the internal and external stimuli are basically chemical or neural and act as inputs to the central nervous system and may be transduced into neural inputs. The spinal cord, brain stem, and autonomic reflexes act through effectors to produce automatic, unconscious effects on the body responses. The chemical stimuli in the circulation influence the endocrine glands to produce the appropriate hormone. The responsiveness of target organs or tissues then effects body responses. By some unknown process, the neural inputs are transformed into conscious perceptions in the brain. Eventually, this perception leads to psychomotor choices of response which activate a body response. These bodily responses, brought about through the chemical-neural-endocrine channels, are fed back as additional stimuli to the regulator. (Roy, 1984a, p. 31)

The cognator subsystem also receives input from external and internal stimuli that involve psychological, social, physical, and physiological factors, including regulator subsystem outputs. These stimuli then are processed through cognitive/emotive pathways (Roy, 1984a). More specifically,

> the internal and external stimuli trigger off four kinds of processes: perceptual/information processing, learning, judgment, and emotion. . . . Under perceptual/information processing, we may consider the person's internal activity of selective attention, coding, and memory. Learning involves such processes as imitation, reinforcement, and insight. The judgment process includes problem solving and decision making. Through the emotional pathways, the person uses defenses to seek relief and affective appraisal and attachment. (Roy, 1984a, p. 33)

Regulator and cognator activity is manifested through coping behavior in four adaptive (effector) modes. The four adaptive modes of the Roy Adaptation Model are the physiological mode, the self-concept mode, the role function mode, and the interdependence mode. The regulator subsystem is related primarily to the physiological mode and the cognator subsystem is related to all four modes (Roy & Roberts, 1981).

The four adaptive modes are predicated on the person's need for physiological integrity, psychic integrity, and social integrity (Roy, 1976a). The physiological mode deals with the need for physiological integrity. This mode encompasses five basic physiological needs and four regulator processes. The physiological needs, hierarchically arranged, are oxygenation, nutrition, elimination, activity and rest, and protection. The regulator processes are the senses, fluids and electrolytes, neurological functions, and endocrine functions. "The physiological mode," Andrews and Roy (1986) explained, "is associated with the way the person responds physically to stimuli from the environment. Behavior in this mode is the manifestation of the physiological activities of all the cells, tissues, organs, and systems comprising the human body" (p. 41).

The self-concept adaptive mode focuses on the need for psychic integrity. Self-concept is defined as "the composite of beliefs and feelings that a person holds about himself or herself at a given time" (Andrews & Roy, 1986, p. 42). Self-concept is formed from internal perceptions and perceptions of others and directs the person's behavior. This mode encompasses perceptions of the physical and the personal self. The physical self deals with body sensation and body image. Body sensation "applies to the ability to feel and to experience oneself as a physical being," and body image "applies to how one views oneself physically and one's appearance" (Andrews & Roy, 1986, p. 124). The personal self encompasses self-consistency, self-ideal, and the moral-ethical-spiritual self. "Self-consistency is that continuity of self over time, even though feelings change based on what is occurring in one's life. The self-ideal is what one expects of self and what one wants to accomplish. The moral-ethical[-spiritual] self involves spiritual values, the goodness of personal lives" (Roy, 1987a, p. 40).

The role function mode emphasizes the need for social integrity. Andrews and Roy (1986) regarded role as "the functioning unit of society," and defined the term as "a set of expectations about how a person occupying one position behaves toward a person occupying another position" (p. 42). They pointed out that the role function mode focuses on "the need to know who one is in relation to others so that one can act" (p. 42). Both instrumental and expressive behaviors related to role function are of interest. Roles are classified as primary, secondary, or tertiary in Roy's conceptual model. The primary role "determines the majority of behaviors engaged in by the person during a particular period of life. It is determined by age, sex, and developmental stage" (Andrews & Roy, 1986, p. 136). An example of a primary role is a 25-year-old young adult male. Secondary roles "are those that a person assumes to complete the tasks associated with a developmental stage and primary role. . . . Secondary roles are normally achieved positions and require specific role performance as opposed to primary qualities. They are typically stable and not readily relinquished since they are developed and mastered over a period of time" (Andrews & Roy, 1986, p. 137). Examples of secondary roles are husband, father, worker. Tertiary roles are "related primarily to secondary roles and represent ways in which individuals meet their role-associated obligations. . . . Tertiary roles are normally temporary in nature, freely chosen by the individual, and may include activities such as clubs or hobbies" (Andrews & Roy, 1986, p. 137). An example is the role of Little League baseball coach associated with the role of father.

The interdependence mode also emphasizes the need for social integrity. Interdependence is "a way of maintaining integrity that involves the willingness and ability to love, respect, and value others, and to accept and respond to love, respect, and value given by others" (Roy, 1987a, p. 41). The giving of love, respect, and value in interdependent relationships is called contributive behavior and the receiving of love, respect, and value is called receptive behavior (Andrews & Roy, 1986). The primary focus of the interdependence mode, according to Andrews and Roy (1986), is affectional adequacy, defined as "the feelings of security in nurturing relationships" (p. 43). Significant others and support systems are the two specific relationships of interest.

Environment

Roy (1984a) defined environment as "all conditions, circumstances, and influences surrounding and affecting the development and behavior of persons or groups" (p. 39). Environment is viewed as constantly changing and is divided into internal and external components. Culture, family, and growth and development are "significant factors that act as internal and external environment for the person" (Roy, 1984a, p. 39).

The internal and external environments are sources of inputs into the adaptive system. In this conceptual model, the inputs take the form of stimuli (Roy & Roberts, 1981). Following Helson (1964), Roy identified three classes of stimuli. The focal stimulus is "the one most immediately confronting the person and the one to which the person must make an adaptive response" (Roy, 1984a, p. 52). Contextual stimuli are "those contributing to the behavior caused or precipitated by the focal stimulus. They are all other stimuli present that affect the behavior being observed" (Roy, 1984a, p. 52). The residual stimuli are "factors that may be affecting behavior but whose effects are not validated" (Roy, 1984a, p. 54). Residual stimuli, such as beliefs, attitudes, traits, and cultural determinants, have an immeasurable effect on a situation.

Person and Environment

Further discussion of the environment requires consideration of the interaction between the person and the environment. Andrews and Roy (1986) explained,

> The changing environment stimulates the person to make adaptive responses. For human beings, life is never the same. It is constantly changing and representing new challenges. The person has the ability to make new responses to these changing conditions. As the environment changes, the person has the opportunity to continue to grow and develop and to enhance the meaning of life for self and others. (p. 7)

Roy (1984a) claimed that "the person's ability to respond positively, or to adapt, depends on the degree of change taking place and the state of the person coping with the change" (p. 37). She equated the degree of change with the focal stimulus, and the person's ability to respond positively with adaptation level. Drawing from Helson's (1964) work, Roy defined adaptation level as "a constantly changing point . . . which represents the person's own standard of the range of stimuli to which one can respond with ordinary adaptive responses" (pp. 27–28). Adaptation level is determined by the pooled effect of focal, contextual, and residual stimuli. Roy drew from Peak's (1955) work to explain that the adaptation level sets up a zone of adaptation, such that any stimuli falling within it will lead to a positive or adaptive response by the person, and any stimuli falling outside the zone will lead to a negative or ineffective response.

Roy (1984a) described adaptive responses as "those that promote the integrity of the person in terms of the goals of the human system: survival, growth, reproduction, and mastery" (p. 35). Ineffective responses are those "that do not contribute to these goals" (p. 49). Adaptive and ineffective responses, which are considered outputs from the adaptive system, encompass behaviors of the person that show coping mechanism activity (Andrews & Roy, 1986). In a cyclical manner, the responses then act as feedback, which is further input for the system (Roy & Roberts, 1981). Figure 9–1 illustrates the components of the person as an adaptive system.

Health

Health is defined by Roy (1984a) as "a state and a process of being and becoming an integrated and whole person" (p. 39). A whole per-

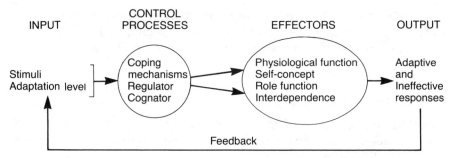

Figure 9–1. The person as an adaptive system. (From Roy, C. (1984): Introduction to nursing. An adaptation model (2nd ed., p. 30). Englewood Cliffs, NJ: Prentice-Hall, with permission.)

son, according to Andrews and Roy (1986), "is one with the highest possible fulfillment of human potential" (p. 8). They went on to explain that "a lack of integration" is "a lack of health" (p. 8).

Roy's definition of health is based on the notion that "adaptation is a process of promoting integrity, [which in turn] implies soundness or an unimpaired condition that can lead to completeness or unity" (Roy, 1984a, p. 39). Health then, "is a reflection of adaptation" (Andrews & Roy, 1986, p. 50).

Health is viewed as a dynamic concept, a process of being and becoming an integrated and whole person, in this conceptual model. Roy (1987a) maintained that her view of health is not consistent with the notion of the health-illness continuum, because "it is a limited view and reflects a given point in time on a continuum" (p. 42). She noted that being and becoming integrated and whole may occur throughout life. Even "dying individuals are going through that process of final being and becoming where they are integrating themselves" (pp. 42–43).

Roy's categorization of the person's responses to the changing environment as adaptive or ineffective indicates that health is viewed as a dichotomy. This point is underscored when taking into account the definition of adaptive responses as those promoting integrity of the person and the definition of ineffective responses as those not contributing to integrity.

Nursing

Roy (1976a) defined nursing as "a theoretical system of knowledge which prescribes a process of analysis and action related to the care of the ill or potentially ill person" (p. 3). Roy's conceptual model stipulates that a nurse is needed "when unusual stresses or weakened coping mechanisms make the person's usual attempts to cope ineffective" (Roy & Roberts, 1981, p. 45).

Roy distinguished nursing from medicine by noting that medicine focuses on biological systems and the person's disease, but nursing focuses on the person as a total being who responds to internal and external environmental stimuli (Roy, 1970; Roy & Roberts, 1981). This distinction is elaborated further when the goals of medicine and nursing are compared. According to Roy (1970), the physician's goal is "to move the patient along the continuum from illness to health" (p. 43). The goal of nursing "is to promote adaptation by the use of the nursing process, in each of the adaptive modes, thus contributing to health, quality of life, and dying with dignity" (Roy, 1987a, p. 43). Furthermore, "nursing aims to increase the person's adaptive response and to decrease ineffective responses" (Roy, 1984a, p. 37).

The goal of nursing was placed within the context of the overall goal of the health team in the following manner:

> The projected outcome [of nursing] is an adapted state in the patient which frees him to respond to other stimuli. This freeing of energy makes it possible for the goal of nursing to contribute to the overall goal of the health team, high-level wellness. When energy is freed from inadequate coping attempts, then it can promote healing and wellness. (Roy & Roberts, 1981, p. 45)

The Roy Adaptation Model includes a detailed nursing process, which was defined as "a problem-solving procedure for gathering data, identifying problems, selecting and implementing approaches, and evaluating results in relation to care of the ill or potentially ill person" (Roy, 1976a, p. 21). The nursing process encompasses six steps: assessment of behaviors, assessment of influencing factors (stimuli), nursing diagnosis, goal setting, selection of intervention approaches, and evaluation.

Assessment of behaviors, or first-level assessment, involves collection of data regarding the person's internal and external behavior. Behavior of particular interest to the nurse is "the person's responses to environmental changes that require further adaptive responses" (Roy, 1984a, p. 46). The methods of assessment were identified as direct observation of behavior; objective measurement of behavior using appropriate tools, such as paper and pencil instruments and measures of physiological parameters; and interviewing to obtain subjective reports (Roy, 1984a). Once the data are collected, the nurse must judge whether the behavior "is of concern to the nurse and/or to the person" (Roy, 1984a, p. 49). Furthermore, "the nurse determines, in collaboration with the person, whether the behavior is adaptive or ineffective" (Roy 1984a, p. 49). Judgments are based on comparison of the person's behavior with known norms signifying adaptation. In areas where norms have not been established, general signs of adaptation difficulty are used as a basis for comparison. These signs, according to Roy

(1984a), are "identified as pronounced regulator activity with cognator ineffectiveness" (p. 50). Some manifestations of pronounced regulator activity are increase in heart rate or blood pressure, tension, excitement, or loss of appetite. Manifestations of cognator ineffectiveness include faulty perceptual/information processing, ineffective learning, poor judgment, and inappropriate affect.

Roy (1984a) maintained that the person should actively participate in the judgment about the effectiveness of behavior. She stated,

> The person is often the best judge of whether or not behavior is effective in coping with a given stimuli. . . . The nurse should always take the person's observations of his or her own behavior into account in making a judgment about whether the behavior is adaptive or ineffective. The range of adaptive responses is wide. Norms are broad and circumstances change the judgment about whether a behavior is adaptive or ineffective. (p. 50)

Assessment of influencing factors, or second-level assessment, involves assessment of the factors that influence the behaviors of concern to the nurse and the person. Ineffective behaviors are of interest because the nurse wants to change these to adaptive behaviors, and adaptive behaviors are of interest because the nurse wants to maintain or enhance them. Furthermore, "in situations where all presenting behaviors appear adaptive, it may be necessary to carry out second-level assessment to identify potential threats to that adaptation" (K. Des Rosiers, cited in Roy, 1984a, p. 51). This step of the nursing process requires the nurse to prioritize the behaviors to be assessed. Roy (1984a) based her priorities on the goals of the adaptive system (survival, growth, reproduction, and mastery) and offered the following hierarchy of importance for assessment of behaviors:

1. Those that threaten the survival of the individual, family, group, or community
2. Those that affect the growth of the individual, family, group, or community
3. Those that affect the continuation of the human race or of society
4. Those that affect the attainment of full potential for the individual or group (p. 58)

Once priorities have been established, second-level assessment involves identification of the focal, contextual, and residual stimuli that influence the behaviors of interest and contribute to adaptive or ineffective responses. Roy (1984a) pointed out that the nurse can presume the influence of residual stimuli from theoretical knowledge and intuitive hunches. Residual stimuli become focal or contextual stimuli when their effects can be validated. Roy (1984a) advocated continued participation of the person in second-level assesment. She suggested using Orlando's (1961) deliberative nursing process to validate the relevant stimuli with the person. Thus, the nurse should share her ideas of influencing factors with the person and receive confirmation or discuss the person's perception of the situation until agreement is reached.

The next step of the nursing process is nursing diagnosis, defined as "the nurse's interpretation of the assessment data that have been compiled" (Roy, 1984a, p. 55). Three approaches to nursing diagnosis were given by Roy (1984a). One method is to cluster the behaviors and influencing factors within each of the adaptive modes and to name each cluster with a label from a beginning typology of adaptation problems identified by Roy (1973, 1976, 1984a). The current typology of adaptation problems is displayed in Table 9–1.

A second method is to again cluster the behaviors and influencing factors within each adaptive mode and to simply state the diagnosis as the behavior of concern with the most relevant influencing factors. This method "allows for the incompleteness of the typology of problems, and . . . it provides more specific indications for nursing interventions" (Roy, 1984a, p. 56). A third method is to summarize all

TABLE 9–1.   Typology of Common Adaptation Problems

Physiologic Mode	Self-Concept Mode
1. Oxygenation	1. Physical self
Hypoxia	Decreased sexual self-concept
Shock	Aggressive sexual behavior
Overload	Loss
2. Nutrition	2. Personal self
Malnutrition	Anxiety
Nausea	Powerlessness
Vomiting	Guilt
3. Elimination	Low self-esteem
Constipation	
Diarrhea	Role Function Mode
Flatulence	Role transition
Incontinence	Role distance
Urinary retention	Role conflict
4. Activity and rest	Role failure
Inadequate physical activity	
Potential disuse consequences	Interdependence Mode
Inadequate rest	Separation anxiety
Insomnia	Loneliness
Sleep deprivation	
Excessive rest	
5. Skin integrity	
Itching	
Dry skin	
Pressure sores	

From Roy, C. (1984). Introduction to nursing. An adaptation model (2nd ed., p. 56). Englewood Cliffs, NJ: Prentice-Hall, with permission.

behaviors across adaptive modes that are affected by the same stimuli. Roy (1984a) maintained that this method "recognizes the holistic functioning of the person and the interrelatedness of the adaptive modes" (pp. 56–57). Roy (1984a) pointed out that nursing diagnosis may be used for both adaptive and ineffective behaviors. She also noted that labels approved by the North American Nursing Diagnoses Association may be used "as they relate to developments within the adaptive modes of the Roy model" (p. 57). Regardless of the method and labels used, diagnoses are placed in a hierarchy of importance, using the priorities identified in the section on second-level assessment.

The fourth step of the nursing process is goal setting. The goal for nursing care is established from the behavioral description of the person's situation developed through first- and second-level assessments and nursing diagnosis. Goals are stated as behavioral outcomes of nursing intervention.

The fifth step of the nursing process is intervention, or selection of approaches. This step involves management of stimuli that were identified as influencing factors to achieve the stated goals for nursing care. Management encompasses increasing, decreasing, maintaining, removing, or otherwise altering or changing relevant focal and/or contextual stimuli (Andrews & Roy, 1986). The focal stimulus is selected for management whenever possible because it is the primary influence on the behaviors of interest. If it is not possible to alter the focal stimulus, contextual stimuli are to be managed to raise the adaptation level. Roy (1984a) advocated using the nursing judgment method outlined by McDonald and Harms (1966) as a basis for selection of which stimuli to change. Roy explained that the McDonald and Harms method

> is a way of listing possible approaches, then selecting the approach with the highest probability of achieving the valued goal. Combining this method with the Roy Adaptation Model, we can say that the various stimuli affecting patient behaviors are listed. Then the consequences of dealing with each stimuli are outlined. The probability of each consequence is determined. In addition, the values of the outcomes of the approach are judged. The approach with the highest probability of reaching the valued goal can then be selected. (p. 60)

The sixth and final step of the nursing process is evaluation of the effectiveness of nursing intervention. The criterion for effectiveness of nursing intervention is whether the desired goal was attained, that is, whether the person exhibited adaptive behavior after the nursing intervention was performed. The end result of this step is an update of the nursing care plan. Roy (1984a) explained the cyclical aspect of the nursing process:

When the nurse determines the effects of intervention, she returns to the first step of the nursing process. The nurse looks more closely at behaviors that continue to be ineffective and reassesses the factors influencing these. For behaviors that have become adaptive, with no threat of returning to ineffective, the nurse may delete this behavior as a priority of nursing concern. For behaviors that are still ineffective, influencing stimuli are reassessed to see if the nursing approach should be modified by managing another stimulus. (p. 61)

Andrews and Roy (1986) pointed out that the nursing process is ongoing, with steps overlapping one another for various behaviors:

> In fact, many of the steps occur simultaneously. The nurse may be assessing behavior in one area while proceeding with a nursing intervention in another area. She may be assessing behavior and stimuli at the same time or discussing goals with the patient while she is evaluating the attainment of goals in another area. (p. 104)

The nursing process for Roy's Adaptation Model is summarized in Table 9–2.

**TABLE 9–2. Summary of the Nursing Process
for Roy's Adaptation Model**

I. Assessment of behaviors (first level assessment)
  A. Methods used to collect data
    1. Observation of the person's responses using all senses (sight, sound, touch, taste, smell)
    2. Objective measurement of the person's responses
    3. Interview the person
  B. Areas of data collection
    1. Physiological mode
      a. Oxygenation
      b. Nutrition
      c. Elimination
      d. Activity and rest
      e. Protection
      f. The senses
      g. Fluid and electrolytes
      h. Neurological functions
      i. Endocrine functions
    2. Self-concept mode
      a. Physical self
      b. Self-consistency
      c. Self-ideal
      d. Moral-ethical-spiritual self
    3. Role function
      a. Primary role
      b. Secondary roles
      c. Tertiary roles

TABLE 9–2. *Continued*

    4. Interdependence mode
      a. Contributive behavior
      b. Receptive behavior
  C. Judgment of behaviors
    1. Adaptive or ineffective responses
    2. Criteria for judgment
      a. Comparison of behavior with norms signifying adaptation
      b. Regulator mechanism activity
      c. Cognator mechanism effectiveness
      d. The person perceives behavior as adaptive or ineffective
II. Assessment of influencing factors (second level assessment)
  A. Use criteria to set priorities for further assessment of the person's behaviors
    1. Behaviors that threaten the survival of the individual, family, group, or community
    2. Behaviors that affect the growth of the individual, family, group, or community
    3. Behaviors that affect the continuation of the human race or of society
    4. Behaviors that affect the attainment of full potential for the individual or group
  B. Methods used to determine influencing factors
    1. Observation
    2. Objective measurement
    3. Interview the person
    4. Validate hunch about relevant stimuli with the person
  C. Influencing factors
    1. Focal stimulus
    2. Contextual stimuli
      a. Genetic makeup
      b. Sex
      c. Developmental stage
      d. Drugs
      e. Alcohol
      f. Tobacco
      g. Self-concept
      h. Role functions
      i. Interdependence
      j. Social interaction patterns
      k. Coping mechanisms and styles
      l. Physical and emotional stress
      m. Cultural orientation and ethnicity
      n. Religion
      o. Physical environment
      p. Socioeconomic standing
      q. Family structure and tasks
    3. Residual stimuli
      a. Beliefs
      b. Attitudes
      c. Traits
      d. Cultural determinants

TABLE 9–2. *Continued*

III. Nursing diagnosis
   A. Three approaches
      1. Cluster behaviors and influencing factors within each adaptive mode and name each cluster using typology of adaptation problems
      2. Cluster behaviors and influencing factors within each adaptive mode and state diagnosis as behavior with most relevant influencing factor(s)
      3. Summarize behaviors across adaptive modes that are affected by the same stimulus(i)
   B. Arrange diagnoses in order of priority using criteria in II.A.
IV. Goal setting
   A. Statement of behavioral outcomes of nursing intervention
   B. Determine that the person agrees with goal
 V. Nursing Intervention
   A. Goal of nursing intervention is to manage stimuli so they fall in the person's zone of adaptation
   B. Forms of management of stimuli
      1. Increase stimuli
      2. Decrease stimuli
      3. Maintain stimuli
      4. Remove stimuli
   C. Priorities
      1. Manage focal stimulus first if possible
      2. Manage contextual next
   D. Selection of nursing intervention approach
      1. List possible approaches
      2. Outline consequences of management of each stimulus
      3. Determine probability for each consequence
      4. Judge value of outcomes of each approach
      5. Share options with the person
      6. Select approach with highest probability of reaching valued goal
VI. Evaluation
   A. Methods used
      1. Observation
      2. Objective measurement
      3. Interview the person
   B. Criteria for judgment of effectiveness of nursing intervention
      1. Goal attained or not attained
      2. Person does or does not manifest behavior stated in goal

Adapted from Roy, C. (1984a). Introduction to nursing. An adaptation model (2nd ed., pp. 42–63). Englewood Cliffs, NJ: Prentice-Hall.

Content of the Model: Propositions

The metaparadigm concepts of person, environment, and health are linked in the following statements:

> The person encounters adaptation problems in changing environments, especially in situations of health and illness. (Roy & Roberts, 1981, p. 45)

> According to the Roy Adaptation Model, the changing environment stimulates the person to make adaptive changes. (Andrews & Roy, 1986, p. 7)

The metaparadigm concepts of person, health, and nursing are linked in the following statements:

> Since the Roy Adaptation Model views the person as an adaptive system, the goal of nursing within this model can be stated most simply as: to promote adaptation. (Roy, 1984a, p. 36)

> Nursing aims to increase the person's adaptive responses and to decrease ineffective responses. (Roy, 1984a, p. 37)

The linkage of all four metaparadigm concepts are presented in this statement:

> Persons or adaptive systems interact with environment and move toward the goal of adaptation and health. The nursing process based on the model influences that movement. (Roy, 1984a, p. 40)

Areas of Concern

The area of concern addressed by Roy's conceptual model is problems in adaptation to the changing environment. A typology of common adaptation problems identified by Roy (1984a) was listed in Table 9–1. The labels for problems presented in Table 9–1 "represent adaptation problems currently identified as commonly recurring according to the Roy Adaptation Model" (pp. 55–56). The sources of problems in adaptation are stimuli from the internal and external environments.

EVALUATION OF ROY'S ADAPTATION MODEL

This section presents an evaluation of Roy's Adaptation Model. The evaluation is based on the results of the analysis of this conceptual model as well as on publications by others who have used or commented on Roy's work.

Explication of Assumptions

Roy has presented the assumptions upon which her conceptual model is based in a clear and explicit manner. Furthermore, she has made clear distinctions between the scientific and philosophical assumptions. It must be pointed out, however, that the scientific assumptions actually are propositions that define, describe, and link the concepts of the conceptual model. Strictly speaking, then, these statements are not assumptions upon which the model was based.

It is obvious that Roy assumes people are integrated wholes capable of action. It also is obvious that Roy values the active participation of persons in their nursing care. She noted that although such action may not always be possible, as in the case of infants and unconscious or suicidal patients, the nurse "is constantly aware of the active responsibility of the patient to participate in his own care when he is able to do so" (Roy & Roberts, 1981, p. 47).

Comprehensiveness of Concepts and Propositions

Roy addressed each of the metaparadigm concepts adequately for the level of abstraction of a conceptual model. Person was fully defined and described. Although some difficulty has been reported in distinguishing the adaptive mode to which a particular behavior belongs, especially in the self-concept, role function, and interdependence modes (Wagner, 1976), recent revisions in the conceptual model have begun to clarify the focus of each adaptive mode. Roy (1987a) explained, "Through many revisions with input from educators, clinicians, and theory critics, the physiological mode has been reorganized, and can now be used for nursing assessment and the organization of curriculum content" (p. 39). She went on to say, "The content changes in the interdependence mode have been significant over the last couple of years. This allows interdependence to be distinguished from self-concept and role function" (p. 41).

Environment was defined sufficiently for a conceptual model. The distinction between the internal and external environments, however, is not always clear. Acknowledging this, Roy and Roberts (1981) commented: "Further clarification of environment as distinct from internal stimuli awaits additional theoretical work on the model" (p. 43). Additional work also is needed to describe the nature of environmental change. Further development of the concept of environment was undertaken by Randall, Poush Tedrow, and Van Landingham (1982). Roy (1982) acknowledged that the introduction of the ideas of transaction and perception in their treatment of environment has expanded her model.

Health is clearly defined and is discussed in terms of adaptation, adaptation level, zone of adaptation, and adaptive and ineffective responses. Given that Roy (1987a) regarded the health-illness continuum as a limited viewpoint, it is not surprising that she gave no explicit definitions of wellness or illness. It must be inferred that adaptive responses signify wellness and ineffective responses signify illness. The exact meaning of these terms with regard to health state needs to be clarified to avoid confusion and misinterpretations. This is especially so as Roy (1984a) has labeled adaptive responses as positive and ineffective responses as negative.

The concept of nursing is defined and described clearly. The goal of nursing is articulated and the nursing process is described in considerable detail. Furthermore, most of the criteria for nursing process established by Walker and Nicholson (1980) have been met. Judgments concerning the adaptability of the person's behavior are based on explicit criteria drawn from existing scientific knowledge. The process is dynamic in that the results of the last step, evaluation, lead to the first step, assessment of behaviors, and updating of the nursing care plan and in that various steps may occur simultaneously as different behaviors are considered. Roy intended that her model, and hence the nursing process, be applicable in a variety of settings and with all recipients of nursing care: individuals, families, groups, communities, and society as a whole. Documentation of this criterion has been provided by the many nurses whose work with Roy's conceptual model are described in the section on social utility. Roy's insistence that the person be an active participant in the decision-making aspects of the nursing process attests to her concern for ethical standards of nursing practice. Furthermore, the nursing process is consistent with the American Nurses' Association Standards of Practice (Roy & Roberts, 1981). Moreover, the Roy Adaptation Model nursing process is consistent with scientific findings on human behavior. This is documented by Roy's (1984a) statement that nursing science provides the knowledge of what behaviors to observe when making assessments. It is also documented by selection of nursing intervention approaches based on information about the probability of their effectiveness.

A major concern in relation to this last criterion is the fact that Roy's model was derived from Helson's (1964) work on adaptation, which was limited to investigation of the responses of the retina of the eye to environmental stimuli. The generalizability of Helson's findings to the person as a totality has not been firmly established. Thus, the credibility of the basic premise of the model—the person as an adaptive system—has not yet been supported.

Logical Congruence

World Views

The Roy Adaptation Model reflects an organismic view of the world. Roy repeatedly emphasized the need to view the person as an holistic adaptive system that "functions as a whole and is more than the mere sum of its parts" (Andrews & Roy, 1986, pp. 21–22). Roy also emphasized the active nature of the person. This is seen in the description of adaptive as meaning that "the human system has the capacity to adjust effectively to changes in the environment and, in turn, affects the environment" (Andrews & Roy, 1986, p. 22). The active nature of the person also is seen in the description of the person's active participation in the nursing process, as noted in the following comment:

> According to this nursing model, the person is to be respected as an active participant in his care. It is the information that the patient shares with the nurse that forms the assessment. The goal arrived at is one of mutual agreement between nurse and patient. Interventions are the options that the nurse provides for the patient. (Roy & Roberts, 1981, p. 47)

Roy and Roberts (1981) have begun to translate the essentially mechanistic idea of adaptation to an organismic viewpoint. They stated, "This notion of adaptation does not negate the fact that humans do not merely respond to stimuli in the environment, but can take the initiative to change the environment" (p. 45). They did acknowledge, however, that further work in this area is needed. Furthermore, Roy (1988) maintained that her conceptual model does not reflect a mechanistic viewpoint. She explained that "the complexities and subtleties of the process whereby the person takes in and responds to the environment preclude such a behavioristic interpretation" of her use of the terms stimuli and behavior (p. 32).

The Roy Adaptation Model also reflects a change view of the world. In fact, Roy (1978a) emphatically denied that the model promotes the status quo or is a static view. She stated, "Coping means the person continually raises his adaptation level." It may be inferred, then, that change is a natural and desirable condition for the person. The continuous nature of change was addressed explicitly in the model's description of life and the environment as constantly changing. The change viewpoint also is reflected in the definition of adaptive responses as those that promote growth. This world view is further demonstrated in Roy's (1978a) assumption that "the person as a totality has great potential for self-actualization."

Classification of the Model

Roy (1980) maintained that her model "can be viewed primarily as a systems model though it also contains interactionist levels of analysis" (p. 179). Examination of the content of the model revealed that this is an accurate classification, although the systems characteristics of the model were not developed in any detail prior to the publication of Roy and Roberts's (1981) book.

The systems model characteristic of system was addressed in the designation of the person as an open adaptive system. The subsystems were identified as the regulator and cognator mechanisms. These two subsystems were linked through the process of perception (Roy & Roberts, 1981).

Environment was addressed in terms of the internal and external environments. The relationship between the adaptive system and its environment was described in terms of the influences of the environment on the adaptive system and the system's capacity to alter the environment.

The systems model characteristic of boundary was not addressed in Roy's conceptual model. The characteristic of tension, stress, strain, and conflict is addressed in the form of focal, contextual, and residual stimuli from the internal and external environments. These stimuli are the adaptive system inputs and represent influences on system behavior. The function of the stimuli was made explicit in Roy and Roberts's (1981) theoretical development of the adaptation. They stated:

> The process of adaptation can be described as stressors, or focal stimuli, being mediated by contextual and residual factors . . . to partially produce the interaction called stress. (p. 55)

Roy and Roberts (1981) went on to explain that the regulator and cognator act as coping mechanisms whose actions result in an adaptive or ineffective response. It may be inferred that the response results in tension reduction, although this point is not clear.

The characteristic of equilibrium was addressed by Roy and Roberts (1981) in the following statement:

> Helson's work points to adaptation as a dynamic state of equilibrium involving both heightened and lowered responses brought about by autonomic and cognitive processes triggered by internal and external stimuli. (p. 54)

Input, output, and feedback characteristics of systems model also were addressed by the Roy Adaptation Model. Inputs to the adaptive system "come both externally from the environment outside the person and internally from the self" (Roy, 1984a, p. 31), in the form of focal, contextual, and residual stimuli. The outputs from the adaptive system are adaptive and ineffective responses. Roy and Roberts (1981) explained that these responses "act as feedback which is further input for the person as a system" (p. 43).

Characteristics of interaction models also are evident in the Roy Adaptation Model. The role function adaptive mode deals with the social integrity of the person. The characteristic of perception was incorporated in the discussion of the regulator and cognator mechanisms. In particular,

> Inputs to the regulator are transformed into perceptions. Perception is a process of the cognator. The responses following perception are feedback into both the cognator and regulator. (Roy & Roberts, 1981, p. 67)

Communication was not directly addressed in the model. Role and self-concept were explicitly addressed through the adaptive modes of role function and self-concept. In fact, these modes were deliberately developed within the context of the interactionist viewpoint (Roy, 1980).

Meleis (1985) placed Roy's conceptual model in her outcomes category. Marriner (1986) placed Roy's model in the systems category. Stevens (1984) regarded Roy's conceptual model as an example of her intervention category. No rationales were given for these categorizations.

Generation and Testing of Theory

Roy's Adaptation Model has generated a general theory of the person as an adaptive system and individual theories of the four adaptive modes: physiological, self-concept, role function, and interdependence. These theories were presented by Roy and Roberts (1981). It should be noted that Roy (1984a, 1987a) has pointed out that her distinctions between conceptual models and theories are based on form and function rather than on levels of abstraction, as is the case in this book. However, the work presented by Roy and Roberts clearly is directed toward development of middle-range theories as defined in this book.

The theory of the person as an adaptive system considers the person holistically. The major concepts are system, adaptation, regulator subsystem, and cognator subsystem (Roy & Roberts, 1981). The regulator and cognator subsystems are explained in considerable detail through sets of propositions. An example of a regulator subsystem proposition is: "Internal and external stimuli are basically chemical or neural; chemical stimuli may be transduced into neural inputs to the central nervous system" (Roy & Roberts, 1981, p. 62). One proposition dealing with the cognator subsystem is: "The optimum amount and clarity of input of internal and external stimuli positively influences the adequacy of selective attention, coding, and memory" (Roy & Roberts, 1981, p. 65).

The theory dealing with the physiological mode applies the propositions from the regulator subsystem to physiological needs. The theory encompasses adaptive and ineffective regulatory responses related to exercise and rest, nutrition, elimination, fluid and electrolytes, oxygen and circulation, temperature, the senses, and the endocrine system. Roy and Roberts (1981) pointed out that by considering regulator activity, they avoided exploration of biological systems, which they viewed as the focus of medicine.

The theories dealing with the psychosocial modes of self-concept, role function, and interdependence consider these modes as systems "through which the regulator and cognator subsystems act to promote adaptation" (Roy & Roberts, 1981, p. 248). Each theory describes the relevant system in terms of its wholeness, subsystems, relation of parts, inputs, outputs, and self-regulation and control.

All four adaptive mode theories were explicated further in a series of propositions. One proposition taken from each theory follows:

> Theory of physiological needs: The magnitude of the internal and external stimuli will positively influence the magnitude of the physiological response of an intact system. (Roy & Roberts, 1981, p. 91)
>
> Theory of self-concept: The level of feelings of adequacy positively influences the quality of presentation of self. (Roy & Roberts, 1981, p. 255)
>
> Theory of role function: The level of adequacy of role taking positively influences the level of role mastery. (Roy & Roberts, 1981, p. 267)
>
> Theory of interdependence: Adequacy of seeking nurturance and nurturing positively influences interdependence. (Roy & Roberts, 1981, p. 277)

Roy and Roberts (1981) derived a sample hypothesis for each theory. For example, the hypothesis derived from the theory of interdependence states: "If the nurse provides time and space for private family visits, the patient will demonstrate more appropriate attention-seeking behavior" (Roy & Roberts, 1981, p. 280). The hypotheses have not yet been tested empirically. However, Roy and Roberts recognized the need for a systematic program of research to test the sample hypotheses as well as other hypotheses that could be derived from the theories. They also recognized the need to further develop and test the general theory of the person as an adaptive system. They noted:

> We must look at the theory of the adaptive person to further explain the interrelatedness of the adaptive modes. In this process we must also search for multivariable and nonlinear relationships. Cognator and regulator processes must be studied to discover the proposed hierarchy of processes. (p. 289)

Furthermore, as Roy and Roberts (1981) pointed out, nursing practice theory must be developed within the context of Roy's Adaptation Model. That is, theories need to be formulated to explain and predict the effects of specific nursing interventions on patients' adaptive responses.

Other aspects of Roy's conceptual model have been subject to scrutiny. Hammond, Roberts, and Silva's (1983) work tested the contention of Roy's conceptual model that both first- and second-level assessments are needed to make accurate nursing diagnoses. Their findings, which supported the hypothesis that nurses who used first-level assessment data would make as many accurate nursing diagnoses as those using both first- and second-level assessment, suggested that Roy's contention may be invalid. However, as Silva (1987a) pointed out, "this conclusion must be tempered by the small sample size and the difficulty in operationally defining accurate nursing diagnoses" (p. 234).

Social Considerations

Social Congruence

Roy's conceptual model is generally congruent with societal expectations of nursing care. Consumers who expect to have input into their nursing care should find this model consistent with their views. Moreover, the model's emphasis on adaptation to a constantly changing environment is congruent with many people's perspective of the world today as a place of turmoil and rapid change. However, as with other conceptual models that include a focus on the well person, Roy's model may not be entirely congruent with some people's expectations of nursing care. This would be especially so when the nurse's action is directed toward reinforcement of already adaptive behaviors.

Social Significance

The social significance of Roy's Adaptation Model is beginning to be established. Mastal, Hammond, and Roberts (1982) reported that use of Roy's model resulted in increased patient satisfaction. Although they did not present empirical evidence to support their claim, they noted that studies designed to determine patient satisfaction with nursing care are in progress. Moreover, Hammond, Hepner, Mastal, and Roberts (personal communication, June 30, 1982) noted that the staff who used the model at the National Hospital for Orthopaedics and Rehabilitation in Arlington, Virginia, "Demonstrate growth in professional practice which can only benefit all health consumers."

Furthermore, Hoch (1987) studied the effects of a treatment protocol derived from Roy's conceptual model on depression and life satisfaction in a sample of retired individuals. She found that the Roy protocol group had lower depression scores and higher life satisfaction scores than a control group who received nursing intervention that was not based on an explicit conceptual model. Although the logical connection between depression and life satisfaction and the adaptive modes of Roy's conceptual model might be questioned, Hoch's study represents the beginning of the empirical work that is needed to determine the credibility of conceptual models of nursing.

Social Utility

The utility of Roy's conceptual model for nursing research, practice, education, and administration is fully documented, as can be seen in the following discussion as well as in the annotated bibliography at the end of this chapter. This conceptual model is being used by nurses throughout the United States and in other countries, including Canada and Switzerland (Roy, personal communication, May 15, 1982). Furthermore, books related to Roy's conceptual model have been published by Randall, Push Tedrow, and Van Landingham (1982) and Rambo (1984).

The Roy Adaptation Model has proved useful as a guide for nursing research. Rules for research are being formulated, as is evident in the following statement by Roy (1987a):

> Research based on the Roy model involves inquiry into basic life processes and how nursing enhances those processes. Research based on the model develops basic science, as well as a practice discipline. The research focuses on persons or groups adapting and on those adaptive processes that affect health status. (p. 44)

Rules for research also are evident in Roy's (1980) discussion of directions for further research related to her model. She stated:

> Some assumptions about the model should be validated, for example, the assumption that the person has four modes of adaptation. Assumed values, particularly the value concerning the uniqueness of nursing, need to be made more explicit, and perhaps should also be supported. The model's goal, patiency, source of difficulty, and intervention in terms of focus and mode are all replete with possibilities for further clarification. A particularly fruitful field for study is the patient's use of adaptive mechanisms and the nurse's support of these in each of the adaptive modes. (p. 188)

Silva and Sorrell (1987) identified several doctoral dissertations related to Roy's Adaptation Model, including those by Beckerman (1984), Cohen (1980), Dahlen (1980), Holcombe (1986), Kiker (1983), Pollock (1982), Scherubel (1986), Schmidt (1983), Trentini (1986), Wilson (1984), and Zonka (1980). Furthermore, Roy's (1977) and Bean's (1988) doctoral dissertations were derived from Roy's conceptual model.

Published reports of research based on Roy's conceptual model include instrument development work, studies of patients' responses to various clinical problems, and studies of the effects of nursing interventions on patients' adaptation. Research instruments that have been derived from Roy's conceptual model include Idle's (1978) tool for measuring self-perceived adaptation level of elderly clients, Roy's (1979b) tools to measure hospitalized patients' perception of powerlessness and their perceptions of their decision-making activities, Lewis, Firsich, and Parsell's (1978, 1979) tool to measure health outcomes of nursing care for adult cancer patients receiving chemotherapy, and Fawcett, Tulman, and Myers's (1988) questionnaire to measure recovery of functional status after childbirth.

Some studies have focused on patients' responses to various clinical situations. Roy (1978b) explored the relationship between patients' adaptation to focal stimuli and their emotional feelings of distress during hospitalization and on the day before discharge. Fawcett (1981b) classified mothers' and fathers' responses to the cesarean birth of their infants according to need deficits and excesses in each of the four adaptive modes. Kehoe (1981) identified and classified the needs of postpartum cesarean birth mothers in the four adaptive modes. Farkas (1981) identified problems in adaptation for elderly persons and their significant others. Smith, Garvis, and Martinson (1983) identified the adaptive strengths of child with cancer and their parents. Francis, Turner, and Johnson (1983) described the effects of domestic animal visitation on nursing home residents' behavior. Pollock (1986) reported patients' physiological and psychosocial responses to chronic illness. Munn and Tichy (1987) reported their findings of nurses' perceptions of stressors in a pediatric intensive care unit. Silva (1987b) identified the needs of spouses of surgical patients. Tulman and Fawcett (1988) described the differences in recovery of functional ability after childbirth for women who had vaginal deliveries and those who had cesarean deliveries.

Other published studies have focused on the effects of nursing interventions on adaptation. Leonard (1975) investigated psychiatric patients' attitudes toward nursing interventions. Nolan (1977) explored the relationship between nursing interventions in the operating room and postoperative patients' reports of the quality of their care. Guzzetta (1979) studied the effect of a teaching program on patient learning. Norris, Campbell, and Brenkert (1982) evaluated the effect of nursing procedures on transcutaneous oxygen tension in premature infants. Fawcett and Burritt (1985) and Fawcett and Henklein (1987) reported the results of field tests of an antenatal education program designed to prepare expectant parents for unplanned cesarean childbirth. Shannahan and Cotrell (1985) and Cottrell and Shannahan (1986, 1987) studied the effects of using a birth chair on duration of second stage labor, as well as maternal and fetal outcomes.

Roy (1987b) has conducted research to determine patients' responses to surgery for acoustic neuroma. The data were analyzed in relation to the four adaptive modes of the Roy conceptual model. Furthermore, Roy (1987b) has developed a theoretical framework of cognitive processing and is conducting research on patients with head injuries to test the theory. One study described cognitive processing in patients with minor and moderate head injuries. Another study tested a nursing intervention protocol for these patients. Roy indicated that future research will focus on descriptions of cognitive processing in patients with severe head injuries and development of intervention protocols for these patients.

The Roy Adaptation Model has documented utility for nursing practice. Roy (1987a) noted that her conceptual model can direct nursing practice. Her statement regarding the influence of the model on practice presents implications for rules for nursing practice. She commented,

> As a practice discipline, nursing focuses on nursing's function of promoting adaptation, that is, nursing diagnoses, interventions, and outcomes for persons or groups. Nursing as a practice discipline can be seen from the point of view of the role of the nurse. Model-based practice helps look at how nursing models are taught. It sheds light on the content of nursing. Implementing the model of nursing care in whole health care systems will require another area of expertise both in implementation and in evaluation of the outcomes. Some of the outcomes are important in relation to what the model does for nursing, such as increasing autonomy, accountability, and professionalism in general, and in changing relationships with other disciplines. (p. 44)

Roy (1971) outlined the use of her model in practice and described its application in the nursing care of a diabetic teenager and a postoperative patient who had had gynecological surgery. Gordon (1974) used Roy's nursing process format in the care of a 70-year-old male patient who had suffered a myocardial infarction. She described a nursing care plan that encompassed the first 2 days of the patient's care in the coronary care unit, structured according to the four adaptive modes. Downey (1974) applied Roy's model to the care of a 27-year-old Mexican-American woman who delivered an infant in respiratory distress. Wagner (1976) described application of Roy's conceptual model in many acute care and outpatient settings. Starr (1980) structured care of the dying client according to Roy's model. She emphasized the need to identify the clients' adaptive behaviors, relevant stimuli, and appropriate nursing interventions for these individuals. Schmitz (1980) applied Roy's conceptual model in a community setting. She described the home nursing care of a family whose members included a 23-year-old mother, her 6-year-old son, 5-year-old twin daughters, a 2-month-old son, and the children's grandmother. Janelli (1980) used the nursing process of Roy's conceptual model to describe nursing care for elderly patients. Kehoe (1981) used Roy's model to identify the nursing care needs of the postpartum cesarean mother. Fawcett (1981a) applied the model to the nursing care of cesarean fathers. Limandri (1986) described the use of Roy's model for care of abused women. Giger, Bower, and Miller (1987) used Roy's conceptual model to guide care of a 23-year-old man who had been severely injured when he was thrown from and pinned under a farm mower. They developed a detailed nursing care plan that reflected the nursing process of Roy's model. Leuze and McKenzie (1987) systematically evaluated the effect of the use of a preoperative assessment tool based on Roy's model on nurses' knowledge of patients' physiological and psychosocial needs. Nash (1987) used Roy's model to develop a nursing care plan for children with Kawasaki disease. Sirignano (1987) explained the nursing care of patients experiencing cardiomyopathy during the peripartum period within the context of Roy's model.

The development of a conceptual-theoretical system of knowledge for nursing practice is illustrated by Galligan's (1979) work. She combined the Roy model with knowledge of child development and children's responses to hospitalization and surgery to formulate a nursing care plan for hospitalized children. A special feature of the care plan was its division into four stages—prehospitalization, preoperative state, postoperative stage, and discharge. Another conceptual-theoretical system of knowledge for nursing practice is illustrated by Miles and Carter's (1983) work. They combined the basic elements of Roy's conceptual model with theories of stress to develop a format for assessment of stress experienced by parents whose children are in intensive care units.

Roy (1983a, 1983b, 1983c) expanded her conceptual model to encompass nursing care of the family. She explained how the model could be used in the care of the expectant family and for a family that included an adolescent with diabetes. Whall (1986) constructed a conceptual-theoretical system of knowledge by reformulating and linking the theory of strategic family therapy with Roy's conceptual model. Roy (1984b) also expanded her model for use in community health nursing.

The utility of Roy's conceptual model for nursing education is well documented and rules for nursing education are beginning to be formulated. Some rules were suggested by Roy (1979) in her discussion of the sequence of content in nursing courses at Mount St. Mary's College Department of Nursing in Los Angeles, California. The curriculum content is based on Roy's conceptual model. The vertical strands of the curriculum focus on theory and practice. The theory strand encompasses content on the adapting person, health/illness, and stress/disruption. The practice strand emphasizes nursing management. The horizontal strands include nursing process and student adaptation/leadership. Additional discussion of curriculum content was presented by Andrews and Roy (1986), who also included suggestions for teaching-learning activities. The Roy Adaptation Model is appropriate for use in hospital-based schools of nursing, community colleges, and universities. Thus, the model may be used to guide curricula for diploma, associate degree, and baccalaureate and higher degree programs. The requirements for admission to the nursing programs in these settings would specify the rule regarding characteristics of students.

The widespread interest in using this model in educational programs is attested to by three conferences that were held for faculty members who planned to use or were already using the model as a basis for curriculum development in their schools. The first and second conferences were held at Alverno College in Milwaukee, Wisconsin, in 1978 and 1979. The third conference was held at Mount St. Mary's College in Los Angeles, California, in 1981.

Roy (personal communication, May 15, 1982) provided a list of schools of nursing where she or a faculty member from Mount Saint Mary's College "have made consultant visits and there is some evidence of follow-through with curriculum development." The nursing programs are at Cerritos Community College in Cerritos, California; Golden West College in Huntington Park, California; Mount St. Mary's College in Los Angeles, California; Point Loma College in San Diego, California; Harbor Community College in San Pedro, California; Wesley Passavant School of Nursing in Chicago, Illinois; Kansas State College in Pittsburg, Kansas; Maryland General Hospital in Baltimore, Maryland; Graceland College in Independence, Missouri; Northwest Missouri State University in Kirksville; William Patterson College in Wayne, New Jersey; Central State College in Edmond, Oklahoma; the University of Tulsa in Tulsa, Oklahoma; the University of Portland in Portland, Oregon; Widener University in Chester, Pennsylvania; Edinboro State College in Edinboro, Pennsylvania; Villa Maria College in Erie, Pennsylvania; Community College of Philadelphia, in Pennsylvania; the University of Texas at Arlington and at Austin; Alverno College and Columbia Hospital in Milwaukee, Wisconsin; Royal Alexander Hospital in Edmonton and the University of Calgary in Calgary, both in Alberta, Canada; Health Sciences Centre in Winnipeg, Manitoba, Canada; Vanier College in Montreal, Quebec, Canada; and Ecole Genevoise D Infirmiere, Le Bon Secours, in Geneva, Switzerland. Roy (personal communication, May 15, 1982) commented that in addition to these schools, "many other schools throughout the United States, Canada and abroad have implemented the Roy Adaptation Model in various ways without our direct consultation." Other schools of nursing that have used Roy's conceptual model were identified by Asay and Ossler (1984). These nursing programs are at California State University in Hayward and in Sacramento; Southern Connecticut State University in New Haven; Florida Agricultural and Mechanical University in Tallahassee; Olivet Nazarene College in Kankakee, Illinois; the University of Evansville in Evansville, Indiana; Fort Hays State University in Hays, Kansas; Pittsburg State University in Pittsburg, Kansas; Michigan State University in East Lansing and Eastern Michigan University in Ypsilanti; Moorhead State University in Moorhead, Minnesota; Mount Saint Mary College in Newburgh, New York; City College of the City University of New York; the University of North Carolina at Greensboro; Minot State College in Minot, South Dakota;

East Central Oklahoma State University in Ada; Millersville University in Millersville, Pennsylvania; Baylor University in Dallas, Texas; Westminster College in Salt Lake City, Utah; the American University in Washington D.C.; and Humacao University College in Humacao, Puerto Rico. Roy's conceptual model also has been used as a curriculum guide at the University of Minnesota School of Nursing in Minneapolis and at the University of North Carolina at Charlotte.

Brower and Baker (1976) described the use of Roy's model in the geriatric nurse practitioner program at the University of Miami in Miami, Florida. The four adaptive modes served as the organizing focus for this 10-month continuing education program. The authors contended that the adaptive modes permitted differentiation of nursing practice from medical practice. They explained,

> If we conceptualize role function, self-concept, and interdependence as existing within the domain of nursing, and pathophysiology and treatment modalities as being domains shared by medicine and nursing and relevant to the physiological mode, we can formulate a nurse practitioner curriculum that provides for both overlap and distinction between the two roles. (p. 687)

Knowlton, Goodwin, Moore, Alt-White, Guarino, and Pyne (1983) described the development of a nursing curriculum based on Roy's conceptual model. They outlined the use of the model for various systems, including the family, groups, communities, and the health care system.

An interesting application of the model in nursing education was presented by Camooso, Greene, and Reilly (1981). These nursing students described their adjustment to graduate school within the context of the four adaptive modes of Roy's model, citing adaptive and ineffective behaviors they exhibited during the course of graduate study.

The utility of Roy's conceptual model for nursing service administration also is documented. Rules for nursing administration were formulated by Fawcett, Botter, Burritt, Crossley, and Frink (in press). They stated,

> The distinctive focus and purpose of nursing in a clinical agency is provision of nursing services designed to promote patient adaptation in the physiological, self-concept, role function, and interdependence modes. The collective nursing staff is viewed as an adaptive system in a constantly changing environment. The department of nursing or the entire health care institution also may be viewed as an adaptive system. The settings for nursing services are not clearly delineated in Roy's model, although review of the literature indicates that it has been used successfully in most types of clinical agencies and in most specialty practice areas. Management strategies emphasize promotion of staff, departmental, or institutional adaptation to constantly changing environmental stimuli.

Roy (personal communication, May 15, 1982) reported that her conceptual model has been used as a basis for nursing practice at the National Hospital for Orthopaedics and Rehabilitation in Arlington, Virginia; Children's Hospital of Orange County in Orange, California; Waukesha Memorial Hospital in Waukesha, Wisconsin; and the Centre Hospitalier Pierre Janet in Hull, Quebec, Canada. The Roy model also has been used by nurses at the South Coast Medical Center in South Laguna, California; Shawnee Mission Medical Center in Shawnee Mission, Kansas (Blue, Brubaker, Papazian, & Riester, 1986; Roy, 1985); and at Santa Monica Hospital Medical Center in Santa Monica, California.

Mastal, Hammond, and Roberts (1982) described the use of the model as the structure for nursing practice at National Hospital for Orthopaedics and Rehabilitation in Arlington, Virginia. Commenting on the use of Roy's model at that agency, Hammond, Hepner, Mastal, and Roberts (personal communication, June 30, 1982) stated that the model "provides a more scientific rationale for nursing care and is contributing to the development of a distinct body of nursing knowledge by our staff. Further, we are realizing it has value for structuring our agency's nursing administrative practice."

Tremblay (personal communication, August 4, 1982) reported on the development and use of a nursing history and diagnosis form based on Roy's model at the Centre Hospitalier Pierre Janet in Hull, Quebec, Canada. She stated that nurses thought the tool "helped them to have a global approach to their nursing care" and most patients found the tool "not only permitted them to tell their personal history but also helped [them] to relate to the nurse in a special way." Interestingly, Tremblay noted that "patients stayed longer in the hospital" after the nursing history tool was implemented. She went on to say that research is planned to determine if there is a causal relationship between use of the tool and length of hospital stay.

Further documentation of the utility of the model in nursing service administration comes from McGlone, Sowden, and Hoffmans (personal communication, September 8, 1982), who described the use of Roy's conceptual model at Children's Hospital of Orange County in Orange, California. Age-related nursing history and discharge planning forms are organized according to the four adaptive modes. The nursing flow sheets and the patient Kardex include data related to the physiological mode. Nurses new to the agency "complete a class on the Roy model and . . . are instructed how to utilize the data obtained in the nursing history to develop a nursing care plan based on the model." An age-related nursing history based on the model also is used in the Orofacial, Cystic Fibrosis, and Neonatal High Risk outpatient clinics at Children's Hospital.

Kloepfel (personal communication, July 9, 1982) reported on a pilot project to use Roy's model on one unit at Waukesha Memorial Hospital in Waukesha, Wisconsin. She noted that the time constraints imposed by use of the model, turnover in the Head Nurse and Clinical Director positions on the project unit, and other factors led to discontinuation of use of the model. Kloepfel went on to say, "it is our objective to continue the use of a nursing model in delivering professional nursing care as an integral part of the health care team patient care plan. For many nurses at Waukesha Memorial, the medical model is no longer sufficient."

Torosian, DeStefano, and Dietrick-Gallagher (1985) described the development of a day gynecologic chemotherapy unit at the Hospital of the University of Pennsylvania in Philadelphia. They used Roy's conceptual model as the basis for nursing interventions and identification of patient outcomes.

Laros (1977) used the model to develop outcome criteria for patients with chronic obstructive pulmonary disease at Providence Hospital in Oakland, California. The evaluation tool listed the criteria for each adaptive mode, in a progressive sequence of days following admission to the hospital. Riegel (1985) described a method of presenting intershift report based on Roy's conceptual model and the nursing process. Furthermore, Roy and Martinez (1983) presented a conceptual framework for clinical specialist nursing practice based on Roy's work and systems notions. Moreover, Roy and Anway (in press) discussed theories and hypotheses for nursing administration derived from the Roy Adaptation Model, and DiIorio (in press) described the application of the conceptual model to nursing administration.

Contributions to Nursing Knowledge

Roy's conceptual model makes a significant contribution to nursing knowledge by focusing attention on the nature of the person's adaptation to a changing environment. Roy's perspective of adaptation goes beyond that presented by other disciplines by placing it within the context of the person as a totality. Thus, this model presents a distinctive view of the person, one that developed within the discipline of nursing.

Roy and others (e.g., Randall, et al., 1982) have continued to develop the various concepts of the conceptual model, so that only a few gaps and omissions are apparent at this time. In fact, this work appeared to anticipate the questions raised by the analysis and evaluation framework used in this book. Speaking in this vein, Roy (1980) commented, "The Roy adaptation model has been developed as a nursing model and can thus be more easily analyzed according to the characteristics of models" (p. 187).

Roy and Roberts's (1981) work to develop a theory of the person as an adaptive system is especially noteworthy. This has resulted in construction of the beginnings of a logically congruent conceptual-theoretical system of nursing knowledge that can be used for nursing activities. The importance of the theory of the person as an adaptive system to nursing was summarized by Roy and Roberts (1981):

> Investigation of adaptive systems is evident in the literature of a number of fields including genetics, biology, physiology, physics, psychology, anthropology, and sociology. All of these approaches can be helpful in conceptualizing the adaptive system. Yet each approach views the person or the group from the perspective of that discipline. The nursing model directs that the nurse view the patient holistically. We need a theory of the holistic person as an adaptive system. Since the basic sciences do not provide nurses with a single working theory, the nurse using the adaptation model must create one for herself. This . . . is a beginning effort to do this—to create a theory of the holistic person as an adaptive system. (p. 49)

Given the importance of this work, it is unfortunate that programs of research designed to systematically test propositions have not yet been developed.

The Roy Adaptation Model encompasses an extensive vocabulary with many new words. Furthermore, even familiar words such as adaptation have been given new meanings in Roy's attempt to translate mechanistic ideas into organismic ones. Thus, the first step in the use of this conceptual model should be mastery of the vocabulary.

In conclusion, Roy's conceptual model has been adopted enthusiastically by many nurse educators and clinicians. Although such enthusiasm about the model could result in its uncritical application, Roy has attempted to guard against this by pointing out areas of the model needing further clarification and development.

REFERENCES

Abdellah, F.G., Beland, I., Martin, A., & Matheney, R. (1960). Patient-centered approaches to nursing. New York: Macmillan.

Andrews, H.A., & Roy, C. (1986). Essentials of the Roy Adaptation Model. Norwalk, CT: Appleton-Century-Crofts.

Asay, M.K., & Ossler, C.C. (Eds.). (1984). Conceptual models of nursing. Applications in community health nursing. Proceedings of the Eighth Annual Community Health Nursing Conference. Chapel Hill: Department of Public Health Nursing, School of Public Health, University of North Carolina.

Bean, C.A. (1988). Needs and stimuli influencing needs of adult cancer patients. Dissertation Abstracts International, 48, 2259B.

Beckerman, A. (1984). The impact of Roy's model of adaptation on nursing students' generation of patient data: A comparison study. Dissertation Abstracts International, 45, 513B.

Blue, C.L., Brubaker, K.M., Papazian, K.R., & Riester, C.M. (1986). Sister Callista Roy. Adaptation model. In A. Marriner, Nursing theorists and their work (pp. 297–312). St. Louis: CV Mosby.

Brower, H.T.F., & Baker, B.J. (1976). Using the adaptation model in a practitioner curriculum. Nursing Outlook, 24, 686–689.

Camooso, C., Greene, M., & Reilly, P. (1981). Students' adaptation according to Roy. Nursing Outlook 29, 108–109.

Cohen, B.J. (1980). The perception of patient adaptation to hemodialysis: A study of registered nurses and hemodialysis patients. Dissertation Abstracts International, 41, 129B–130B.

Cottrell, B., & Shannahan, M. (1986). Effect of the birth chair on duration of second stage labor and maternal outcome. Nursing Research, 35, 364–367.

Cottrell, B., & Shannahan, M. (1987). A comparison of fetal outcome in birth chair and delivery table births. Research in Nursing and Health, 10, 239–243.

Dahlen, R.A. (1980). Analysis of selected factors related to the elderly person's ability to adapt to visual prostheses following senile cataract surgery. Dissertation Abstracts International, 41, 894B.

DiIorio, C. (in press). Applying Roy's model to nursing administration. In B. Henry, M. DiVincenti, C. Arndt, & A. Marriner (Eds.), Dimensions of nursing administration. Theory, research, education, and practice. Boston: Blackwell Scientific Publications.

Downey, C. (1974). Adaptation nursing applied to an obstetric patient. In J.P. Riehl & C. Roy, Conceptual models for nursing practice (pp. 151–159). New York: Appleton-Century-Crofts.

Farkas, L. (1981). Adaptation problems with nursing home aplication for elderly persons: An application of the Roy Adaptation Nursing Model. Journal of Advanced Nursing, 6, 365–368.

Fawcett, J. (1981a). Assessing and understanding the cesarean father. In C.F. Kehoe (Ed.), The cesarean experience. Theoretical and clinical perspectives for nurses (pp. 143–156). New York: Appleton-Century-Crofts.

Fawcett, J. (1981b). Needs of cesarean birth parents. Journal of Obstetric, Gynecologic, and Neonatal Nursing, 10, 371–376. (b)

Fawcett, J., Botter, M.L., Burritt, J., Crossley, J.D., & Frink, B. B. (in press). Conceptual models of nursing and organization theories. In B. Henry, M. DiVincenti, C. Arndt, & A. Marriner (Eds.), Dimensions of nursing administration. Theory, research, education, and practice. Boston: Blackwell Scientific Publications.

Fawcett, J., & Burritt, J. (1985). An exploratory study of antenatal preparation for cesarean birth. Journal of Obstetric, Gynecologic, and Neonatal Nursing, 14, 224–230.

Fawcett, J., & Henklein, J. (1987). Antenatal education for cesarean birth: Extension of a field test. Journal of Obstetric, Gynecologic, and Neonatal Nursing, 16, 61–65.

Fawcett, J., Tulman, L., & Myers, S. (1988). Development of the Inventory of Functional Status after Childbirth. Manuscript submitted for publication.

Francis, G., Turner, J.T., & Johnson, S.B. (1985). Domestic animal visitation as therapy with adult home residents. International Journal of Nursing Studies, 22, 201–206.

Galligan, A.C. (1979). Using Roy's concept of adaptation to care for young children. American Journal of Maternal Child Nursing, 4, 24–28.

Giger, J.A., Bower, C.A., & Miller, S.W. (1987). Roy adaptation model: ICU application. Dimensions of Critical Care Nursing, 6, 215–224.

Gordon, J. (1974). Nursing assessment and care plan for a cardiac patient. In J.P. Riehl & C. Roy, Conceptual models of nursing practice (pp. 144–151). New York: Appleton-Century-Crofts.

Guzzetta, C. (1979). Relationship between stress and learning. Advances in Nursing Science, 1(4), 35–49.

Hammond, H., Roberts, M., & Silva, M. (1983, Spring). The effect of Roy's first level and second level assessment on nurses' determination of accurate nursing diagnoses. Virginia Nurse, 14–17.

Helson, H. (1964). Adaptation-level theory. New York: Harper & Row.

Henderson, V. (1960). Basic principles of nursing care. London: International Council of Nurses.

Hoch, C.C. (1987). Assessing delivery of nursing care. Journal of Gerontological Nursing, 13, 10–17.

Holcombe, J.K. (1986). Social support, perception of illness, and self-esteem of women with gynecologic cancer. Dissertation Abstracts International, 47, 1928B.

Idle, B.A. (1978). SPAL: A tool for measuring self-perceived adaptation level appropriate for an elderly population. In E.E. Bauwens (Ed.), Clinical nursing research: Its strategies and findings. (Monograph series 1978: Two, pp. 56–63). Indianapolis: Sigma Theta Tau.

Janelli, L. (1980). Utilizing Roy's adaptation model from a gerontological perspective. Journal of Gerontological Nursing, 6, 140–150.

Kehoe, C.F. (1981). Identifying the nursing needs of the postpartum cesarean mother. In C.F. Kehoe (Ed.), The cesarean experience. Theoretical and clinical perspectives for nurses (pp. 85–141). New York: Appleton-Century-Crofts.

Kiker, P.M. (1983). Role adequacy of pediatric outpatients undergoing surgery. Dissertation Abstracts International, 44, 1782B.

Knowlton, C., Goodwin, M., Moore, J., Alt-White, A., Guarino, S., & Pyne, H. (1983). Systems adaptation model of nursing for families, groups and communities. Journal of Nursing Education, 22, 128–131.

Laros, J. (1977). Deriving outcome criteria from a conceptual model. Nursing Outlook, 25, 333–336.

Leonard, C. (1975). Patient attitudes toward nursing interventions. Nursing Research, 24, 335–339.

Leuze, M., & McKenzie, J. (1987). Preoperative assessment. Using the Roy Adaptation Model. AORN Journal, 46, 1122–1134.

Levine, M.E. (1966). Adaptation and assessment: A rationale for nursing intervention. American Journal of Nursing, 66, 2450–2453.

Lewis, F., Firsich, S.C., & Parsell, S. (1978). Development of reliable measures of patient health outcomes related to quality nursing care for chemotherapy patients. In J.C. Krueger, A.H. Nelson, & M.O. Wolanin, Nursing research. Development, collaboration, utilization (pp. 225–228). Germantown, MD: Aspen.

Lewis, F.M., Firsich, S.C., & Parsell, S. (1979). Clinical tool development for adult chemotherapy patients: Process and content. Cancer Nursing, 2, 99–108.

Limandri, B. (1986). Research and practice with abused women: Use of the Roy Adaptation Model as an exploratory framework. Advances in Nursing Science, 8(4), 52–61.

Marriner, A. (1986). Nursing theorists and their work. St. Louis: CV Mosby.

Mastal, M.F., Hammond, H., & Roberts, M.P. (1982). Theory into hospital practice: A pilot implementation. Journal of Nursing Administration, 12(6), 9–15.

McCain, R.F. (1965). Nursing by assessment—not intuition. American Journal of Nursing, 65(4), 82–84.

McDonald, F.J., & Harms, M. (1966). Theoretical model for an experimental curriculum. Nursing Outlook, 14(8), 48–51.

Meleis, A.I. (1985). Theoretical nursing: Development and progress. Philadelphia: JB Lippincott.

Miles, M.S., & Carter, M.C. (1983). Assessing parental stress in intensive care units. American Journal of Maternal Child Nursing, 8, 354–359.

Munn, V.A., & Tichy, A.M. (1987). Nurses' perceptions of stressors in pediatric intensive care. Journal of Pediatric Nursing, 2, 405–411.

Nash, D.J. (1987). Kawasaki disease: Application of the Roy Adaptation Model to determine interventions. Journal of Pediatric Nursing, 2, 308–315.

Nightingale, F. (1859). Notes on nursing. What it is, and what it is not. London: Harrison. (Reprinted by JB Lippincott, 1946.)

Nolan, M. (1977). Effects of nursing intervention in the operating room as recalled on the third postoperative day. In Communicating nursing research in the bicentennial year (Vol. 9, pp. 41–50). Boulder, CO: Western Interstate Commission for Higher Education.

Norris, S., Campbell, L., & Brenkert, S. (1982). Nursing procedures and alterations in transcutaneous oxygen tension in premature infants. Nursing Research, 31, 330–336.

Orlando, I.J. (1961). The dynamic nurse-patient relationship. New York: GP Putnam's Sons.

Peak, H. (1955). Attitude and motivation. In M.R. Jones (Ed.), Nebraska symposium on motivation (pp. 149–189). Lincoln: University of Nebraska Press.

Peplau, H. (1952). Interpersonal relations in nursing. New York: GP Putnam's Sons.

Pollock, S. (1982). Level of adaptation: An analysis of stress factors that affect health status. Dissertation Abstracts International, 41, 4364B.

Pollock, S. (1986). Human responses to chronic illness: Physiologic and psychosocial adaptation. Nursing Reseach, 35, 90–95.

Rambo, B. (1984). Adaptation nursing: Assessment and intervention. Philadelphia: WB Saunders.

Randall, B., Poush Tedrow, M., & Van Landingham, J. (1982). Adaptation nursing. The Roy conceptual model applied. St. Louis: CV Mosby.

Riegel, B. (1985). A method of giving intershift report based on a conceptual model. Focus on Critical Care, 12(4), 12–18.

Riehl, J.P., & Roy, C. (1974). Conceptual models for nursing practice. New York: Appleton-Century-Crofts.

Riehl, J.P., & Roy, C. (1980). Conceptual models for nursing practice (2nd ed.). New York: Appleton-Century-Crofts.

Roy, C. (1970). Adaptation: A conceptual framework for nursing. Nursing Outlook, 18(3), 42–45.

Roy, C. (1971). Adaptation: A basis for nursing practice. Nursing Outlook, 19, 254–257.

Roy, C. (1973). Adaptation: Implications for curriculum change. Nursing Outlook, 21, 163–168.

Roy, C. (1974). The Roy Adaptation Model. In J.P. Riehl & C. Roy, Conceptual models for nursing practice. New York: Appleton-Century-Crofts.

Roy, C. (1976a). Introduction to nursing: An adaptation model. Englewood Cliffs, NJ: Prentice-Hall.

Roy, C. (1976b). Comment. Nursing Outlook, 24, 690–691.

Roy, C. (1977). Decision-making by the physically ill and adaptation during illness. Unpublished doctoral dissertation, University of California, Los Angeles.

Roy, C. (1978a, December). Adaptation model. Paper presented at Second Annual Nurse Educator Conference, New York. (Cassette recording)

Roy, C. (1978b). The stress of hospital events: Measuring changes in level of stress (Abstract). In Communicating nursing research. Vol. 11: New approaches to communicating nursing research (pp. 70–71). Boulder, CO: Western Interstate Commission for Higher Education.

Roy, C. (1979a). Health-illness (powerlessness) questionnaire and hospitalized patient decision-making. In M.J. Ward & C.A. Lindeman (Eds.), Instruments for measuring nursing practice and other health care variables (Vol. 1, pp. 147–153). Hyattsville, MD: U.S. Department of Health, Education, and Welfare.

Roy, C. (1979b). Relating nursing theory to education: A new era. Nurse Educator, 4(2), 16–21.

Roy, C. (1980). The Roy Adaptation Model. In J.P. Riehl & C. Roy, Conceptual models for nursing practice (2nd ed., pp. 179–188). New York: Appleton-Century-Crofts.

Roy, C. (1982). Foreword. In B. Randall, M. Poush Tedrow, & J. Van Landingham, Adaptation nursing. The Roy conceptual model applied (pp. vii–viii). St. Louis: CV Mosby.

Roy, C. (1983a). The expectant family. Analysis and application of the Roy Adaptation Model. In I.W. Clements & F.B. Roberts, Family health, A theoretical approach to nursing care (pp. 298–303). New York: John Wiley & Sons.

Roy, C. (1983b). The family in primary care. Analysis and application of the Roy Adaptation Model. In I.W. Clements & F.B. Roberts, Family health, A theoretical approach to nursing care (pp. 375–378). New York: John Wiley & Sons.

Roy, C. (1983c). Roy Adaptation Model. In I.W. Clements & F.B. Roberts, Family health. A theoretical approach to nursing care (pp. 255–278). New York: John Wiley & Sons.

Roy, C. (1984a). Introduction to nursing: An adaptation model. (2nd ed.). Englewood Cliffs, NJ: Prentice-Hall.

Roy, C. (1984b). The Roy Adaptation Model: Applications in community health. In M.K. Asay & C.C. Ossler (Eds.), Conceptual models of nursing. Applications in community health nursing. Proceedings of the Eighth Annual Community Health Nursing Conference (pp. 51–73). Chapel Hill: Department of Public Health Nursing, School of Public Health, University of North Carolina.

Roy, C. (1985, August). Sr. Callista Roy's framework. Application to practice, research, and education. Paper presented at conference on Nursing Theory in Action, Edmonton, Alberta, Canada. (Cassette recording)

Roy, C. (1987a). Roy's Adaptation Model. In R.R. Parse, Nursing science. Major paradigms, theories, and critiques (pp. 35–45). Philadelphia: WB Saunders.

Roy, C. (1987b, May). Roy's model. Paper presented at Nurse Theorist Conference, Pittsburgh, PA. (Cassette recording)

Roy, C. (1988). An explication of the philosophical assumptions of the Roy adaptation model. Nursing Science Quarterly 1, 26–34.

Roy, C., & Anway, J. (in press). Theories and hypotheses for nursing administration. In B. Henry, M. DiVincenti, C. Arndt, & A. Marriner (Eds.), Dimensions of nursing administration. Theory, research, education, and practice. Boston: Blackwell Scientific Publications.

Roy, C., & Martinez, C. (1983). A conceptual framework for CNS practice. In A. Hamric & J. Spross (Eds.), The clinical nurse specialist in theory and practice (pp. 3–20). New York: Grune & Stratton.

Roy, C., & Roberts, S.L. (1981). Theory construction in nursing. An adaptation model. Englewood Cliffs, NJ: Prentice-Hall.

Scherubel, J.C.M. (1986). Description of adaptation patterns following an acute cardiac event. Dissertation Abstracts International, 46, 2627B.

Schmidt, C.S. (1983). A comparison of the effectiveness of two nursing models in decreasing depression and increasing life satisfaction of retired individuals. Dissertation Abstracts International, 43, 2856B.

Schmitz, M. (1980). The Roy Adaptation Model: Application in a community setting. In J.P. Riehl & C. Roy, Conceptual models for nursing practice (2nd ed., pp. 193–206). New York: Appleton-Century-Crofts.

Shannahan, M., & Cottrell, B. (1985). Effect of the birth chair on duration of second stage labor, fetal outcome, and maternal blood loss. Nursing Research, 34, 89–92.

Silva, M.C. (1987a). Conceptual models of nursing. In J.J. Fitzpatrick & R.L. Taunton (Eds.), Annual review of nursing research (Vol. 5, pp. 229–246). New York: Springer.

Silva, M.C. (1987b). Needs of spouses of surgical patients: A conceptualization within the Roy Adaptation Model. Scholarly Inquiry for Nursing Practice: An International Journal, 1, 29–44.

Silva, M.C., & Sorrell, J.M. (1987, April). Doctoral dissertation research based on five nursing models: A select bibliography. January 1952 through February 1987. (Available from M.C. Silva, George Mason University School of Nursing, Fairfax, VA)

Sirignano, R.G. (1987). Peripartum cardiomyopathy: An application of the Roy Adaptation Model. Journal of Cardiovascular Nursing, 2, 24–32.

Smith, C., Garvis, M., & Martinson, I. (1983). Content analysis of interviews using a nursing model: A look at parents adapting to the impact of childhood cancer. Cancer Nursing, 6, 269–275.

Starr, S.L. (1980). Adaptation applied to the dying client. In J.P. Riehl & C. Roy. Conceptual models for nursing practice (2nd ed., pp. 189–192). New York: Appleton-Century-Crofts.

Stevens, B.J. (1984). Nursing theory. Analysis, application, evaluation (2nd ed.). Boston: Little, Brown & Co.

Strickler, M., & LaSor, B. (1970). Concept of loss in crisis intervention. Mental Hygiene, 54, 301–305.

Torosian, L.C., DeStefano, M., & Dietrick-Gallagher, M. (1985). Day gynecologic chemotherapy unit: An innovative approach to changing health care systems. Cancer Nursing, 8, 221–227.

Trentini, M. (1986). Nurses' decisions in dialysis patient care: An application of the Roy Adaptation Model. Dissertation Abstracts International, 47, 575B.

Tulman, L., & Fawcett, J. (1988). Return of functional ability after childbirth. Nursing Research, 37, 77–81.

Wagner, P. (1976). Testing the adaptation model in practice. Nursing Outlook, 24, 682–685.

Walker, L.O., & Nicholson, R. (1980). Criteria for evaluating nursing process models. Nurse Educator, 5(5), 8–9.

Whall, A.L. (1986). Strategic family therapy: Nursing reformulations and applications. In A.L. Whall, Family therapy theory for nursing. Four approaches (pp. 51–67). Norwalk, CT: Appleton-Century-Crofts.

Wilson, F.S. (1984). The Roy Adaptation Model of Nursing: Implications for baccalaureate nursing education. Dissertation Abstracts International, 45, 91A.

Zonka, B.J. (1980). The effects of a formal in-hospital patient education program on anxiety in postmyocardial infarction patients. Dissertation Abstracts International, 41, 1418A.

ANNOTATED BIBLIOGRAPHY

Aggleton, P., & Chalmers. H. (1984). The Roy Adaptation Model. Nursing Times, 80(40), 45–48.
A brief overview of Roy's conceptual model is given in this article, as well as a discussion of how the model can be applied to practice through its nursing process.

Andrews, H.A., & Roy, C. (1986). Essentials of the Roy Adaptation Model. Norwalk, CT: Appleton-Century-Crofts.
This book highlights the essential elements of Roy's conceptual model and provides an overview and description of key concepts.

Blue, C.L., Brubaker, K.M., Papazian, K.R., & Riester, C.M. (1986). Sister Callista Roy. Adaptation model. In A. Marriner, Nursing theorists and their work (pp. 297–312). St. Louis: CV Mosby.
This book chapter presents a brief overview of Roy's conceptual model.

Brower, H.T.F., & Baker, B.J. (1976). Using the adaptation model in a practitioner curriculum. Nursing Outlook, 24, 686–689.
Roy's conceptual model is used as the guide for a geriatric nurse practitioner program. Each of the adaptive modes is related to nursing care of the aging. The application of the model to the curriculum is described. The authors found the model useful for curriculum planning, as well as helpful in students' development of a nursing identity.

Camooso, C., Greene, M., & Reilly, P. (1981). Students' adaptation according to Roy. Nursing Outlook, 29, 108–109.
Roy's model is used to analyze and explain the authors' experiences in graduate school.

DiIorio, C. (in press). Applying Roy's model to nursing administration. In B. Henry, M. DiVincenti, C. Arndt, & A. Marriner (Eds.), Dimensions of nursing administration. Theory, research, education, and practice. Boston: Blackwell Scientific Publications.
This book chapter describes the application of Roy's conceptual model to the administration of nursing services.

Downey, C. (1974). Adaptation nursing applied to an obstetric patient. In J.P. Riehl & C. Roy, Conceptual models for nursing practice (pp. 151–159). New York: Appleton-Century-Crofts.
A case study of an obstetric patient is pesented and an assessment based on the Roy model is described. A detailed nursing care plan is included.

Farkas, L. (1981). Adaptation problems with nursing home application for elderly per-

sons: An application of the Roy Adaptation Nursing Model. Journal of Advanced Nursing, 6, 363–368.
The article reports the findings of a study designed to identify adaptation problems of elderly people and their significant others that were associated with applications for nursing home placement.

Fawcett, J. (1981). Assessing and understanding the cesarean father. In C.F. Kehoe (Ed.), The cesarean experience. Theoretical and clinical perspectives for nurses (pp. 143–156). New York: Appleton-Century-Crofts.

Fawcett, J. (1981). Needs of cesarean birth parents. Journal of Obstetric, Gynecologic, and Neonatal Nursing, 10, 371–376.
The adaptive modes of Roy's conceptual model are used to classify survey data dealing with mothers' and fathers' responses to the cesarean birth of their children. Need deficits and excesses in each adaptive mode are identified. Suggestions for the nursing care of these parents are identified.

Fawcett, J., Botter, M.L., Burritt, J., Crossley, J.D., & Frink, B.B. (in press). Conceptual models of nursing and organization theories. In B. Henry, M. DiVincenti, C. Arndt, & A. Marriner (Eds.), Dimensions of nursing administration. Theory, research, education, and practice. Boston: Blackwell Scientific Publications.
This book chapter presents an overview of Roy's model and explains how the model can be modified for nursing service administration. A conceptual-theoretical system of knowledge to assist nurse administrators to more fully understand what structural arrangements will promote the highest level of organizational performance is created by linking the model with contingency theory.

Fawcett, J., & Burritt, J. (1985). An exploratory study of antenatal preparation for cesarean birth. Journal of Obstetric, Gynecologic, and Neonatal Nursing, 14, 224–230.

Fawcett, J., & Henklein, J. (1987). Antenatal education for cesarean birth: Extension of a field test. Journal of Obstetric, Gynecologic, and Neonatal Nursing, 16, 61–65.
These articles report the findings of two studies designed to determine the utility of an antenatal program of information about cesarean birth. Roy's model was used to structure the educational program.

Fawcett, J., Tulman, L., & Myers, S. (1988). Development of the Inventory of Functional Status after Childbirth. Manuscript submitted for publication.
The investigators describe the development of the Inventory of Functional Status after Childbirth, a questionnaire designed to measure functional status after childbirth. Functional status is regarded as a theoretical representative of the role function adaptive mode of Roy's conceptual model.

Fitzpatrick, J.J., Whall, A.L., Johnston, R.L., & Floyd, J.A. (1982). Nursing models and their psychiatric mental health applications. Bowie, MD: Brady.
This book presents a brief analysis of Roy's conceptual model, among others. Reformulated theoretical approaches, consistent with Roy's model, in individual psychotherapy and family therapy are discussed.

Francis, G., Turner, J.T., & Johnson, S.B. (1985). Domestic animal visitation as therapy with adult home residents. International Journal of Nursing Studies, 22, 201–206.
The investigators describe the results of their study to determine the effect of exposure of residents of an adult care home to visits by puppies once a week. Roy's conceptual model provided the conceptual frame of reference for the study. Outcome variables included social interaction, psychosocial function, life satisfaction, mental function, depression, social competence, psychological well-being, personal neatness, and health self-concept.

Galbreath, J.G. (1980). Sister Callista Roy. In Nursing Theories Conference Group, Nursing theories. The base for professional nursing practice (pp. 199–212). Englewood Cliffs, NJ: Prentice-Hall.

Galbreath, J.G. (1985). Sister Callista Roy. In Nursing Theories Conference Group, Nursing theories. The base for professional nursing practice (2nd ed., pp. 300–318). Englewood Cliffs, NJ: Prentice-Hall.
An overview of Roy's conceptual model is presented. Key terms are defined and each of the adaptive modes is delineated. Examples of clinical situations examined

from the perspective of Roy's model are given. Strengths and weaknesses of the model are discussed.

Galligan, A.C. (1979). Using Roy's concept of adaptation to care for young children. American Journal of Maternal Child Nursing, 4, 24–28.
   The adaptation model is applied to the care of hospitalized children. Stages of hospitalization are identified as prehospitalization, preoperative, postoperative, and discharge. Adaptive needs are identified for each stage. A detailed acount of behavior in each adaptive mode during each stage is given.

Germain, C.P. (1984). Power and powerlessness in the adult hospitalized cancer patient. In Proceedings of the 3rd International Conference on Cancer Nursing (pp. 158–162). Melbourne, Australia: The Cancer Institute/Peter MacCallum Hospital and the Royal Melbourne Hospital.
   Roy's conceptual model and French and Raven's theory of power are used as a basis for discussion of power and powerlessness in the cancer patient. Coercive power, reward power, referrent power, and expert power are described using examples from the author's ethnographic study of an adult cancer unit.

Germain, C.P. (1984). Sheltering abused women: A nursing perspective. Journal of Psychosocial Nursing, 22(9), 24–31.
   This article is a partial report of an ethnographic study of a residential shelter for abused women and children. Findings related to common health problems are discussed. The investigator contends that use of a conceptual model would enhance the ability of nurses to identify abused women and refer them for appropriate care. Roy's model is briefly reviewed.

Giger, J.A., Bower, C.A., & Miller, S.W. (1987). Roy Adaptation Model: ICU application. Dimensions of Critical Care Nursing, 6, 215–224.
   This article presents a case study using Roy's model to guide nursing care of a trauma victim.

Goodwin, J.O. (1980). A cross-cultural approach to integrating nursing theory and practice. Nurse Educator, 5(6), 15–20.
   A general model of the nursing process is outlined. Roy's model is presented as one example of integration of a conceptual model with the general nursing process model. Use of the combined model in a French nursing school is described. Modifications in the model for the French culture and nursing practice are identified.

Gordon, J. (1974). Nursing assessment and care plan for a cardiac patient. In J.P. Riehl & C. Roy, Conceptual models for nursing practice (pp. 144–151). New York: Appleton-Century-Crofts.
   Roy's model is applied to the care of a cardiac patient. Nursing assessments and diagnoses based on the model are discussed.

Guzzetta, C. (1979). Relationship between stress and learning. Advances in Nursing Science, 1(4), 35–49.
   The concept of adaptation was selected to provide the framework for the investigation reported in this article. Study subjects were male patients with a diagnosis of acute myocardial infarction. Findings indicate that formal cardiac teaching improves patients' knowledge of illness and related health care issues and that time period of teaching is not an important consideration.

Hammond, H., Roberts, M., & Silva, M. (1983, Spring). The effect of Roy's first level and second level assessment on nurses' determination of accurate nursing diagnoses. Virginia Nurse, 14–17.
   This paper reports the findings of a study designed to determine whether nurses need both first- and second-level assessment data to make accurate nursing diagnoses. Findings indicated no significant difference in accuracy of nursing diagnoses between the group who used both first- and second-level assessment data and the group who used only first-level assessment data.

Hoch, C.C. (1987). Assessing delivery of nursing care. Journal of Gerontological Nursing, 13, 10–17.
   This article presents a report of a study designed to compare outcomes of nursing intervention directed by Neuman's conceptual model, Roy's model, and a control

treatment directed by no explicit model. Study subjects were retired persons attending a senior citizen center. Sixteen subjects were in each of the three study groups. Findings indicated that the Neuman and Roy groups had higher life satisfaction and lower depression scores than the control group. There were no differences, however, between the Neuman and Roy groups.

Huch, M.H. (1987). A critique of the Roy Adaptation Model. In R.R. Parse, Nursing science. Major paradigms, theories, and critiques (pp. 47–66). Philadelphia: WB Saunders.

This book chapter is the publication of the critique of Roy's conceptual model presented at the Nurse Theorist conference held in Pittsburgh, Pennsylvania, in May 1985.

Idle, B.A. (1978). SPAL: A tool for measuring self-perceived adaptation level appropriate for an elderly population. In E.E. Bauwens (Ed.), Clinical nursing research: Its strategies and findings (Monograph series 1978: Two, pp. 56–63). Indianapolis: Sigma Theta Tau.

Roy's model is used to guide development of a tool to measure elderly patients' perceptions of their adaptation to life events.

Janelli, L. (1980). Utilizing Roy's adaptation model from a gerontological perspective. Journal of Gerontological Nursing, 6, 140–150.

This article presents a description of the benefits of using Roy's conceptual model when working with elderly clients. A clinical application of Roy's nursing process is included.

Kehoe, C.F. (1981). Identifying the nursing needs of the postpartum cesarean mother. In C.F. Kehoe (Ed.), The cesarean experience. Theoretical and clinical perspectives for nurses (pp. 85–141). New York: Appleton-Century-Crofts.

Roy's model is used to classify exploratory study data regarding the needs of the postpartal cesarean mother, and as a guide for the nursing care of this patient population. Detailed nursing care plans are included.

Kehoe, C.F., & Fawcett, J. (1981). An overview of the Roy Adaptation Model. In C.F. Kehoe (Ed.), The cesarean experience. Theoretical and clinical perspectives for nurses (pp. 79–83). New York: Appleton-Century-Crofts.

Roy's conceptual model is reviewed.

Knowlton, C., Goodwin, M., Moore, J., Alt-White, A., Guarino, S., & Pyne, H. (1983). Systems adaptation model for nursing for families, groups and communities. Journal of Nursing Education, 22, 128–131.

This article presents an overview of the development of a nursing curriculum based on Roy's Adaptation Model and general system theory at The Catholic University of America School of Nursing. A description is given of how the model is applied to the systems of family, groups, community, nursing, and the health care system along with an explanation of each system's placement within the curriculum.

Laros, J. (1977). Deriving outcome criteria from a conceptual model. Nursing Outlook, 25, 333–336.

Roy's conceptual model is used as the framework for identification of evaluation criteria. Outcome criteria are developed for each adaptive mode for a patient with chronic obstructive pulmonary disease. Use of the model to guide staff development programs is discussed.

Leonard, C. (1975). Patient attitudes toward nursing interventions. Nursing Research, 24, 335–339.

This article reports the findings of a study of psychiatric inpatients' attitudes toward nursing interventions during three periods of administrative changes. Roy's emphasis on contextual stimuli is discussed.

Leuze, M., & McKenzie, J. (1987). Preoperative assessment using the Roy Adaptation Model. AORN Journal, 46, 1122–1134.

This article reports the findings of a study designed to test the hypothesis that circulating nurses involved with patients who have had preoperative nursing assessments based on the Roy Adaptation Model would demonstrate increased knowledge of the patient's psychosocial needs over those who do not. The hypothesis was supported.

Lewis, F.M., Firsich, S.C., & Parsell, S. (1978). Development of reliable measures of patient health outcomes related to quality nursing care for chemotherapy patients. In J.C. Krueger, A.H. Nelson, & M.O. Wolanin, Nursing research. Development, collaboration, and utilization (pp. 225–228). Germantown, MD: Aspen.

Lewis, F.M., Firsich, S.C., & Parsell, S. (1979). Clinical tool development for adult chemotherapy patients: Process and content. Cancer Nursing, 2, 99–108.

The Roy Adaptation Model is used to guide development of items for an instrument designed to assess health outcomes of nursing care of adult cancer patients receiving chemotherapy. Psychometric evaluation of the instrument supported its content validity, interrater reliability, test-retest reliability, and internal consistency reliability.

Limandri, B. Research and practice with abused women: Use of the Roy Adaptation Model as an exploratory framework. Advances in Nursing Science, 8(4), 52–61.

This article presents a discussion of the use of Roy's conceptual model in research and practice with abused women. Suggestions for modifications in the model for this client population are given.

Mastal, M.F., & Hammond, H. (1980). Analysis and expansion of the Roy Adaptation Model: A contribution to holistic nursing. Advances in Nursing Science, 2(4), 71–81.

Roy's model is analyzed to elucidate basic assumptions, concepts, and propositions. One basic concept, health-illness, is described in detail and expanded from the original conception. Points along the health-illness continuum are defined throroughly so as to clarify nursing assessment areas. Propositions that may facilitate development of hypotheses are suggested.

Mastal, M.F., Hammond, H., & Roberts, M.P. (1982). Theory into hospital practice: A pilot implementation. Journal of Nursing Administration, 12(6), 9–15.

The authors describe a project designed to implement Roy's conceptual model on one unit of a small community hospital. The article describes the administrative tasks needed to realize the project, the process of staff education, and outcomes.

Miles, M.S., & Carter, M.C. (1983). Assessing parental stress in intensive care units. American Journal of Maternal Child Nursing, 8, 354–359.

This article presents a conceptual-theoretical system of nursing knowledge that links Roy's conceptual model with theories of stress. The knowledge system was developed as a guide for assessment of stress experienced by parents whose children are in intensive care units.

Munn, V.A., & Tichy, A.M. (1987). Nurses' perceptions of stressors in pediatric intensive care. Journal of Pediatric Nursing, 2, 405–411.

The authors report the findings of their study of factors identified by 10 nurses as stressful to school-aged children and adolescents who are patients in a pediatric intensive care unit.

Nash, D.J. (1987). Kawasaki disease: Application of the Roy Adaptation Model to determine interventions. Journal of Pediatric Nursing, 2, 308–315.

This article presents a nusing care plan based on Roy's conceptual model for children with Kawasaki disease.

Nolan, M. (1977). Effects of nursing intervention in the operating room as recalled on the third postoperative day. In M.V. Batey (Ed.), Communicating nursing research in the bicentennial year (Vol. 9, pp. 41–50). Boulder, CO: Western Interstate Commission for Higher Education.

The relationship between the quality of nursing care given by operating room nurses and the quality of care as reported by postoperative patients was examined in this study. Use of Roy's conceptual model is discussed.

Norris, S., Campbell, L., & Brenkert, S. (1982). Nursing procedures and alterations in transcutaneous oxygen tension in premature infants. Nursing Research, 31, 330–336.

Holloway, E., & King, I. (1983). Re: "What's going on here?" (Letter to the editor). Nursing Research, 32, 319.

Berkemeyer, S.N., & Campbell, L.A. (1983). To the editor. (Letter to the editor). Nursing Research, 32, 319–329.

Roy, C. (1983). To the editor. (Letter to the editor). Nursing Research, 32, 320.

Norris, Campbell, and Brenkert report the results of their study of the effect of nursing procedures on transcutaneous oxygen tension in premature infants. The study was derived from Roy's concepts of focal, contextual, and residual stimuli and physiological adaptation.

Holloway and King critique the Norris, et al. study and point out that the investigators used a secondary source when they cited Roy's writings about stimuli. They maintained that the primary source was Helson.

Berkemeyer (nee Norris) and Campbell defend their use of Roy's interpretation of Helson's work on stimuli,

Roy's response to Holloway and King's letter indicates her support for Norris, et al.'s use of Roy as a primary source for their study.

Pollock, S.E. (1984). Adaptation to stress. Texas Nursing, 58(10), 12–13.

Pollock, S.E. (1984). The stress response. Critical Care Quarterly, 6(4), 1–14.

Pollock, S.E. (1986). Human responses to chronic illness: Physiologic and psychosocial adaptation. Nursing Research, 35, 90–95.

The author describes the development of a framework for research derived from Roy's conceptual model and theories of stress and hardiness and reports the findings of her study of the relationship between hardiness and adaptive behavior among persons with diabetes mellitus, hypertension, and rheumatoid arthritis.

Porth, C.M. (1977). Physiological coping: A model for teaching pathophysiology. Nursing Outlook, 25, 781–784.

The author presents a teaching model that facilitates students' abilities to look for physiological cues and apply relevant knowledge in patient care. The model operationalizes the physiological adaptive mode of Roy's conceptual model.

Rambo, B. (1984). Adaptation nursing: Assessment and intervention. Philadelphia: WB Saunders.

This textbook presents an explanation of the adaptation model of nursing and the nursing process. Assessment of the physiological and psychosocial modes is explained in detail, and an assessment tool and two nursing care plans are included in the appendix.

Randall, B., Poush Tedrow, M., & Van Landingham, J. (1982). Adaptation nursing. The Roy conceptual model applied. St. Louis: CV Mosby.

The book presents the authors' interpretation of Roy's conceptual model and expands several concepts. Examples are given to illustrate application of the model and related theoretical knowledge in several clinical situations.

Riegel, B. (1985). A method of giving intershift report based on a conceptual model. Focus on Critical Care, 12(4), 12–18.

This article describes a systematic method of giving intershift report based on Roy's conceptual model and the nursing process, within the context of the ANA definition of nursing. The report method increases the amount and quality of nursing information without ignoring the medical information required for patient care.

Roy. C. (1970). Adaptation: A conceptual framework for nursing. Nursing Outlook, 18, 42–45.

Roy presents the basic concepts of her conceptual model. Adaptation theory is described and applied to nursing. Use of the model to facilitate the independent role of the nurse is discussed.

Roy, C. (1971). Adaptation: A basis for nursing practice. Nursing Outlook, 19, 254–257.

Roy presents additional elements of her model and elaborates on the nursing process. Clinical examples are given to illustrate use of the model in nursing practice.

Roy, C. (1973). Adaptation: Implications for curriculum change. Nursing Outlook, 21, 163–168.

Roy discusses the use of her model as a guide for curriculum development at the baccalaureate level. A typology of adaptation problems is presented and a specific design for curriculum is included. An example of a teaching model based on Roy's conceptual model is given.

Roy, C. (1974). The Roy Adaptation Model. In J.P. Riehl & C. Roy, Conceptual models for nursing practice (pp. 135–144). New York: Appleton-Century-Crofts.

Roy presents the elements of her conceptual model and identifies basic assumptions. Areas of future study to validate aspects of the model are suggested.

Roy, C. (1976). Comment. Nursing Outlook, 24, 690–691.
Roy responds to the Brower and Baker and the Wagner articles and discusses points to consider in the implementation of her model in nursing practice.

Roy, C. (1976). Introduction to nursing: An adaptation model. Englewood Cliffs, NJ: Prentice-Hall.
The book provides a detailed explication of the Roy model. Contributing authors present each of the adaptive modes in detail, including assessment processes and appropriate nursing interventions. Use of the model with minority groups is discussed. The book was written as a first-level nursing text for undergraduate students.

Roy, C. (1979). Health-illness (powerlessness) questionnaire and hospitalized patient decision making. In M.J. Ward & C.A. Lindeman (Eds.), Instruments for measuring nursing practice and other health care variables (Vol. 1, pp. 147–153). Hyattsville, MD: U.S. Department of Health, Education, and Welfare.
The research instruments used by Roy in her doctoral dissertation are described.

Roy, C. (1979). Relating nursing theory to education: A new era. Nurse Educator, 4(2), 16–21.
Roy describes the use of her model to guide the curriculum of a baccalaureate nursing program. Strands and course sequence are identified and course content is summarized.

Roy, C. (1980). The Roy Adaptation Model. In J.P. Riehl & C. Roy, Conceptual models for nursing practice (2nd ed., pp. 179–188). New York: Appleton-Century-Crofts.
Further refinements in Roy's model are presented.

Roy, C. (1981). A systems model of nursing care and its effect on quality of human life. In G.E. Lasker (Ed.), Applied systems and cybernetics. Vol. 4. Systems research in health care, biocybernetics and ecology (pp. 1705–1714). New York: Pergamon Press.
Roy reviews the major ideas of her conceptual model of nursing and presents clinical examples that suggest use of the model may have enhanced the quality of the patients' lives.

Roy, C. (1983). Roy Adaptation Model. In I.W. Clements & F.B. Roberts, Family health. A theoretical approach to nursing care (pp. 255–278). New York: John Wiley & Sons.
Roy presents a discussion of the philosophical and theoretical basis of her conceptual model and explains how the family can be viewed as an adaptive system.

Roy, C. (1983). The expectant family. Analysis and application of the Roy Adaptation Model. In I.W. Clements & F.B. Roberts, Family health. A theoretical approach to nursing care (pp. 298–303). New York: John Wiley & Sons.
A case study of an older couple expecting their first child is analyzed within the context of Roy's model. The nursing process is outlined in a table.

Roy, C. (1983). The family in primary care. Analysis and application of the Roy Adaptation Model. In I.W. Clements & F.B. Roberts, Family health. A theoretical approach to nursing care (pp. 375–378). New York: John Wiley & Sons.
An adolescent with diabetes mellitus and her family are the subjects of a case study analyzed within the context of Roy's model and the nursing process is outlined in a table.

Roy, C. (1984). Introduction to nursing: An adaptation model (2nd ed.). Englewood Cliffs, NJ: Prentice-Hall.
Refinements in Roy's conceptual model are presented in this book.

Roy, C. (1984). The Roy Adaptation Model: Applications in community health. In M.K. Asay & C.C. Ossler (Eds.), Conceptual models of nursing. Applications in community health nursing. Proceedings of the Eighth Annual Community Health Nursing Conference (pp. 51–73). Chapel Hill: Department of Public Health Nursing, School of Public Health, University of North Carolina.
Roy presents a discussion of the use of her conceptual model in community health nursing.

Roy, C. (1987). Roy's Adaptation Model. In R.R. Parse, Nursing science. Major paradigms, theories, and critiques (pp. 35–45). Philadelphia: WB Saunders.
This book chapter is the publication of Roy's presentation at the Nurse Theorist Conference held in Pittsburgh, Pennsylvania, in May 1985.

Roy, C. (1988). An explication of the philosophical assumptions of the Roy Adaptation Model. Nursing Science Quarterly, 1, 26–34.
Roy identifies the philosophical assumptions upon which her conceptual model is based.

Roy, C., & Anway, J. (in press). Theories and hypotheses for nursing administration. In B. Henry, M. DiVincenti, C. Arndt, & A. Marriner (Eds.), Dimensions of nursing administration. Theory, research, education, and practice. Boston: Blackwell Scientific Publications.
This book chapter presents a discussion of the use of Roy's conceptual model as a guide for nursing administration.

Roy, C., & Martinez, C. (1983). A conceptual framework for CNS practice. In A. Hamric & J. Spross (Eds.), The clinical nurse specialist in theory and practice (pp. 3–20). New York: Grune & Stratton.
This book chapter presents a conceptual framework for clinical specialist practice and provides a frame of reference for subsequent chapters. A systems framework for clinical specialist practice is described and illustrated with an example from a psychiatric nursing practice.

Roy, C., & Obloy, M. (1978). The practitioner movement—toward a science of nursing. American Journal of Nursing, 78, 1698–1702.
The nurse practitioner is identified as an important user of nursing models and derived theories. Several nursing models and theories are discussed. A clinical situation involving an ill child in which the Roy model was used to guide nursing practice is presented.

Roy, C., & Roberts, S.L. (1981). Theory construction in nursing. An adaptation model. Englewood Cliffs, NJ: Prentice-Hall.
Roy's model is reviewed. A general theory of the person as an adaptive system is put forth, as are individual theories of the adaptive modes. Testable hypotheses derived from each theory are identified.

Sato, M.K. (1986). The Roy Adaptation Model. In P. Winstead-Fry (Ed.), Case studies in nursing theory (pp. 103–125). New York: National League for Nursing.
This book chapter presents an overview of Roy's conceptual model and a case study of a 28-year-old woman expecting her first child using Roy's nursing process.

Schmitz, M. (1980). The Roy Adaptation Model: Application in a community setting. In J.P. Riehl & C. Roy, Conceptual models for nursing practice (2nd ed., pp. 193–206). New York: Appleton-Century-Crofts.
Roy's model is modified for use in a home care setting. A detailed case study of nursing care of a newborn is presented. Nursing care plans for mothers of infants with various disorders are included.

Shannahan, M., & Cottrell, B. (1985). Effect of the birth chair on duration of second stage labor, fetal outcome, and maternal blood loss. Nursing Research, 34, 89–92.

Cottrell, B., & Shannahan, M. (1986). Effect of the birth chair on duration of second stage labor and maternal outcome. Nursing Research, 35, 364–367.

Cottrell, B., & Shannahan, M. (1987). A comparison of fetal outcome in birth chair and delivery table births. Research in Nursing and Health, 10, 239–243.
These articles report the findings of studies that examined the effects of use of a birth chair on maternal and fetal outcome. The studies were guided by Roy's conceptual model. Findings revealed that the birth chair is a safe alternative delivery method, although maternal blood loss was increased when the birth chair was used and second stage labor was not shorter than with the traditional delivery position.

Silva, M.C. (1987b). Needs of spouses of surgical patients: A conceptualization within the Roy Adaptation Model. Scholarly Inquiry for Nursing Practice: An International Journal, 1, 29–44.

Roy, C. (1987). Response to "Needs of spouses of surgical patients: A conceptualization within the Roy Adaptation Model." Scholarly Inquiry for Nursing Practice: An International Journal, 1, 45–50.

Silva reports the findings of her study of needs of 75 spouses whose husbands or wives had had surgery. Factor analysis of data revealed that needs reflected the four adaptive modes of Roy's conceptual model, but in a slightly different pattern. Factors were labeled psychosocial needs, physiological needs, staff support/confidence in care needs, and information needs.

Roy presents a discussion and critique of Silva's study. She points out that Silva conducted her study prior to publication of Roy's 1984 text, which purposefully omitted the concept of need.

Sirignano, R.G. (1987). Peripartum cardiomyopathy: An application of the Roy Adaptation Model. Journal of Cardiovascular Nursing, 2, 24–32.

This article describes the use of Roy's conceptual model to guide care of patients experiencing cardiomyopathy during the peripartum period.

Smith, C., Garvis, M., & Martinson, I. (1983). Content analysis of interviews using nursing model: A look at parents adapting to the impact of childhood cancer. Cancer Nursing, 6, 269–275.

Roy's conceptual model was used for the content analysis of interviews of parents of children with cancer. The results suggest that questions that elicit needs in the adaptive modes facilitate parents' identification of their own and their children's adaptive strengths.

Starr, S.L. (1980). Adaptation applied to the dying client. In J.P. Riehl & C. Roy, Conceptual models for nursing practice (2nd ed., pp. 189–192). New York: Appleton-Century-Crofts.

Roy's model is used to guide the nursing care of the dying patient. Nursing interventions in each of the adaptive modes are presented.

Torosian, L.C., DeStefano, M., & Dietrick-Gallagher, M. (1985). Day gynecologic chemotherapy unit: An innovative approach to changing health care systems. Cancer Nursing, 8, 221–227.

The development of a day gynecologic chemotherapy unit is described in this article. Health care reimbursement issues, analysis of patient needs, unit develoment, the role of the GYN-Oncology Clinical Specialist, and evaluation of the unit and patient outcomes are discussed. The authors claim that the use of Roy's model as a guide for practice was associated with positive patient outcomes.

Tiedeman, M.E. (1983). The Roy Adaptation Model. In J.J. Fitzpatrick & A.L. Whall, Conceptual models of nursing: Analysis and application (pp. 157–180). Bowie, MD: Brady.

This book chapter presents a review of Roy's conceptual model.

Tulman, L., & Fawcett, J. (1988). Return of functional ability after childbirth. Nursing Research, 37, 77–81.

This article reports the findings of a retrospective exploratory study of women's recovery of full functional ability after childbirth. Comparisons are made between vaginally and cesarean delivered women. Although not noted explicitly, functional ability is regarded as a theoretical representative of the role function adaptive mode of Roy's conceptual model.

Wagner, P. (1976). Testing the adaptation model in practice. Nursing Outlook, 24, 682–685.

The author reports graduate students' experiences in the use of Roy's conceptual model in several clinical settings, including general medical-surgical, maternity, intensive care, and psychiatric in-patient units; physicians' offices; medical-surgical, psychiatric, and pediatric orthopedic outpatient clinics; industrial health centers; and nurse-clinician hypertension clinics.

Whall, A.L. (1986). Strategic family therapy: Nursing reformulations and applications. In A.L. Whall, Family therapy theory for nursing. Four approaches (pp. 51–67). Norwalk, CT: Appleton-Century-Crofts.

Whall explains how the theory of strategic family therapy can be reformulated for nursing and links the reformulated theory with Roy's conceptual model.

10

Conceptual Models and Theories Revisited_____

This chapter expands the discussion of conceptual models of nursing and nursing theories that began in Chapter 1, with emphasis on implications of conceptual models for nursing practice. Here, issues related to numbers of conceptual models needed by the discipline are explored and methods for determination of the credibility of conceptual-theoretical systems of nursing knowledge are outlined. The chapter concludes with a discussion of directions for future work with conceptual models of nursing and nursing theories.

KEY TERMS_____

Multiple Conceptual Models	Implications for Nursing
Unified Conceptual Model	Education
Matching Conceptual Models to	Credibility of Conceptual
Clinical Agencies	Models of Nursing
Matching Conceptual Models to	Informal Determination of
Clinical Specialties	Credibility
Matching Conceptual Models to	Formal Determination of
Patients' World Views	Credibility
	Directions for the Future

SINGLE VERSUS MULTIPLE CONCEPTUAL MODELS OF NURSING

A major issue related to conceptual models of nursing is the need for several different perspectives versus the need for a single unified approach to nursing. Advocates of several different conceptual models base their position on the following three main points:

First, most disciplines have several conceptual models that present diverse views of their metaparadigm phenomena. This allows members of the discipline to explore phenomena in a variety of ways and avoids a restrictive viewpoint. Second, as Feldman (1980) noted, several conceptual models permit "the profession to view nursing from many perspectives, thereby increasing understanding of its nature and scope" (p. 87). Third, multiple conceptual models avoid the problem of "premature closure on options for the discipline" and foster development of the "full scope to the inherent potential of the discipline" (Stevens, 1981, pp. 38, 43). The third point may be extended to include not only premature closure for the discipline but in turn for the individual clinician. Kristjanson, Tamblyn, and Kuypers (1987) pointed out that use of just one conceptual model "prematurely closes the perceptions of the practitioner" (p. 525). They then noted the limitations of premature closure, stating,

> If perception is limited to only those phenomena which are congruent with the model employed, then recognition of dissonant phenomena in a situation will be limited. The associated opportunity to explore and/or develop alternate, potentially more relevant, theoretical constructs will similarly be stifled. The resulting mental block represents a serious obstacle to an evolution of theory relevant to nursing. The rigidity of this congruent-seeking mental set is a potential barrier to the practitioner's ability to adapt to changes in contexts and constructs relevant to practice specifically. This affects the practice situation specifically but it also affects health care more generally. (p. 525)

In contrast to the position of multiple conceptual models, Riehl and Roy (1980) advocated a single unified conceptual model of nursing. They suggested that such a model would lend stability to the discipline of nursing and maintained that concepts and propositions from various conceptual models could be combined in summary statements related to the person, the goals of nursing, and the nursing process. Recently, however, Riehl-Sisca (personal communication, July 23, 1987) indicated that a single conceptual model of nursing would not be appropriate.

Riehl and Roy's (1980) earlier position was a simplistic solution to a difficult problem that must take into account the fact that each conceptual model is based on distinctive philosophical assumptions and presents a different view of metaparadigm phenomena. The differences between conceptual models frequently are irreconcilable, as Kuhn (1970) explained in the following comments:

> To the extent . . . that two scientific schools disagree about what is a problem and what a solution, they will inevitably talk through each

other when debating the relative merits of their respective paradigms. (p. 109)

The proponents of competing paradigms will often disagree about the list of problems that any candidate for paradigm must resolve. Their standards or their definitions of science are not the same. (p. 148)

The proponents of competing paradigms practice their trades in different worlds. . . . Practicing in different worlds, the two groups of scientists see different things when they look from the same point in the same direction. (p. 150)

In addition, as Stevens (1981) pointed out, any attempt at synthesis of several conceptual models fails to recognize that meanings of concepts arise within the context of a particular model, that propositions of different models are contradictory and cannot be subsumed under a more inclusive model, and that it is unrealistic to assume that contradictory positions will synthesize.

Furthermore, those who advocate a unified conceptual model of nursing fail to consider that any short term gains from a single approach, such as ease of mobility from educational program to clinical practice setting or from one clinical agency to another, could be offset by long term losses. For example, what if use of the conceptual model resulted in negative effects on patients' health states? What if the conceptual model was not appropriate in certain clinical settings or for certain clinical problems? Would those settings and problems be given up by nursing and handed over to another discipline? And what if the conceptual model was not appropriate for certain cultural groups? Would nurses not care for members of those cultural groups?

Moreover, advocates of a unified conceptual model of nursing apparently have failed to consider that disciplines that relied on a single model experienced scientific revolutions when empirical data did not conform to the propositions of the prevailing perspective (Kuhn, 1970). Although scientific revolutions certainly have advanced knowledge in some disciplines, the price paid by many scholars has been very high in terms of acceptance of their work and career advancement. Consider, for example, the long period of time when Barbara McClintock's research on gene transposition was not valued because she worked outside the predominant paradigm in biology (Keller, 1983).

It may, of course, be possible to combine essentially similar models or to use certain concepts and propositions from one model to supplement those of another. Procedures for combining conceptual models of nursing may be extracted from Laudan's (1977) discussion of integrating research traditions. One procedure involves the grafting of one model onto another without modifying the content of either one. Another procedure involves the elimination of the components of two or more models that have been refuted through empirical research or logical analysis and combining the remaining components in a new way. It is important to point out that these procedures should be used only after a detailed examination of the models that are to be combined, with emphasis on the logical congruence of the different viewpoints.

A word of caution must be interjected here. In nursing, the still limited experience with conceptual models provides no basis for knowing which parts of which models most profitably could be included in a unified model, or in a combination of a few models (Stevens, 1981). Combining models is particularly dangerous at this time in the evolution of the discipline of nursing because any concept that would be excluded from the unified model most likely would fall into disuse. Thus, there is a danger of turning down a blind alley. Before all nurses follow the same path, the competition of multiple models is needed to determine the superiority of one or more of them. Such superiority can be determined only when many nurses have worked with all of the models enough to know which of them leads to problems and solutions that are deemed significant for nursing. It is important to point out, however, that although the use of different models requires different ways of thinking, they may not always lead to different nursing actions. This seems to be especially so in the case of nursing interventions. The fact that significantly different nursing interventions have not been derived from each conceptual model may be because different conceptual models simply do not lead to substantially different interventions or because of the fundamental nature of the many interventions used by nurses that are driven by principles from the basic sciences, physician orders, or biomedical technology. Or, in some cases, it may be because nurses are reluctant to give up their usual ways of caring for people. If this last reason is responsible for lack of distinct interventions stemming from different conceptual models, the commitment of nurses to more than "lip service" use of conceptual models must be questioned.

Finally, as Johnson (1974) pointed out, "the question of whether any model is right or wrong for nursing is a social decision" (p. 376). Thus, superiority of one model over all others, although not likely to emerge, would be determined in the main by agreement of the members of the discipline and by recipients of nursing care.

In conclusion, close examination of various conceptual models of nursing may lead to identification of areas of overlap and congruence, and thus to some consolidation. It is, however, unlikely that there ever will be one unified conceptual model of nursing. It seems that given the complexity of nursing activities and the variety of situations in which nurses function, it is much more desirable at present that a number of conceptual models be considered in a variety of clinical situations with diverse patient populations and in various functional areas, including clinical practice, nursing research, nursing education, and nursing administration. This so-called pluralism in conceptual models of nursing is growing in acceptance. Dickoff and James (1978, 1986) have recommended a purposeful pluralism of conceptual models rather than a search for a unified conceptual model. Story and Ross (1986) maintained that the demands of increasingly complex and varied nursing situations mandate pluralism in the curricula of basic nursing education programs. They stated,

> Given the increasing complexity of nursing practice in our ever chang- ing society, and given the fact that the setting in part determines the nature of nursing in that setting, it does not seem reasonable to assume that one conceptual framework is adequate to prepare students for be- ginning professional practice in a variety of situations. (p. 77)

Kristjanson, Tamblyn, and Kuypers (1987) also advocated plural- ism of conceptual models of nursing and identified its advantages. They maintained,

> When a practitioner or practice profession acknowledges that there are a range of choices available in any given practice situation, a corollary notion is accepted. This associated notion is that there is no one solu- tion to a particular clinical situation. Practitioners make different choices and in so doing, select a standard against which to decide what is correct. While it is nevertheless essential that practitioners at- tempt to make informed choices by paying attention to current relevant research developments, the dominant feature of any helping profession is that the choices made within the interaction are internally directed choices rooted in the practitioner-client exchange. (p. 528)

Single Versus Multiple Conceptual Models of Nursing for Clinical Agencies

The discussion of the issue of single versus multiple conceptual models of nursing has thus far emphasized the number of models needed by the discipline of nursing as a whole. Another aspect of this issue is the need for one or many conceptual models within a clinical agency.

Clinical agencies that provide service to just one category of pa- tients or encompass just one specialty area should not have difficulty using one conceptual model to guide all nursing practice activities. General purpose agencies, however, may encounter difficulties if the conceptual model selected does not readily guide practice for all spe- cialty areas and all categories of patients. But use of more than one conceptual model within an agency may pose problems for a nurse who works on different units as well as for patients who are moved from unit to unit as their health states change. Guidelines for deci- sions regarding the number of conceptual models within a particular clinical agency have not yet been developed, although Schmieding (1984) offered her unsubstantiated opinion that adopting a single conceptual model for nursing practice in a clinical agency "can help nurses work together for quality nursing care" (p. 759).

The literature associated with the seven conceptual models included in this book suggests that each model is appropriate in a wide range of specialties and for many different categories of patients. Aggleton and Chalmers (1985) pointed out that the literature "might encourage some nurses to feel that it does not really matter which model of nursing is chosen to inform nursing practice within a particular care setting" (p. 39). They also pointed out that this literature might "encourage the view that choosing between models is something one does intuitively, as an act of personal preference. Even worse, it might encourage some nurses to feel that all their everyday problems might be eliminated were they to make the 'right choice' in selecting a particular model for use across a care setting" (p. 39). Critical appraisals of the literature have not yet revealed the extent to which the "fit" of the conceptual model to particular categories of patients and particular specialties was forced. In fact, the issue of "forced fit" has not yet been addressed in the literature. Furthermore, little attention has been given to the extent to which a particular conceptual model is modified by an individual or group to fit a given situation (C.P. Germain, personal communication, October 21, 1987). Although modifications certainly are acceptable, they should be acknowledged and a decision should be made with regard to retaining or changing the name of the conceptual model to indicate that modifications have been made. Clearly, systematic exploration of the specialty practice implications of various conceptual models, coupled with more practical experience with each model in a variety of settings, is required.

Conceptual Models of Nursing and Specialty Practice

An issue related to the number of conceptual models used in a clinical agency and to the possibility of the "forced fit" of existing conceptual models in certain situations is formulation of additional conceptual models for particular clinical practice settings. Avant and Walker (1984) claimed that none of the existing conceptual models is appropriate for all practice settings and, therefore, advised clinicians to construct their own nursing models to meet their particular needs.

Avant and Walker's advice fails to consider the limitations of conceptual models that are constructed for particular clinical specialty areas. What are the advantages of such models over models that might be more general? Indeed, how would specialty areas be identified? Would nursing continue to use traditional medical specializations as the basis for nursing specialties?

Avant and Walker's advice also fails to consider the facts that clinicians have always constructed their own models, and that most of these have remained implicit private images of nursing practice that draw heavily from medicine (Johnson, 1987; Reilly, 1975). There is no guarantee that new personal models would be more explicit, public, or focused on nursing phenomena. Furthermore, Avant and Walker's advice fails to consider the difficulty and time required for construction of a concise, logical, and innovative conceptual model. As is evident from the descriptions of their historical development in this book, the models developed by Johnson, King, Levine, Neuman, Orem, Rogers, and Roy took many years to construct and have been revised and refined many times. And many of the refinements have come about as a result of suggestions and constructive criticism by others. Orem, for example, has worked with the Nursing Development Conference Group for almost 20 years on revisions in her conceptual model. Roy has collaborated with colleagues at Mount St. Mary's College and elsewhere for more than 10 years on the development and refinement of her model.

The position taken here is that several good general conceptual models "introduce more order and are more parsimonious of everyone's time than a thousand limited, specific ones" (Nye & Berardo, 1981, p. xxv). Admittedly, the validity of the position supporting multiple public conceptual models, in contrast to multiple personal models or a single unified one, is not yet established. It is, therefore, incumbent on nurses to continue to systematically evaluate use of the conceptual models of nursing and report their findings at conferences and in widely circulated peer-reviewed journals.

Conceptual Models of Nursing and Patients' World Views

Still another aspect of the issue of single versus multiple conceptual models is the relationship of the patient's view of the world with that reflected in various conceptual models. McLane (1983) highlighted the importance of matching the conceptual model to the patient's view of the world. She maintained that "it is time to put the client into the decision about models of nursing and to consider the impact such a decision would have on practice, teaching and research" (p. 15). McLane then pointed out that "partial answers to the question of which model for which client can be found in the models themselves and in the unique cultural characteristics of groups of clients" (p. 15). McLane's position implies that many different conceptual models would be needed to accommodate the diversity of patients to whom nursing care is directed.

Moreover, McLane's position requires even further evaluation of the generality of various conceptual models than was done in this book. Her suggestion to more closely examine the models for implications regarding appropriateness for categories of patients is amplified by Aggleton and Chalmers's (1985) work. They presented the following four questions that represent a format for systematic evaluation of the appropriateness of a particular conceptual model for a given clinical situation:

1. Did the nursing model provide guidelines on assessment that enabled the patient's problems to be clearly identified?
2. Did the planning of care and the setting of goals match the patient's expectations for care?
3. Did the model suggest a range of nursing interventions which were practical within that particular care setting?
4. Did the nursing interventions enable the nurse to provide a standard of care acceptable both to herself and to her patient? (p. 39)

Implications for Nursing Education

The outcome of more systematic determination of the appropriateness of various conceptual models for different clinical agencies, specialties, and patients has implications for the education of nurses with regard to conceptual models. If it is determined that conceptual models of nursing are not generalizable across various situations, then nurses would have to be proficient in the use of several models or the patient would have to be referred to the nurse who was proficient in the use of the model that was appropriate for that patient. In either case, programs of nursing education would have to include one or more courses that include content about and clinical practice related to several conceptual models of nursing. This is already being done at the University of Ottawa School of Nursing in Ontario, Canada, where pluralism in conceptual models is "a major underpinning for curricular development and implementation" (Story & Ross, 1986, p. 77). This curriculum includes first-year content dealing with health of individuals that is based on Roy's (1984) Adaptation Model. Second-year content deals with health of expanding and childrearing families and also is based on Roy's conceptual model. Third-year content focuses on biophysical and psychosocial health and illness of individuals and families. Various elements of this content are based on Roy's conceptual model, Orem's (1985) general theory of nursing, and Neuman's (1982) Systems Model. Fourth-year content emphasizes health and illness of individuals, groups, and the community and is based on Neuman's conceptual model.

CREDIBILITY OF CONCEPTUAL MODELS OF NURSING

Another major issue related to conceptual models of nursing is determination of their credibility. Credibility determination is necessary to avoid the danger of uncritical acceptance and adoption of conceptual models. Uncritical use of conceptual models could easily lead to their use as ideologies, a situation that must be avoided if nursing is to continue its evolution as a professional discipline. Credibility determination also is needed to establish the social significance of conceptual models, that is, the effect of use of a conceptual model on patients' health status.

The credibility of a conceptual model cannot be determined directly. Rather, the abstract and general concepts and propositions of the conceptual model must be linked with the more specific and concrete concepts and propositions of a middle-range theory to determine credibility. The resulting conceptual-theoretical system of nursing knowledge then is used to guide nursing activities and the results of use are examined. Thus, credibility of conceptual models is determined through tests of conceptual-theoretical systems of nursing knowledge. More specifically, credibility is determined by comparing the propositions of a conceptual-theoretical system of nursing knowledge with empirical data, including outcomes of nursing care and research findings. The nursing care outcomes and research findings represent indirect evidence of the credibility of the conceptual model. If outcomes and findings conform to expectations that are raised by the conceptual model propositions and made more specific by the propositions of the theory, the theory and the conceptual model may be considered credible. If, however, outcomes and findings do not conform to expectations, the credibility of the theory and the conceptual model must be questioned.

Examination of the outcomes of nursing care guided by conceptual-theoretical systems of nursing knowledge constitutes informal determination of the credibility of a conceptual model. This is accomplished in three steps. First, prototype conceptual-theoretical systems of nursing knowledge are developed for each clinical specialty area or each nursing department and for various patient populations. Next, individualized systems of knowledge are developed by each nurse for particular patients. Nursing care then is carried out in accordance with the nursing process of the selected conceptual model which is amplified by logically consistent middle-range theories. Finally, the results of the evaluation step of this process provide data that may be used to determine credibility of the knowledge system. The conceptual-theoretical system of knowledge is considered credible if patient outcomes are in accordance with expectations. If, however, patient outcomes are not in accordance with expectations, the credibility of the knowledge system, and hence the conceptual model, must be questioned.

Hoch's (1987) work is an example of a systematic approach to informal determination of conceptual model credibility. She conducted a small-scale study of the effects of three treatment protocols on depression and life satisfaction in a sample of retired individuals. One group (N = 16) received nursing care guided by a treatment protocol derived from Neuman's (1982) Systems Model. Another group (N = 16) received nursing care guided by a treatment protocol derived from Roy's (1984) Adaptation Model. Still another group (N = 16), which served as the control group, received nursing care that was not based on an explicit conceptual model of nursing. Study findings revealed that the groups whose care was derived from Neuman's and Roy's conceptual models had lower depression scores and higher life satisfaction scores than the control group. Interestingly, there were no statistically significant differences in the depression or life satisfaction scores between the Neuman and Roy groups. Hoch acknowledged the limitations of her prelimiary work with a small sample but concluded that her findings suggested that "planned, purposeful nursing intervention based on a [conceptual] framework was more effective in decreasing [depression] and increasing life satisfaction among retirees than the absence of planned nursing intervention" (p. 17).

Another example of informal credibility determination is the project described by Roy, Kirk, and Wu (1985). They explained that the clinical utility of Orem's, Rogers's, and Roy's conceptual models is being determined in the areas of acute medical-surgical, community health, primary ambulatory care, and gerontological nursing at five different sites across the United States.

Examination of the findings of research guided by conceptual-theoretical systems of nursing knowledge constitutes formal determination of the credibility of a conceptual model. Conceptual models function as research traditions that include "(i) a set of [statements] about what sorts of entities and processes make up the domain of inquiry and (ii) a set of epistemic and methodological norms about how the domain is to be investigated, how theories are to be tested, how data are to be collected, and the like" (Laudan, 1981, p. 151). The statements and norms of research traditions are specified in the rules for research given in Chapter 1 of this book. Laudan (1981) explained the relationships between conceptual models as research traditions, theories, and empirical testing. He stated,

> Research traditions are not directly testable, both because their ontologies are too general to yield specific predictions and because their methodological components, being rules or norms, are not straightforwardly testable assertions about matters of fact. Associated with any active research tradition is a family of theories. . . . The theories . . . share the ontology of the parent research tradition and can be tested and evaluated using its methodological norms. (p. 151)

Formal determination of the credibility of a conceptual model by means of examination of empirical research findings is accomplished in two steps. First, the influence of the conceptual model on the research process must be evaluated through application of the following criteria, which were adapted from work by Silva (1986):

- The conceptual model of nursing is explicitly identified as the underlying guide for the research.
- The conceptual model of nursing is discussed in sufficient breadth and depth so that the relationship between the model and the study purpose and research question(s) is clear.
- The linkages between conceptual model concepts and propositions and middle-range theory concepts and propositions are stated explicitly.
- The study methodology reflects the conceptual model.
- The study subjects are drawn from a population that is appropriate for the focus of the conceptual model.
- The instruments are appropriate measures of phenomena encompassed by the conceptual model.
- The study design clearly reflects the focus of the conceptual model.
- The statistical techniques are in keeping with the world view reflected by the conceptual model.
- Discussion of study results includes conclusions regarding the credibility of both the middle-range theory and the conceptual model of nursing.

The systematic application of these criteria is especially important because some researchers do little more than cite a particular conceptual model in the study report (Silva, 1987). If a research report satisfies these criteria, determination of credibility may proceed to the second step. This step involves comparing the research findings with the propositions of the conceptual-theoretical system of nursing knowledge that was used to guide the research. If the research findings support the theory, then it is likely that the conceptual model is credible. If, however, the research findings do not support the theory, the credibility of both the theory and the conceptual model must be questioned.

The ultimate aim of determination of the credibility of conceptual models of nursing is to ascertain which conceptual models are appropriate for use in which clinical settings and with which patients. It is likely that determination of credibility will either support or refute the current impression that *any* conceptual model "can explain or guide any nursing intervention in any setting, and that all [models] are equally relevant for guiding the practice of nursing" (See, 1986, p. 355). Confirmation or refutation of this impression through both informal and formal determination of the credibility of conceptual models is crucial if nursing is to continue to advance as a respected discipline characterized by excellence in scientific and clinical scholarship.

DIRECTIONS FOR THE FUTURE

Articulation of conceptual models is a critical step in the continuing evolution of nursing as a discipline. Each conceptual model presents a distinctive view of the phenomena of interest to the discipline, which are capsulized in the four metaparadigm concepts: person, environment, health, and nursing. Each model, therefore, outlines a comprehensive body of nursing knowledge.

The next step in the evolution of the discipline of nursing must be development of theories that address the person, the environment, health, and nursing, within the context of each conceptual model. Progress is apparent. Theories have been derived from several of the conceptual models reviewed in this book. These theories and their parent conceptual models are discussed in the preceding chapters. Each of these theories now must be tested empirically.

Although several theories already have been directly derived from conceptual models of nursing, many more theories are needed to fully specify the concepts and propositions of the models. Thus, future work should be directed not only toward testing theories already derived from conceptual models of nursing, but also toward generation of middle-range theory level descriptions of phenomena identified by the conceptual models and subsequent testing of the new theories. Generation and testing of theories derived from conceptual models of nursing will require researchers to direct their efforts toward development of operational definitions of the concepts of the theories, development of appropriate instruments, formulation of testable hypotheses, development of appropriate statistical techniques, and the design of research programs that ultimately will test the effects of nursing actions derived from each conceptual model on patients' health states.

Another step in the evolution of nursing as a discipline should be continued efforts directed toward systematic informal and formal determination of the credibility of conceptual-theoretical systems of nursing knowledge. Future work should emphasize use of the credibility criteria to evaluate published reports of nursing practice and nursing research guided by conceptual models of nursing. Furthermore, the criteria for formal determination of credibility should be used as a checklist when designing research projects and preparing reports of findings.

CONCLUSION

This chapter identified major issues surrounding the use and further development of conceptual models of nursing. The beliefs that conceptual models of nursing, rather than conceptual models of other disciplines, are proper guides for nursing activities and that the conceptual model of nursing that is used to guide the nurse's actions should be explicit have permeated the discussion. This author is convinced that the existing conceptual models of nursing have made a substantial contribution to nursing. That contribution has been recognized with increasing frequency in recent years. Yet we must not be satisfied with this contribution as it now stands. Much more work is needed to determine the credibility of each conceptual model, to discard those conceptual models that do not stand up to credibility checks, and to continue to refine those models that are credible by means of logical analysis and further empirical work.

REFERENCES

Aggleton, P., & Chalmers, H. (1985). Critical examination. Nursing Times, 81(14), 38–39.

Avant, K.C., & Walker, L.O. (1984). The practicing nurse and conceptual frameworks. American Journal of Maternal Child Nursing, 9, 87–88, 90.

Dickoff, J., & James, P. (1978, December). New view of traditional roles: Theoretic pluralism and matrix of models. Paper presented at Nurse Educator Conference, New York. (Cassette recording)

Dickoff, J., & James, P. (1986, August). Overview of the concept of theoretical pluralism. Paper presented at Nursing Theory Congress. "Theoretical Pluralism: Direction for a Practice Discipline." Toronto, Ontario, Canada. (Cassette recording)

Feldman, H.R. (1980). Nursing research in the 1980s: Issues and implications. Advances in Nursing Science, 3(1), 85–92.

Hoch, C.C. (1987). Assessing delivery of nursing care. Journal of Gerontological Nursing, 13, 10–17.

Johnson, D.E. (1974). Development of theory: A requisite for nursing as a primary health profession. Nursing Research, 23, 372–377.

Johnson, D.E. (1987). Guest Editorial: Evaluating conceptual models for use in critical care nursing practice. Dimensions of Critical Care Nursing, 6, 195–197.

Keller, E.F. (1983). A feeling for the organism. The life and work of Barbara McClintock. New York: WH Freeman.

Kristjanson, L.J., Tamblyn, R., & Kuypers, J.A. (1987). A model to guide development and application of multiple nursing theories. Journal of Advanced Nursing, 12, 523–529.

Kuhn, T.S. (1970). The structure of scientific revolutions (2nd ed.). Chicago: University of Chicago Press.

Laudan, L. (1977). Progress and its problems: Towards a theory of scientific growth. Berkeley: University of California Press.

Laudan, L. (1981). A problem-solving approach to scientific progress. In I. Hacking (Ed.), Scientific revolutions (pp. 144–155). New York: Oxford University Press.

McLane, A. (1983). Book review of Fawcett, J. Analysis and evaluation of conceptual models of nursing. The Leading Edge (Newsletter of Delta Gamma Chapter of Sigma Theta Tau), 3(2), 15–16.

Neuman, B. (1982). The Neuman Systems Model. Application to nursing education and practice. Norwalk, CT: Appleton-Century-Crofts.

Nye, F.I., & Berardo, F.N. (Eds.). (1981). Emerging conceptual frameworks in family analysis. New York: Macmillan.

Orem, D.E. (1985). Nursing: Concepts of practice. New York: McGraw-Hill.

Reilly, D.E. (1975). Why a conceptual framework? Nursing Outlook, 23, 566–569.

Riehl, J.P., & Roy, C. (1980). Conceptual models for nursing practice. New York: Appleton-Century-Crofts.

Roy, C. (1984). Introduction to nursing. An adaptation model (2nd ed.). Englewood Cliffs, NJ: Prentice-hall.

Roy, C., Kirk, L., & Wu, R. (1985, June). Defining and measuring the impact of three nursing models on four specialties of advanced nursing practice. Paper presented at the Measurement of Clinical and Educational Nursing Outcomes Conference, New Orleans, LA.

Schmieding, N.J. (1984). Putting Orlando's theory into practice. American Journal of Nursing, 84, 759–761.

See, E.M. (1986). Book review of George, J. (Ed.). Nursing theories. The base for nursing practice (2nd ed.). Research in Nursing and Health, 9, 355–356.

Silva, M.C. (1986). Research testing nursing theory: State of the art. Advances in Nursing Science, 9(1), 1–11.

Silva, M.C. (1987). Conceptual models of nursing. In J.J. Fitzpatrick & R.L. Taunton (Eds.), Annual Review of Nursing Research (vol. 5, pp. 229–246). New York: Springer.

Stevens, B.J. (1981). Nursing theories: One or many? In J.C. McCloskey & H.K. Grace, Current issues in nursing (pp. 35–43). Boston: Blackwell Scientific Publications.

Story, E.L., & Ross, M.M. (1986). Family centered community health nursing and the Betty Neuman Systems Model. Nursing Papers, 18(2), 77–88.

ANNOTATED BIBLIOGRAPHY

Aggleton, P., & Chalmers, H. (1985). Critical examination. Nursing Times, 81(14), 38–39.

The authors present the following questions as a method of evaluating the appropriateness of a conceptual model for a particular clinical situation:

Did the nursing model provide guidelines on assessment that enabled the patient's problems to be clearly identified?

Did the planning of care and the setting of goals match the patient's expectations for care?

Did the model suggest a range of nursing interventions which were practical within that particular care setting?

Did the nursing interventions enable the nurse to provide a standard of care acceptable both to herself and to her patient?

Avant, K.C., & Walker, L.O. (1984). The practicing nurse and conceptual frameworks. American Journal of Maternal Child Nursing, 9, 87–90.

The authors outline the advantages of using a conceptual model to guide nursing practice. They maintain that nurses need to construct conceptual models that are relevant and specific to their practices.

Baldwin, S. (1983). Nursing models in special hospital settings. Journal of Advanced Nursing, 8, 473–476.

The author discusses the advantages of using a nursing model in a hospital that serves mentally handicapped persons. The medico-legal model, the moral-attribution model, and the educational model are presented as frameworks that are used to deliver nursing care to this population.

Beck, C.T. (1985). Theoretical frameworks cited in Nursing Research from January 1974–June 1985. Nurse Educator, 10(6), 36–38.
The article presents the results of a review of the theoretical frameworks cited in Nursing Research for 11½ years. Stress, role theory, and social learning theory were the most frequently cited frameworks. Johnson's and Rogers's were the only unique nursing conceptual models that were cited.

Carveth, J.A. (1987). Conceptual models in nurse-midwifery. Journal of Nurse-Midwifery, 32, 20–25.
The author presents a rationale for using conceptual models of nursing to guide nurse-midwifery practice, research, and education.

Fitzpatrick, J.J., & Whall, A.L. (1984). Should nursing models be used in psychiatric nursing practice? Journal of Psychosocial Nursing and Mental Health Services, 22(6), 44–45.
Fitzpatrick argues that psychiatric nursing practice should be guided by conceptual models of nursing. Whall argues that a variety of approaches should be used and that to rely solely on nursing models may hinder development of a body of practice-based theory.

Green, C. (1985). An overview of the value of nursing models in relation to education. Nurse Education Today, 5, 267–271.
This article identifies the value of nursing models and presents implications for nursing education.

Hoch, C.C. (1987). Assessing delivery of nursing care. Journal of Gerontological Nursing, 13, 10–17.
This article reports the findings of a study that compared the effects of using nursing protocols derived from Neuman's conceptual model, Roy's conceptual model, and no explicit model on the retired person's life satisfaction and depression. Results indicated that the Neuman and Roy groups did not differ, although subjects in both groups had higher life satisfaction and lower depression scores than the no model group.

Jackson, M. (1986). On maps and models. Senior Nurse, 5(4), 24–26.
This article presents a discussion of the similarities between a map and a conceptual model.

Jacobs, M.K. (1986). Can nursing theory be tested? In P.L. Chinn (Ed.), Nursing research methodology. Issues and implementation (pp. 39–53). Rockville, MD: Aspen.
The author contends that nursing must carefully evaluate its theoretical endeavors and continually examine how well theory advances practice. The chapter presents a discussion of problems and issues related to testing theory and reconceptualization of traditional scientific theory as a means toward testable theory.

Kinney, M. (1984). Nursing models. Focus on Critical Care, 11(6), 5–6.
In this editorial, Kinney supports the use of conceptual models in critical care nursing. She states that critical care nurses have been accused of doing nothing more than implementing the medical regimen, although in actuality these nurses do much more than care for the physical needs of the patient. Adoption of a nursing model could help these nurses conceptualize and define their knowledge of nursing.

Kotaska, J., Hooperfer, D., & Moir, V. Yes: Nursing models can help. RNABC News, 18(5), 23–27.

Craig, J. No: Model mania, RNABC News, 18(5), 23–27.
The authors present the pros and cons of nursing models.

Kristjanson, L.J., Tamblyn, R., & Kuypers, J.A. (1987). A model to guide development and application of multiple nursing theories. Journal of Advanced Nursing, 12, 523–529.
The authors advocate the use of multiple conceptual models and present a framework that allows nurses to examine various models in relation to their applicability to a given client situation. The following three questions constitute the major focus of the framework:
What is the ideal? (Health)

What error is preventing the ideal state from occurring?
What change should occur to achieve the ideal?

Laudan, L. (1977). Progress and its problems. Berkeley: University of California Press.

Laudan, L. (1981). A problem-solving approach to scientific progress. In I. Hacking (Ed.), Scientific revolutions (pp. 144–155). New York: Oxford University Press.
   Laudan presents his philosophy of science and discusses the functions of research traditions. Procedures for combining research traditions are given in the 1977 publication.

Levine, M.E. (1988). Antecedents from adjunctive disciplines: Creation of nursing theory. Nursing Science Quarterly, 1, 16–21.
   Levine maintains that the metaparadigm concepts, person, environment, health, and nursing, are the commonplaces essential for discussions of nursing. She further maintains that adjunctive concepts, that is, those used in development of nursing knowledge that are from other disciplines, are antecedent to nursing knowledge and must not be misused when incorporated in a nursing theory. Levine suggests that determination of the correct use of these concepts should be part of the analysis and evaluation of nursing knowledge.

Lundh, U., Söder, M., & Waerness, K. (1988). Nursing theories: A critical view. Image: Journal of Nursing Scholarship, 20, 36–40.
   The authors raise questions about the utility of abstract nursing knowledge for nursing practice, education, and research. They point out that such knowledge is normative and concentrates on result-oriented instrumental rationality. These features, the authors claim, pose difficulties when one is trying to learn to ask fruitful questions that are relevant and interesting for the concrete problems of nursing situations.

Martin, L., & Glasper, A. (1986). Core plans: Nursing models and the nursing process in action. Nursing Practice, 1, 268–273.
   This article presents a discussion of the need for core nursing care plans, which are care plans based on explicit conceptual models of nursing that deal with particular nursing problems or needs and are often allied to an agreed policy or procedure discussed with physicians.

Reed, P.G. (1986). A model for constructing a conceptual framework for education in the clinical specialty. Journal of Nursing Education, 25, 295–299.

Reed, P.G. (1987). Constructing a conceptual framework for psychosocial nursing. Journal of Psychosocial Nursing and Mental Health Services, 25, 24–28.
   The author describes her Process Model, which is an approach to developing and refining conceptual frameworks for clinical specialty education by borrowing concepts from selected nursing models. The model is based on the metaparadigm concepts person, environment, health, and nursing practice.
   In her 1987 article, Reed explains how the Process Model was used to construct a framework for psychiatric mental health nursing from concepts from works by Nightingale, Rogers, Parse, Newman, Peplau, King, and Orem.

Silva, M.C. (1986). Research testing nursing theory: State of the art. Advances in Nursing Science, 9(1), 1–11.

Silva, M.C. (1987). Conceptual models of nursing. In J.J. Fitzpatrick & R.L. Taunton (Eds.), Annual review of nursing research (vol. 5, pp. 229–246). New York: Springer.
   In her 1986 publication, Silva reports the results of her review of nursing journals from 1952 to 1985 with regard to use of works by Johnson, Neuman, Orem, Rogers, and Roy to guide research. Just 62 articles were found that focused on tests of nursing models. Using her criteria for use of conceptual models in research, Silva found that 24 of the 62 articles made only minimal use of the models. The 1987 publication presents a review and critique of the 62 articles.

Sirra, E. (1986). Using nursing models for nursing practice. Nursing Journal of India, 77, 301–304.
   This article presents an overview of the definition, content, and functions of a conceptual model of nursing.

Smith, L. (1986). Issues raised by the use of nursing models in psychiatry. Nurse Education Today, 6, 69–75.

The author maintains that the use of nursing models in psychiatric nursing practice can be beneficial. An example of merging a nursing model with a psychiatric model of care is presented.

Waters, K. (1986). Editorial. Nursing Practice, 1, 201.

The author maintains that the move to nursing models in nursing practice may be premature.

Webb, C. (1986). Nursing models: A personal view. Nursing Practice, 1, 208–212.

This article presents a discussion of the intellectual status of nursing models.

Appendix_____

AUDIO AND VISUAL MATERIALS

Audio Productions

The Second Annual Nurse Educator Conference.
    Audio tapes available from Teach 'em, Inc., 160 E. Illinois Street, Chicago, IL 60611.
    Audio tapes of the papers presented at the Nurse Educator Conference held in New York, New York, in December 1978. Presentations are by Johnson, King, Leininger, Levine, Newman, Orem, Paterson and Zderad, Rogers, and Roy. A presentation by Dickoff and James also is included.

Nurse Theorist Conference
    Audio tapes available from Kennedy Recordings, RR5, Edmonton, Alberta, Canada T5P 4B7.
    Audio tapes of the papers presented at the Nurse Theorist Conference held in Edmonton, Alberta, Canada, in August 1984. Presenters include King, Levine, Newman, Rogers, and Roy.

Nursing Theory in Action
    Audio tapes available from Kennedy Recordings, RR5, Edmonton, Alberta, Canada T5P 4B7.
    Audio tapes of the papers and concurrent sessions on applications to practice, research, and education presented at the Nursing Theory in Action conference held in Edmonton, Alberta, Canada, in August 1985. Presenters include King, Levine, Neuman, Newman, Orem (presented by S. Taylor), Parse, Rogers, and Roy. The Roper/Logan/Tierney Framework also is presented.

Nursing Theory Congress
    Audio tapes available from Audio Archives of Canada, 100 West Beaver Creek Road, Unit #18, Richmond Hill, Ontario, Canada L4B 1H4.
    Audio tapes of the papers and concurrent sessions on applications to practice, research, and education presented at the Nursing Theory Congress, "Theoretical Plu-

ralism: Direction for a Practice Discipline," held in Toronto, Ontario, Canada, in August 1986. Presentations focus on models by Johnson (adaptation of the model presented by B. Holaday), King, Levine, Neuman, Orem (presented by S. Taylor), Rogers, and Roy. Presentations by Dickoff and James on theoretical pluralism and by Kritek on nursing theory and nursing diagnosis are included.

Video Productions

Care with a Concept
> Video tape available from Health Sciences Consortium, 201 Silver Cedar Court, Chapel Hill, NC 27514.
> Mary Hale and Gates Rhodes of the University of Pennsylvania School of Nursing produced this video tape documenting the use of Orem's Self-Care Framework at Children's Seashore House in Atlantic City, New Jersey.

The Nurse Theorists. Portraits of Excellence
> Video tapes available from Studio Three, Samuel Merritt College of Nursing, 370 Hawthorne Avenue, Oakland, CA 94609.
> A series of video tapes, produced with a grant from the Helene Fuld Health Trust, depicting major events and incidents in the lives of 14 nurse theorists. Interviews are by Jacqueline Fawcett. When complete, the series will include video tapes of Henderson, Johnson, King, Leininger, Levine, Neuman, Nightingale, Orem, Orlando, Peplau, Rogers, Roy, Rubin, and Watson.

Nursing Theory. A Circle of Knowledge
> Video tape available from National League for Nursing, Ten Columbus Circle, New York, NY 10019–1350.
> Patricia Moccia interviews several nurse theorists, including Benner, Henderson, Orem, Rogers, Roy, and Watson. Discussion emphasizes philosophy of science.

Audio and Video Productions

Nurse Theorist Conference
> Audio and video tapes available from Meetings Internationale, 1200 Delor Avenue, Louisville, KY 40217.
> Audio and video tapes of the presentations, critiques and responses, and panel discussion at the Nurse Theorist Conference held in Pittsburgh, Pennsylvania, in May 1985. Presenters include King, Orem, Parse, Rogers, and Roy. The presentations and critiques are published in Parse, R.R. (1987). Nursing science. Major paradigms, theories, and critiques. Philadelphia: WB Saunders. An address by Peplau also is included.

Nurse Theorist Conference
> Audio and video tapes available from Meetings Internationale, 1200 Delor Avenue, Louisville, KY 40217.
> Audio and video tapes of the presentations, small group sessions, and panel discussion at the Nurse Theorist Conference held in Pittsburgh, Pennsylvania in May 1987. Presenters include King, Leininger, Parse, Rogers, Roy, and Watson. An address by Peplau, "Art and science of nursing: Similarities, differences, and relations," and one by Schlotfeldt, "Nursing science in the 21st century," are included.

Rogers, M.E. Science of unitary man
> Audio and video tapes available from Media for Nursing, Inc., P.O. Box 2467, Brooklyn, NY 11202.
> Tape I. Unitary man and his world: A paradigm for nursing.
>> Rogers discusses the development of nursing science, the uniqueness of nursing, the terminology of her conceptual model, and her view of unitary man and the environment.
> Tape II. Developing an organized abstract system: Synthesis of facts and ideas for a new product.

Rogers discusses the need for an organized abstract system of nursing knowledge. She presents the building blocks of her model, including energy fields, open systems, pattern and organization, and four dimensionality, and synthesizes these into a conceptual system for nursing.

Tape III. Principles and theories: Directions for description, explanation and prediction.

Rogers presents and explains the principles of homeodynamics, including helicy, resonancy, and complementarity. She describes such correlates of unitary human development as wave patterns and rhythms.

Tape IV. Theories of accelerating evolution, paranormal phenomena and other events.

Rogers describes her theories and cites life events that lend support to her propositions.

Tape V. Health and illness: New perspectives.

Rogers discusses the meaning of health and illness within the context of her conceptual model. She re-examines pathology from the perspective of the model. She also compares individual variations in behavior with normative data.

Tape VI. Interventive modalities: Translating theories into practice.

Rogers discusses nursing intervention within the context of the conceptual model and describes alternative forms of healing, including therapeutic touch. She identifies aging and dying as developmental processes. She also discusses the promotion of health versus prevention of disease.

Index

A "t" following a page number indicates a table. A page number in *italics* indicates a figure.